Clinical Maternal-Fetal Nutrition

To Edward Wallach MD
mentor – colleague and
friend – with thanks for the
opportunity to share time
under the dome
Tim
Baltimore
5/93

Maternity dress from the 18th century. (From G. J. Witowski. *Anecdotes & Curiosites historiques sur les Accouchements*. Paris: G. Steinheil, 1892.)

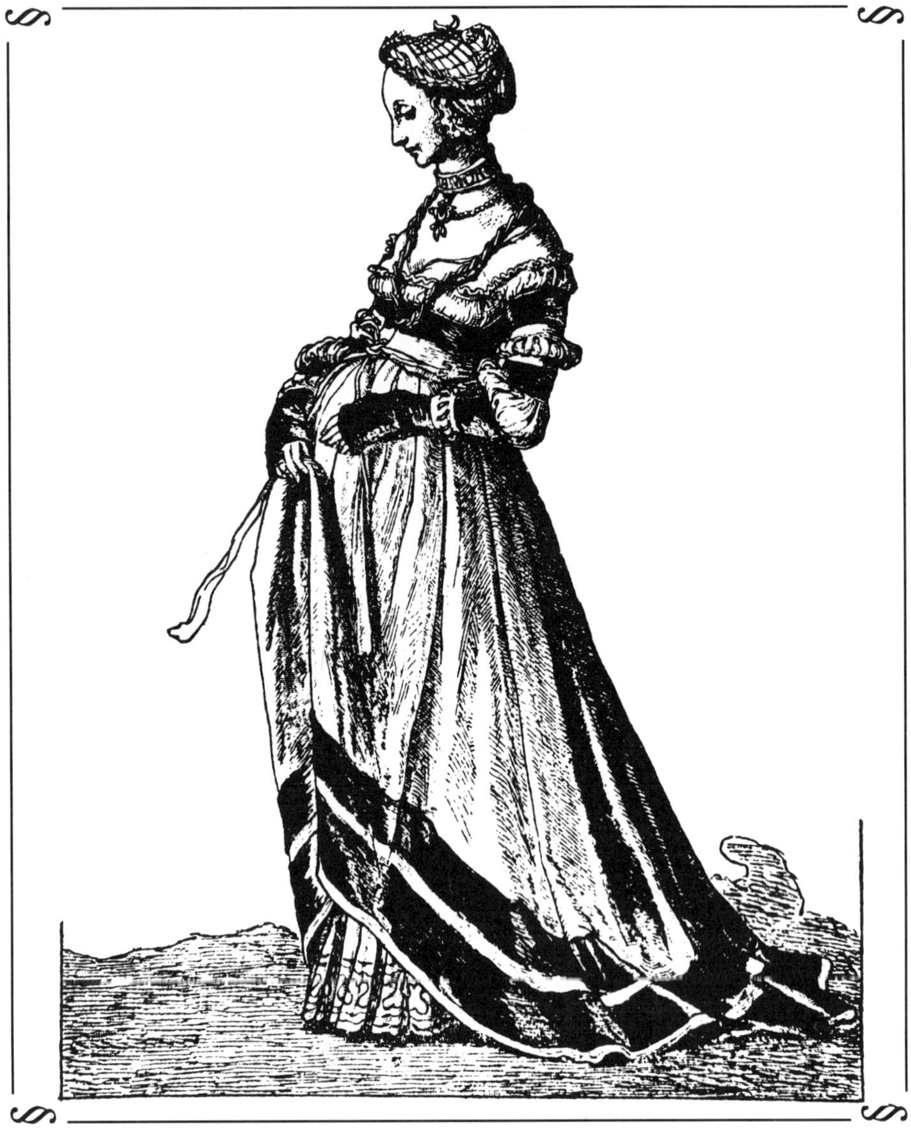

Clinical Maternal-Fetal Nutrition

Barbara Luke, Sc.D., M.P.H., R.D.
Director, Section of Reproductive and Perinatal Epidemiology, and Assistant Professor, Department of Obstetrics and Gynecology and Department of Preventive Medicine, Rush-Presbyterian-St. Luke's Medical Center, Chicago

Timothy R. B. Johnson, M.D.
Associate Professor of Gynecology and Obstetrics and Pediatrics, Johns Hopkins University School of Medicine, and Department of Maternal-Child Health, Johns Hopkins University School of Hygiene and Public Health; Director, Division of Maternal-Fetal Medicine, Department of Gynecology and Obstetrics, The Johns Hopkins Hospital, Baltimore

Roy H. Petrie, M.D., Sc.D.
Professor and Chairman, Department of Obstetrics and Gynecology, St. Louis University School of Medicine; Chief, Obstetrical and Gynecological Service, St. Mary's Health Center, St. Louis

Little, Brown and Company
Boston/Toronto/London

First Edition

Library of Congress Cataloging-in-Publication Data

Luke, Barbara.
Clinical maternal-fetal nutrition / Barbara Luke, Timothy R.B. Johnson, Roy H. Petrie.
p. cm.
Includes bibliographical references and index.
ISBN 0-316-53614-8
1. Pregnancy—Nutritional aspects. I. Johnson, Timothy R. B. II. Petrie, Roy H., 1940– . III. Title.
[DNLM: 1. Fetal Development. 2. Maternal-Fetal Exchange. 3. Nutrition—in pregnancy. WQ 175 L954c]
RG559.L835 1993
618.2'4—dc20
DNLM/DLC
for Library of Congress 92-48905
CIP

Printed in the United States of America
EB-M

Sponsoring Editor: **Susan Pioli**
Production Editor: **Kellie Cardone**
Copyeditor: **Libby Dabrowski**
Indexer: **Julia Figures**
Production Supervisor: **F. David Bell**
Designer: **F. David Bell**
Cover Designer: **Linda Dana Willis**

To Selma Taffel in recognition of her many outstanding contributions in perinatal research

To my beloved husband, Louis *B.L.*

Contents

Preface

During the second half of the 20th century, the fields of obstetrics and nutrition have experienced great changes. Innovations include regionalization of prenatal care, development of neonatal intensive care units, refinement of antepartum testing, and widespread use of artificial reproductive technology. In recent years, the central role of diet therapy in the prenatal management of maternal phenylketonuria and in the prevention of neural tube defects has been recognized. As the age of viability is pushed back to limits never imagined even a decade ago, prenatal nutrition has become a valued therapeutic modality in maximizing the growth potential of the unborn child.

This book presents an overview of the field of maternal nutrition, with its modern roots extending back through the 17th century and promising applications demonstrated daily through clinical trials and epidemiologic research. Although some contemporary problems facing today's obstetricians, such as drug addiction and AIDS, may not be amenable to dietary interventions, nutrition as a component of prenatal management may potentiate the efficacy of medical therapies. *Clinical Maternal-Fetal Nutrition* presents the most current theoretical basis of maternal nutrition and the means by which the theory can be applied to clinical practice. The interrelationships between maternal nutritional status and fetal growth under optimal and compromised conditions are discussed; these conditions include maternal undernutrition and malnutrition, anemia, diabetes, phenylketonuria, adolescence, smoking, alcohol, and multiple gestations. The effects of pregnancy on maternal health are also presented, with discussions of calcium and iron metabolism, delayed menarche, and athletics. The influence of anthropometric and sociodemographic characteristics, singly and in combination, on reproductive performance, including prematurity, are discussed, as are methods for assessment and clinical recommendations.

Clinical Maternal-Fetal Nutrition represents a new era in obstetrics and nutrition: the application of preventive medicine at the very beginning of life, the enrichment of the prenatal environment to optimize the genetic potential of the fetus, and assurance of the best health for the mother. Such interventions lay the foundation for better growth and development for generations to come.

In closing, the historical drawings that appear in *Clinical Maternal-Fetal Nutrition* were obtained through special assistance from librarians and photographers at the Galter Health Sciences Library of Northwestern University, Chicago, Illinois and the Institute of the History of Medicine, Johns Hopkins University School of Medicine, Baltimore, Maryland. We would like to acknowledge the scholarly assistance of Mr. James Shedlock, Director of the Galter Health Sciences Library, librarians Ramune Kubilius, Eric Albright, and Sylvia Nicholas, along with photographers Steven Harp and Donald Smith at Northwestern University. We wish to give special thanks for the extraordinary help of librarian Linda Bright and photographer Victor Raspa at the Institute of the History of Medicine. We would also like to acknowledge the assistance of the Center of Study for Multiple Birth in Chicago, Illinois.

Because of the creative talents of their staff, Little, Brown has published many innovative and scholarly texts. We would like to acknowledge the special efforts of longtime friend and Executive Editor of Medical Books, Susan Pioli, Production Editor, Kellie Cardone, and Production Supervisor, F. David Bell.

B.L.
T.R.B.J.
R.H.P.

Clinical Maternal-Fetal Nutrition

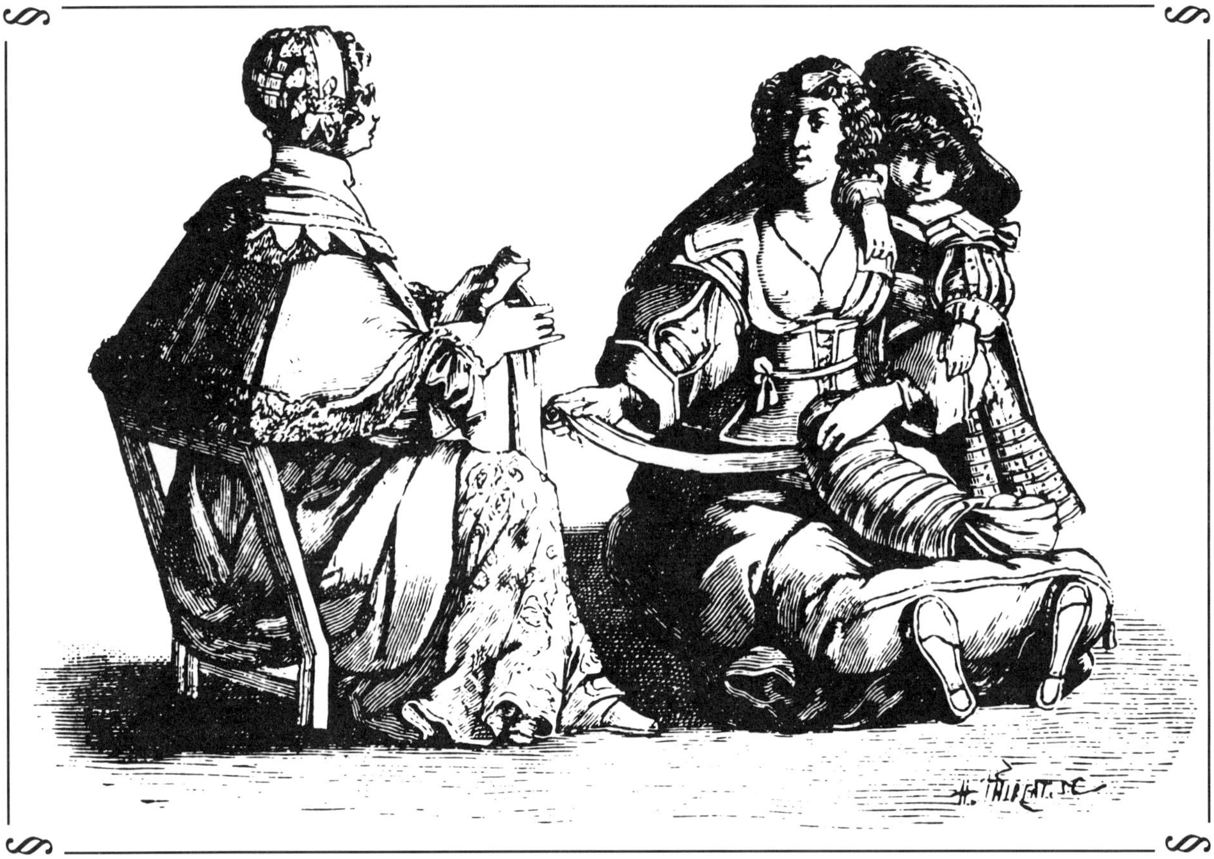

A woman swaddling her baby. An 18th-century engraving.

1

The Historical Basis of Maternal Nutrition Recommendations

Childhood Rickets and the Contracted Pelvis

Although records regarding specific advice on the composition of the prenatal diet date back thousands of years, the history of gestational weight gain recommendations is of fairly recent origin. The value of both weighing the newborn and quantifying and monitoring gestational weight gain has been recognized only within the past 150 years. In 1861, Gassner [1] first advised the routine weighing of pregnant women at each prenatal visit, and in 1852, Guillot [2] first advised the routine weighing of the newborn as part of the overall evaluation of physical and nutritional development at birth.

The belief in the importance of both of these measures, gestational weight gain and the weight of the newborn, stems from one of the overwhelming problems faced by obstetricians for centuries: the adult contracted or rachitic pelvis resulting from childhood rickets. The origin of the adult rachitic pelvis was not insufficient calcium intake during childhood, although this may have been a contributing factor, but rather inadequate vitamin D, which permits intestinal absorption of this mineral that is so vital to bone health. Most vitamin D is synthesized in the skin by exposure to sunlight. Childhood rickets, later manifested in the adult woman as a rachitic or contracted pelvis, stemmed from the generally held belief that exposure to "drafts" caused colds and that it was dangerous to take infants outside in the cold air. The historian Edward Shorter [3] noted that "of the child-rearing practices that kept children from the sun, most hurtful was 'swaddling' in which the infant is wrapped mummylike in a long linen bandage and kept in it for the first half-year of life." During the 17th and 18th centuries, this was almost a universal phenomenon among children. In the 19th century, child-rearing practices began to change, but rickets became a disease of the industrial environment, of keeping children in factories, schools, and cities, where sunlight was blocked by soot and smoke.

Mild rickets, which healed by age two, would generally result in a "flat" or "rachitic-flat" pelvis. During labor the child's head would have difficulty engaging, but once it was inside the pelvis, birth could progress. Severe rickets would result in a "generally contracted" or "generally contracted flat" pelvis, in which the entire pelvis, not just the front-to-back diameter, was too small. William Smellie, the famed British obstetrician and founder of the practice of pelvimetry, was one of the first to associate infantile rickets with pelvic deformities in adults. In his *Treatise on the Theory and Practice of Midwifery* [4], published in 1752, he concluded that, "most of those who have been rickety in their infancy, whether they continue little and deformed, or, recovering of that disease, grow up to be tall, stately women, are commonly narrow and distorted in the pelvis and consequently subject to tedious and difficult labours, for, as the pelvis is more or less distorted, the labour is more or less dangerous and difficult." As recently as 50 years ago, the contracted pelvis was a common obstetric problem in the United States. In a 1926 study by J. Whitridge Williams and K. C. Sun of 11,630 women delivering at the Johns Hopkins Hospital between 1896 and 1924, the incidence of contracted pelvis was estimated to be 27 percent, including 14 percent among whites and 43 percent among blacks [5].

Options for Delivery Before 1900

The Surgical Option

Difficulty in vaginal delivery has been recorded from the beginning of written history. References to surgical delivery (cesarean section) have also been documented in humanity's earliest writings, most frequently with dire results for both mother and child until recent decades of the 20th century. From the 16th through the 19th centuries, there was much opposition to cesarean section from the leading obstetricians of the day. For example, the 19th-century French obstetrician Baudelocque was labeled an assassin for advocating cesarean section in extreme contraction of the pelvis (his record was 42 deaths in 73 operations) [6]. Velpeau, a medical contemporary of Baudelocque, reported a maternal mortality of 50 percent [6].

A second surgical option entailed cutting the pelvic girdle to enlarge the pelvic cavity in all its diameters. Section at or near the symphysis pubis allowed the bones to separate 2.0 to 2.5 cm, and as much as 6 to 7 cm when the fetal head passed through, although not without some danger. Because the separation of the lower portions of the pelvis was less than in the upper, this operation was not useful in cases of contraction of the pelvic outlet. Symphysiotomy (section through the symphysis pubis) was replaced almost entirely by hebosteotomy, the sawing through of the ramus pubis alongside of the joint. In 1913, DeLee [7] cited mortality from symphysiotomy of 3 to 12 percent for the mother and 9 to 19 percent for the infant. Complications included severe hemorrhage from the wound (particularly when varicose veins were present), extensive injury to the anterior vaginal wall and perineum, tearing of the levator ani muscle from the ramus pubis, tearing of the bladder and urethra, overstretching of the sacroiliac joints, rupture of the anterior ligaments, and hematomas around the joints. Convalescence was frequently complicated by wound infection, poor healing, and thromboembolism, as well as limited motion for 2 to 8 months after delivery.

The third surgical alternative, used only in extreme cases in which the fetus had already died in utero or when there was a clear possibility of death for both mother and child, was that of fetal destructive operations. These procedures, which included craniotomy, embryotomy, evisceration, or decapitation, resulted in killing and dismembering the unborn child and often caused lacerations, hemorrhage, infection, or even death for the mother. All of these options contributed to puerperal infection and hemorrhage, the leading causes of maternal mortality in the United States for many decades. It was not until after World War II, with the perfection of surgical techniques and the availability of antibiotics and safe blood transfusions, that dramatic declines in maternal mortality began to take place.

The Prematurity Option

One of the most common options to facilitate delivery through a contracted pelvis was the induction of premature labor. The infant's head is its largest component, and at term the circumference ranges from about 32.5 to 37.5 cm (5th–95th percentiles) [8]. In theory, premature delivery could result in a smaller head circumference, approximately 0.3 cm per week [9], thereby permitting vaginal delivery through a contracted pelvis. In practice, however, this gain may have been short-sighted, due to the high neonatal mortality associated with prematurity until only recent decades of the 20th century. For example, in 1916, LaFetra [10] reported 85 percent mortality among premature infants born at Bellevue Hospital in New York City.

The Dietary Option (The Prochownick Diet)

Another option developed as a humane alternative to destructive operations or premature or surgical delivery was that of manipulating the maternal diet to produce a much smaller child who could be delivered vaginally at term, even in the presence of a contracted pelvis. The concept of manipulating the prenatal diet to influence the size of the infant is credited to Prochownick, a German obstetrician [11]. His first paper, published in 1889 and based on three cases, outlined a diet high in protein (130–160 gm), low in carbohydrates (100 gm), and severely restricted in fluids (<500 ml). The major purpose of the diet, which was intended to be implemented during the last 2 months of pregnancy, was to minimize the amount of fat accumulated by the fetus and to maximize the mobility of the fetal skull bones to improve the likelihood of vaginal delivery through a contracted pelvis at term without imposing any lasting adverse effects on the newborn. Fluid intake was also restricted, because it was believed that a high intake increased the deposition of fat and that restriction inhibited it.

That the contracted pelvis continued to be an obstetric problem in the United States until relatively recently is shown by the following quote from the American obstetrician Joseph Klein [12], writing in 1946:

> Most physicians who supervise prenatal care caution their patients against excessive weight gain during pregnancy. Their reasons for doing so are multiple. It is the opinion of many that the size of the fetus may thus be controlled. Prevention of overgrowth of the baby, especially in the presence of a pelvic contracture, would reduce the incidence of disproportion with its attendant hazards.

Early Research on Gestational Weight Gain (1920–1950)

As a result of the writings of Gassner [1], Prochownick [11, 13], and others, quantifying and monitoring gestational weight gain became an integral part of prenatal care in the United States during the early decades of the 20th century. In the nearly 70 years since the American obstetrician C. Henry Davis [14] pointed out the value of routine weighing of pregnant women, interest in the association between maternal nutrition and perinatal outcome has resulted in voluminous amounts of research. Of varying scientific merit, and frequently based on small series, case reports, or merely personal opinion, research on gestational weight gain has centered around three major themes: (1) **influencing the size of the newborn and facilitating delivery**, (2) **preventing maternal obesity after delivery**, and (3) **detecting and preventing pregnancy-induced hypertension (preeclampsia and toxemia)**. Comparison and interpretation of published studies in all three areas are hampered by their frequent omission of important variables, such as maternal height, pregravid weight, and pregravid weight-for-height; gestational age; maternal race; social class; smoking habits; and illnesses that could influence both gestational weight gain or intrauterine growth, or both (i.e., diabetes, tuberculosis, premature rupture of membranes, sexually transmitted diseases, and other infections). Although data were typically presented in terms of mean values, more often than not neither the cell size nor the standard deviation was reported, so that it is not retrospectively possible to evaluate the range or to determine the statistical significance of the reported differences between groups.

Another body of medical literature also developed in parallel to the three general themes just mentioned. This research examined the association between the quality of the maternal diet and subsequent perinatal outcome during these years. Many obstetricians formulated specific dietary recommendations, most of which were without scientific basis. For example, in 1925, Hannah [15] recommended a high-carbohydrate diet during the first trimester, followed by a carbohydrate-restricted diet during the second and third trimesters. He also recommended the liberal intake of lettuce, green vegetables, and fruits, and the limited intake of meats and milk, offering the following rationale:

> An excessive diet of carbohydrates and fats, and low in vitamines causes intestinal stasis, provides a field for putrefaction and growth of intestinal flora, from which toxins are absorbed. These toxins cause extra work for the liver and kidneys and other vital organs. Intestinal stasis encourages lesions of the colon, and later on infection of the various organs of the body. In my opinion, this is the reason the pregnant woman frequently complains of pain in the intestinal tract, especially in the right lower quadrant, oftentimes confused with pathology of the appendix. If the patient is permitted to gain in weight and improper or poorly selected food is partaken of, lesions are formed in the tract through which parasites enter the blood stream and infect the various organs of the body.

Slemons and Fagan [16], writing in 1927, made specific dietary recommendations for pregnancy, which included the generous intake of water and the elimination of milk from the diet after quickening occurred. In 1932, Bingham [17] advocated the liberal intake of fruits and vegetables while recommending moderate intake of meat, eggs, and milk. McIlroy and Rodway [18] recommended in 1937 that the prenatal diet be restricted in carbohydrates such as bread and potatoes, and severely restricted in salt. In 1943, Robinson and associates [19] also advocated restriction of carbohydrates and fats during pregnancy. Although it has subsequently been shown that physiologic requirements during pregnancy result in increased carbohydrate demands, this restrictive philosophy remained ingrained in obstetrical thinking for decades, as shown by the following quote from the 10th edition of *Browne's Antenatal Care*, published in 1970 [20]:

> There is no doubt however that carbohydrates, the cheapest form of food, tend to be eaten in excess especially by women frustrated by the

> separation from their normal social contacts at work, and with little mental resources. Excessive consumption of carbohydrate is the commonest cause of excessive weight gain in pregnancy, and it is well to anticipate this by advocating moderate restriction.

For the purposes of this chapter, the review that follows focuses mainly on the research that has evaluated patterns and total amounts of gestational weight gain. It is important to keep in mind that much of this early research, and the resulting conclusions and recommendations, were "ex cathedra dicta," without scientific basis. Because of these reasons, most of this work should be considered historical.

Influencing Birthweight and Facilitating Delivery

Williams, in the first edition of his textbook on obstetrics, published in 1903 [21], stated that women normally gain weight only during the last 3 months of gestation, amounting to about three to five pounds per month. He concluded that "this (weight gain) is not entirely due to the increased size of the uterus and its contents, but to a considerable extent results from an additional deposit of fat in the other portions of the body." In cases of contracted pelvis, or in patients who had previously given birth to excessively large children, Williams advised the use of a calorically restricted diet during the last 2 to 3 months of pregnancy. He stated that, as "Prochownick pointed out, a diet poor in carbohydrates and fluids exerts a marked influence upon the weight of the child without otherwise affecting it, and in not a few cases these precautionary measures may obviate a difficult delivery, or even do away with the necessity for the induction of premature labour."

Not all practitioners agreed with Prochownick's conclusions, however, that the result of his restrictive diet, that is, lower birthweights, had no adverse effect on the newborn. Using the animal model of guinea pigs subjected to adequate or restricted diets during gestation, Paton [22], a British physician and physiologist, showed a strong relationship between gestational weight gain, delivery weight of the mother, and both litter size and birthweight of the offspring. Paton published his study in 1903, concluding that:

> The size of the offspring depends very directly upon the diet and nutrition of the mother during pregnancy. While this explains the very easy labours among the healthy lower classes and confirms Prochownick's conclusions that by dieting the mother the children of rickety women may be so reduced in size as to be viable, it also probably helps to explain the very high infant mortality among the very poor. The infant starts life at a low level and readily succumbs to the hardships to which it is too often subjected.

Hugo Ehrenfest [23], an American obstetrician writing in 1919, reviewed the then current literature on maternal nutrition and documented the general acceptance of the Prochownick diet. He also provided substantial evidence from clinical and animal studies that refuted the efficacy of the Prochownick regimen, stating that "this diet may actually become responsible for toxemic conditions which proper prenatal diet so assiduously attempts to avoid." His opinion was not only clearly in the minority, but it failed to influence succeeding generations of clinicians, who severely restricted the maternal diet and gestational weight gain long after the contracted pelvis ceased to be an important factor in prenatal management.

The Prochownick diet, which purported to have no lasting adverse effects on the resulting smaller infant born at term, triggered a way of thinking that remained in the medical literature for many years. From Prochownick's conclusions many writers inferred that the developing fetus could effectively obtain needed nutrients from the mother, regardless of her dietary intake or nutritional status, in a parasite-like relationship. Although studies during the early decades of the 20th century presented strong evidence to the contrary, specifically, that a poor nutritional state of the mother (including inadequate gestational weight gain) adversely influenced perinatal outcome [23, 24], numerous American obstetricians held to the fetus-as-parasite theory, as reflected by their justifications for limiting gestational weight gain. DeLee, in the 1913 edition of his textbook on obstetrics [7], wrote about the Prochownick diet, stating, "My experiences with it have been absolutely negative, and, indeed, daily observations in other cases, for example, tuberculosis, carcinoma, hyperemesis gravidarum, show that the nutrition of the mother has little effect on the growth of the child, which is, in fact, a parasite." Kerwin, writing in 1926 [25], concluded that

> it is not advisable so to restrict the diet that the fetus is deprived of ingredients necessary for its development, although there is some doubt as to whether these products are procured through the diet of the mother, or can be obtained in sufficient quantity from the mother's tissues. Figures compiled during the starvation period of the war suggest that the fetus is capable of normal development regardless of the mother's diet.

Slemons and Fagan, writing only one year later [16], concluded that "in cases where there is a small gain, no gain at all, or an actual loss, it is certain that the mother's own tissues supply the fetus with more or less of the material normally provided by her food."

Preventing Maternal Obesity After Delivery

The obstetric presumption during the first half of the 20th century that the fetus was an effective parasite was reflected by gestational weight gain recommendations during these years. The focus of research was not on birthweight or length of gestation, but instead centered around assuring rapid return of the mother's pregravid body weight after delivery and the avoidance of maternal obesity, albeit from a man's aesthetic point of view. Writing in 1931, Toombs [26] voiced the prevailing beliefs of the day regarding pregnancy weight gains and the subsequent development of maternal obesity:

> Every middle-aged man has had the saddening experience of meeting, after an interval of many years, some "slip of a girl" he had known in adolescence, only to find her as broad as she was long, and quite indifferent to her own lost grace of proportion because of her pride in her well-set-up sons and daughters. These women just seem to get that way often despite their own conscientious efforts to follow their physicians' instructions as regards diet, exercise and so on.

Chesley [27], after comprehensively reviewing the medical literature on gestational weight gain, concluded in 1944 that, "Many patients fail to return to their pre-pregnancy weights, and the greater the gain during pregnancy (excluding water-gainers), the greater is the net gain left to the maternal organism. This constitutes a good reason for limiting the weight gain in pregnancy to about 20 pounds, as many a husband who married a slip of a girl could testify."

As noted previously, reports on gestational weight gain published during the first half of the 20th century were based on small series, case reports, or personal opinion. As was common during this time, "premature" was used to indicate a birthweight of less than 5.5 lb as often as it was to describe a gestational age of greater than 25 days before the expected date of confinement. Thus, it was difficult to differentiate between an outcome of lowered birthweight versus shortened gestation. Data frequently were presented as a range of values, without documenting the total number of cases, and rarely were stratified by important maternal factors, such as race, parity, height, pregravid weight, or pregravid weight-for-height. When mean values were presented, standard deviations were not. Application of statistical tests to measure the magnitude of reported differences did not appear in the obstetric nutrition literature until 1943 [28], and even then were inconsistently used and inaccurately reported.

Based on 150 of his own patients and observations regarding weight loss after delivery, in 1923, Davis [14] recommended a total weight gain not to exceed 20 lb for women of normal pregravid weight and as much as 30 lb for women who had been underweight before conception. In evaluating gestational weight gain in 236 of his own patients in 1925, Hannah [15] concluded that a gain of 14 lb for women of normal pregravid weight was appropriate. He further concluded that in women with gestational weight gains of 15 lb or less breast-feeding was more successful, birthweight was less, and the duration of labor was shortened by several hours. In 1926, Kerwin [25] evaluated gestational weight gain from the third month of pregnancy to delivery at term in 147 normal patients and concluded that the average gain was 16.5 lb, including 7.5 lb from the 24th week of gestation to delivery. He warned that obesity was "pathologic in pregnancy as well as in the nonpregnant state," and that it should be controlled through diet and exercise. Further, he concluded that excessive weight gain was detrimental to both the mother and child, and that "more consideration should be given to the future health and physique of the pregnant woman. Improvement in these conditions can be obtained through the control of pregnancy fat."

Randall, writing in 1925 [29], reported an average gestational weight gain of 23.2 lb for the 200 normal primiparas and 21 lb for the 100 normal multiparas in his study. In 1927, Slemons and Fagan [16] considered 12 lb to be the normal increase in weight during pregnancy attributable to the products of conception, and concluded that 15 lb was the upper limit of normal gain. These authors warned that higher gains would result in "overgrowth of the fetus," prolongation of labor, development of maternal toxemia, and failure to return quickly to the pregravid weight. Slemons and Fagan then concluded that, "It is advisable to stress the importance of diet-control during pregnancy because this method represents the only one at command for influencing the size of the fetus."

In Bingham's 1932 study [17] of 599 normal primiparas and 689 normal multiparas, he concluded that the average woman of medium size should not gain more than 15 to 20 lb during pregnancy, with overweight patients restricted to gaining less and tall women permitted to gain more. He concluded that such limits resulted in less toxemia and anemia, as well as making labor easier "by reducing the amount of fat in the pelvis." He also deduced that the weight of the infant was as much influenced by the amount the patient exercised as by the amount of food she ate.

In 1933, Siddall and Mack [30] published one of the first studies to consider maternal age and parity in evaluating gestational weight gain. They reported data on 624 normal patients who had been weighed at the 24th, 28th, 32nd, 34th, 36th, 38th, and 40th weeks of gestation. Average gain was calculated for each of these intervals and reported to be 4.4 lb for weeks 24 to 28; 3.9 lb for weeks 28 to 32; 2.0 lb each for weeks 32 to 34, 34 to 36, and 36 to 38, and 1.3 lb for weeks 38 to 40. Mean total gain was 16.1 lb for primiparas, compared to 15.7 lb for women having their second child, and 14.3 lb for those pregnant for the third time or more. Overall, younger women and those with lower pregravid weights and lower parity tended to gain more than older women and those of higher pregravid weights and higher parity. McIlroy and Rodway, writing in 1937 [18], also found that gestational weight gain increased with older maternal age and higher parity. They concluded that increasing gestational weight gain resulted in higher birthweights. In his 1933 study of 1000 private patients, Cummings [31] reported an average gain of less than half a pound in the first trimester and about 13.0 and 10.5 lb, respectively, during the second and third trimesters, with a total average gain of about 24 lb. Mean infant birthweight was 7.7 lb.

Other investigators reported contrary findings. In 1938, Bray [32] concluded that age, parity, and pregravid weight-for-height were not factors in differences in mean gestational weight gain, or in mean weight loss within the first 8 days after delivery. In their 1943 study, Robinson and associates [19] reported a mean gestational gain of 24.4 lb, with no significant differences by maternal parity.

Stander and Pastore [33] constructed a gestational weight gain curve based on 2502 normal pregnancies, including 1097 multiparas and 1227 primiparas in their 1940 study. Overall mean pregravid weight averaged 128.25 lb, with a mean of 126 lb for primiparas and 133 lb for multiparas. Mean gestational weight gain between 6 and 40 weeks of gestation did not differ by parity and averaged 30.7 lb. These investigators noted that changes in gestational weight gain were proportional to the original (pregravid) weight of the patient: The heavier the patient at the onset of pregnancy, the more marked the increase in weight. Because of this, Stander and Pastore proposed that weight changes be characterized by the percentage of gain or loss, so that comparisons across pregravid weight groups could be made. Based on a change in body weight of 24.1 percent between 6 and 40 weeks of gestation for normal pregnancies, a percent change for each week of gestation was calculated. Curves of gain were suggested for women with pregravid weights of 40 kg (88 lb), 60 kg (132 lb), and 80 kg (176 lb). In contrast, Robinson and associates [19], in their 1943 study of 484 private patients, found the amount of gestational weight gain to be inversely related to the mother's pregravid weight.

In his 1942 study, Waters [34] reported on observations of 3230 patients. Average weight gain was 23.2 lb and average fetal weight was 7.4 lb. He found that older women tended to have higher pregravid weights and to gain less during gestation. He concluded that gestational weight gain did not influence birthweight or duration of labor.

One of the first studies to control for maternal parity, antepartum illness, and length of gestation was published in 1943 by Kerr [28]. He studied gestational weight gain in 500 normal primiparas with term pregnancies. Mean gain from the third month of pregnancy to delivery was 22.9 lb and mean birthweight was 7.25 lb. He concluded that increased weight gain was associated with increased birthweight, that larger women tended to gain more and to give birth to larger infants, and that increasing weight gain had no influence on the duration of labor.

In his 1946 study of 567 singleton normal term pregnancies, Klein [12] reported a mean gestational weight gain of 21.05 lb and mean birthweight of 7.38 lb. Although the data from his tables showed an increase in birthweight with increasing maternal weight gain, as well as higher gains among multiparas and higher birthweights for their children, he concluded that there was no correlation between pregravid weight, parity, weight gain, and birthweight.

Detecting and Preventing Pregnancy-Induced Hypertension

Zangemeister [35], writing in 1916 as one of the earliest proponents of routine prenatal weights, demonstrated the value of these periodic measures, particularly to detect edema and impending preeclampsia. Pregnancy-induced hypertension (PIH), in all of its forms from mild to severe (preeclampsia, eclampsia, and toxemia), was among the leading causes of maternal morbidity and mortality during the first half of the 20th century. For example, in a study of maternal mortality in New York City between 1930 and 1932, the toxemias of pregnancy were the second leading cause of maternal mortality, after puerperal septicemia [36]. Pregnancy toxemia accounted for 14.8 percent of all maternal deaths, exclusive of abortions and ectopic gestations.

Specific Dietary Recommendations for PIH. In addition to restricting weight gain to produce smaller infants, during the early decades of the 20th century many practitioners advised strict dietary regimens as part of the therapy of PIH. Many of these recommendations were without any scientific basis. For example, in the 1903 edition of Williams' *Obstetrics* [21], the treatment of PIH included not only the restriction of gestational weight gain, but also the elimination of strong vegetables and meats from the daily diet. In order to achieve these restrictions, Williams suggested that the patient depend solely on milk (2 qt/24 hr), both for its nutritional qualities and its value as an "efficient diuretic." Also allowed were small quantities of lettuce salad, bread and butter, and herring roe, as well as considerable quantities of water, Buffalo lithia water, or cream of tartar lemonade.

Support of such restrictions was given by a small news item, entitled "Eclampsia Rare on War Diet in Germany," in the March 3, 1917, issue of the *Journal of the American Medical Association* [37]. This news item concluded that the "restriction of fat and meat tends to ward off eclampsia." Both admonitions led to generations of obstetricians not only restricting gestational weight gain, but also excluding red meat from the prenatal diet during the last half of pregnancy. As late as 1923, Davis, an American obstetrician [14], wrote:

> The marked decrease in eclampsia in Central Europe during the period of war rationing led us to realize that eclamptics are usually women who have gained weight rapidly during pregnancy. Is excessive eating one of the factors in the breakdown of metabolism and the development of this toxemia? Careful regulation of the diet, checked by routine weight records, may give valuable information in this particular.

In addition to limiting total gestational weight gain to 15 lb or less and advocating daily exercise, in 1932, Bingham [17] also advised specific dietary recommendations to prevent toxemia. During the first 3 months, when there is little weight gain, liberal intake of carbohydrates was advised, while meat, eggs, milk, and fruit were to be taken in moderation. After the first 3 months, Bingham recommended that carbohydrates be cut down but that fruits and vegetables be increased (apparently this author was unaware of the true composition of fruits and vegetables). A moderate amount of milk was to be taken, depending on the previous amount of weight gain. Red meats were to be omitted during the last 6 weeks of pregnancy. If after the third month of pregnancy the woman had gained 4 lb or more, she was to restrict her intake of starchy foods. If weight gain continued to increase too rapidly despite this moderate diet and exercise regimen, Bingham recommended discontinuing regular meals every other day and substituting instead one glass of milk and one cracker every 3 hours from 8 AM to 8 PM. Two oranges, one green vegetable, and a cup of coffee were also permitted daily. This regimen of dietary restrictions and exercise to prevent the onset of toxemic symptoms was also advocated in 1937 by McIlroy and Rodway [18], who recommended alternative-day restrictions limited to milk, biscuits, and apples or oranges, supplemented with fresh vegetables and additional fruits.

Role of Gestational Weight Gain in PIH. Higher gestational weight gains had long been anecdotally associated with PIH. As a result, much of the research on gestational weight gain during the early decades of the 20th century sought to clarify the cause-and-effect relationship between weight gain and the development of this condition. Many studies evaluated the total weight gain during pregnancy and erroneously concluded that higher gains were the cause rather than the result of toxemia. Rapid weight gain during the eighth and ninth months of pregnancy was believed by many to be the result of fluid retention, and in such cases fluid intake was typically limited and additional dehydration effected with the use of glucose and saline laxatives [31].

A sudden weight gain was believed by some to precipitate toxemia [15, 17], while other investigators suggested that inadequate early gain was associated with a higher incidence of the disease [29, 30, 33, 38]. One of the earliest studies to evaluate the pattern of gestational weight gain in normal and toxemic pregnancies was reported in 1925 by Randall [29], based on data on 100 healthy multiparas, 200 healthy primiparas, and 12 primiparas with toxemia. For the healthy women, the average weight gain was 21 lb for the multiparas and 23.2 lb for the primiparas, compared to 44.5 lb for the women in whom toxemia had developed. In addition to noting that more than 50 percent of the weight gained by these toxemic women was put on during the last 8 weeks before delivery, Randall observed that toxemic women tended to lose weight or gain poorly during the first trimester, compared to their healthy counterparts.

Writing in 1933, Siddall and Mack [30] reported that excessive gestational weight gain was noted before the onset of definite signs of toxemia in two fifths of cases, but that such gains were also found to occur with the same frequency in the normal pregnancies in their series. They concluded that, "Excessive weight gain appeared to be of questionable clinical value in the early recognition of impending toxemia." Rhoades [38], in his 1962 study of 50 normal pregnancies, 46 with mild toxemia, 42 with moderate toxemia, 25 with severe toxemia, and 29 with eclampsia, concluded that the more weight a woman gained during pregnancy, the less likely were the more severe grades of toxemia or eclampsia to develop. He found neither the overall weight gain nor the rate of weight gain to be a reliable indicator of the future development of preeclampsia.

Using an evaluation of percentage in weekly change in weight gain, Stander and Pastore [33] evaluated 2502 normal pregnancies and 433 women with preeclampsia and eclampsia. In their 1940 study these investigators concluded that the latter had lower gestational weight gains through 30 weeks of pregnancy. They concluded that "lack of gain during early pregnancy seems to be a significant sign in the eclamptic toxemias." In 1955, Tompkins and associates [39] confirmed this finding in their study, which included 65 patients in whom toxemia developed, that failure to gain an average amount before the third trimester was associated with an increased incidence of toxemia.

More recently, the 1970 National Academy of Sciences' report, *Maternal Nutrition and the Course of Pregnancy* [40], devoted a chapter to the relationship of nutrition to the toxemias of pregnancy. This committee concluded that:

> There is no evidence that prescribed caloric restriction during pregnancy has any effect on the incidence of toxemia, and no evidence that women who gain excessively in fatty tissue are more likely to develop toxemia than women who do not. One must distinguish between weight gain due to deposition of fat and that due to water retention. The following questions are pertinent: Does excessive weight gain cause toxemia? Does toxemia cause excessive weight?

Twenty years later these questions still remain, as voiced in the 1990 National Academy of Sciences' report, *Nutrition During Pregnancy* [41]: "The causal relationship between gestational weight gain and PIH/preeclampsia remains unclear. Low early gains may be a marker, or even a determinant, of subsequent gestational hypertensive disorders, but firmer inferences must await the results of future research."

Role of Pregravid Weight in the Genesis of PIH. Pregravid weight was also thought to be a factor in the etiology of this disease, either alone or in combination with the amount of gestational weight gain. Hannah [15] concluded in 1925 that overweight women who gained more than 14 lb would develop symptoms of preeclampsia. In 1934, Cummings [31] reported that 48 percent of patients in his study who gained more than 30 lb were both overweight before conception and

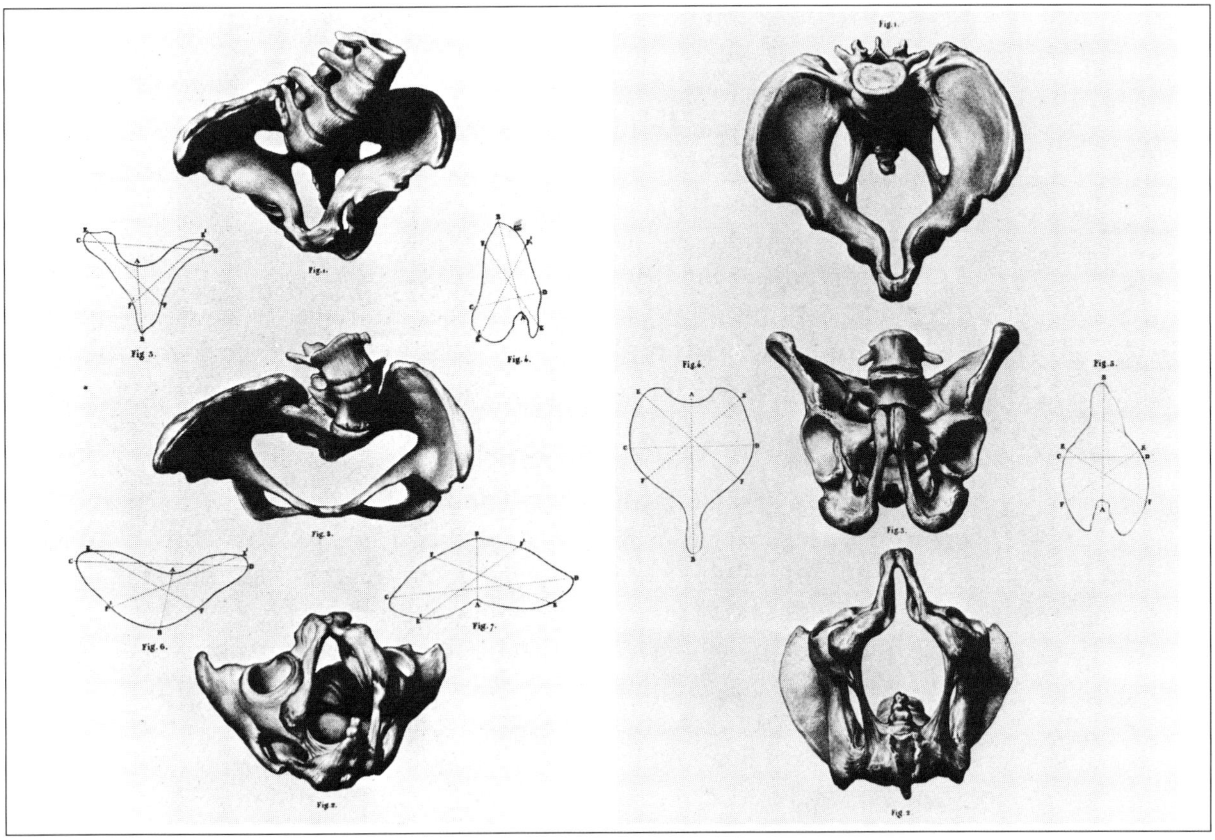

developed toxemia. Writing in 1955, Tompkins and associates [39] reported that both underweight and overweight patients were more likely to develop toxemia than their counterparts of normal weight. In addition, they found that for patients who were 20 percent or more underweight, a weight gain of 9 to 10 lb above the average gain during the first half of pregnancy was associated with the lowest risk of subsequent development of toxemia. Rhoades, writing in 1962 [38], concluded that, "The lighter the patient was for her height, the more likely she was to develop eclampsia."

The Changing Emphasis (1950–1990)

Focus on Birthweight and Length of Gestation

In the late 1940s and early 1950s, research became more sophisticated. Controlling for factors such as gestational age and maternal parity, as well as applying statistical tests to evaluate differences between groups, became common practice. Moreover, the emphasis of research shifted from evaluating the association between prenatal weight gain and maternal body weight postpartum (limiting gain to prevent postdelivery obesity). Instead, the focus centered on both pregravid weight and gestational weight gain as they influenced birthweight and length of gestation. When the association between pregravid weight and birthweight was repeatedly demonstrated, gestational weight gain became viewed as a therapeutic measure to correct the pregravid weight deficit of the mother, reduce antepartum complications such as toxemia and preterm labor, and augment fetal growth with resulting better birthweights.

The studies by Beilly and Kurland [42], Humphreys [43], and Tompkins and associates [39] all clearly demonstrated this focus. Using linear regression, Beilly and Kurland [42] concluded that increases in birthweight paralleled increases in the mother's gestational weight gain. They further concluded that birthweight was influenced by the mother's pregravid weight, with heavier women having larger infants. In addition, they also noted that underweight women tended to gain more than normal-weight or overweight women. In 1954, Humphreys [43] used correlation coefficients, regression equations, and regression coefficients to demonstrate a statistically significant relationship between maternal pregravid weight, gestational weight gain, and birthweight. He reported that women of younger age and lower parity tended to gain more during pregnancy, while women of older age and higher parity had higher pregravid weights (on the average) and tended to give birth to larger infants. Tompkins and associates [39] showed that women who were underweight (>20% below standard weight) gave birth to infants who averaged 11 oz less than the average weight of infants born to women of normal weight (6.69 lb vs. 7.37 lb, respectively). This 1955 study additionally found that the incidence of low birthweight (<2500 gm) was twice as great among infants of underweight women than infants of normal or overweight women.

By the midpoint of the 20th century, the emphasis had changed from inducing preterm labor to preventing it. Birthweight had become an accepted measure of morbidity and predictor of mortality, and research provided evidence demonstrating the association between delivery outcomes (length of gestation and birthweight) with both pregravid weight and gestational weight gain. In 1955, Tompkins and associates [39] reported that preterm labor occurred twice as frequently in the presence of weight loss or less than average gain in the first trimester. Among underweight and overweight patients, preterm labor increased threefold when gestational weight gain was less than average by the end of the second trimester.

The link between obstetric practices and pediatric problems was forged during the early years of the second half of the 20th century.

For example, in 1955, Tompkins and associates [39] stated, "The problem of prematurity is generally considered pediatric rather than obstetric; but, obviously, without premature labor there would not be a premature baby." Although in 1852 Guillot recommended weighing the newborn, it was not until nearly a century later that birthweight first appeared on the birth certificate in the United States. With its inclusion in the 1949 revision of the Standard Certificate of Live Birth, the feasibility of obtaining national statistics on birthweight became possible [44]. The addition of birthweight to the birth certificate also indicated a growing awareness of the importance of this measure of the viability and vitality of the newborn.

The Recommended Daily Allowances and Standards of Care

As a reflection of the emergence of nutrition as a separate science and in recognition of its role in health maintenance, the Food and Nutrition Board of the National Academy of Sciences issued the first edition of the *Recommended Dietary Allowances* (RDAs) in 1943 [45]. Periodically revised (the 10th edition was issued in 1989), the RDAs were formulated as tables with specified levels of selected nutrients by gender and age, and with levels for pregnancy and lactation. They were intended to reflect an interpretation of the current evidence regarding nutrient requirements for healthy individuals and to serve as a guide to good nutrition.

The first two editions (1943 and 1945) did not recommend an increase in caloric intake for pregnant women over nonpregnant levels, and no amount of gestational weight gain was specified. During subsequent revisions, however, recommendations were made for increases in the caloric requirements during pregnancy. These ranged from 200 kcal per day (1964, 1968, and 1974) to 300 kcal per day (1958, 1980, and 1989) to 400 kcal per day (1953). Not only was the amount of caloric increase inconsistent over the years, but so was the recommended implementation period during gestation. For example, caloric increases were recommended for periods ranging from the entire pregnancy in 1968, 1974, and 1980; the last two trimesters only in 1964 and 1989; the last half of pregnancy in 1943, 1945, 1948, and 1958; or only the last trimester in 1953. Recommendations for gestational weight gain also varied over the years, ranging from 22 lb in the fourth and fifth editions (1953 and 1958) to 20 to 25 lb in the seventh edition (1968), to 24 to 27 lb in the eighth and ninth editions (1974 and 1980). Despite these inconsistencies and the lack of scientific data to support most if not all of these changes, the RDAs were accepted by most practitioners as the single most important commentary on nutrition in the United States. As such, the guidelines suggested through the RDAs quickly became integrated into obstetric textbooks and standards of prenatal care.

Also as part of this changing emphasis was a movement away from small studies and personal opinions of private practitioners to large-scale studies and recommendations from national organizations, often in concert with other organizations. A prime example of this change was the Collaborative Perinatal Project (CPP) [46], which studied perinatal data on more than 55,000 women from 12 medical centers throughout the United States between 1959 and 1965. A major focus of this study was "to define parameters of the broad problem of fetal wastage, to identify possible etiologic factors, and to pinpoint possible areas for intervention or for further specific research." Several participating investigators published separate studies using CPP data describing the association between physical characteristics of the mother and birthweight. These studies are now considered the classic investigations that laid the foundation for subsequent higher gestational weight gain recommendations in the United States.

These studies [47–50] were based on term, uncomplicated pregnancies from the CPP. They concluded that increasing pregravid weight and gestational weight gain each independently paralleled increasing birthweight; when acting together, pregravid weight and gestational weight gain became additive in their effects on birthweight [47]. Niswander and associates [49] reported that the association between gestational weight gain and birthweight changed with maternal pregravid weight, that is, increasing pregravid weight diminished the impact of a woman's gestational weight gain on the birthweight of her infant. Using multiple regression, Niswander and Jackson [48] later reported pregravid weight and gestational weight gain to have the strongest association with birthweight, after length of gestation. These authors also demonstrated an inverse relationship between gestational weight gain and perinatal mortality with weight gains up to 30 lb.

Another important CPP paper examined the effect of gestational weight gain on both birthweight and the physical and mental development of the newborn through the first postnatal year. Singer and associates [50] evaluated 10,478 singleton infants at one year of age, using motor and mental scores and neurologic, weight, and height measurements. They found that gestational weight gain was directly related to birthweight, with higher gains paralleling higher birthweights and inversely proportional to the incidence of low birthweight. In addition, they reported a significant relationship between gestational weight gain and birthweight independent of length of gestation. The highest gestational weight gains (36+ lb) were associated with the highest birthweights as well as the best physical and mental development at one year of age. These authors concluded that "abandonment of the traditional practice of keeping weight gain during pregnancy to a minimum might significantly reduce the incidence of prematurity (LBW) and its attendant mortality and morbidity."

Several British investigators also influenced contemporary American recommendations on weight gain during this period. For example, Thomson and Billewicz [51] published an evaluation of weight gain patterns of 4214 obstetric patients delivered at the Aberdeen Maternity Hospital between 1949 and 1954. They evaluated average rates of gain during three periods of gestation, 13 to 20 weeks, 20 to 30 weeks, and 30 to 36 weeks. They found that the highest rates of prematurity (LBW) and perinatal mortality occurred when gestational weight gain was lowest during both mid (20–30 weeks) and late (30–36 weeks) pregnancy. These investigators concluded that a mean rate of weight gain of 1 lb per week from the 20th week of gestation to term was associated with the best outcome.

Hytten and Leitch [52], in the second edition of their text, *The Physiology of Human Pregnancy*, reviewed 35 studies on gestational weight gain published between 1923 and 1968. Because none met their "criteria of acceptability for the establishment of normality," they provided the reader with an analysis of their own data obtained from Aberdeen, Scotland. This analysis later became a standard used in the United States and in many other countries around the world. They evaluated weight gain data on 486 primigravidas 20 to 29 years of age, all of whom were at least 63 in. in height, in good physical health, and with no clinical abnormality, and who delivered at 39 to 41 weeks of pregnancy between 1950 and 1955 at the Aberdeen Maternity Hospital in Aberdeen, Scotland. They reported a mean weekly rate of gain from the 20th week of gestation to delivery of 1.0 lb per week. They concluded that "the best reproductive performance is associated with a weight gain of about 9 kg (about 20 lb) in the last half of pregnancy." They also recommended the following gains: at 10 weeks, 1.5 lb; at 20 weeks, 9 lb; at 30 weeks, 19 lb; and at term, 27.5 lb.

The recommendations from the CPP, the RDAs, and the works of such British investigators as Thomson and Billewicz and Hytten and Leitch ultimately were incorporated into standards of obstetric care in the United States. For example, the American College of Obstetricians and Gynecologists (ACOG), founded in 1951, recommended an evaluation of weight only as part of the initial physical examination of pregnant women in its standards of care issued in 1959 and 1965 [53]. By 1974, however, both the ACOG's *Standards for Ambulatory Obstetric Care* and its *Standards for Obstetric–Gynecologic Services* included sections devoted to nutrition, which advocated nutritional assessment at the start of pregnancy and recommended gains of 22 to 27 lb. Similar guidelines and recommendations are also found in the fifth and sixth editions (1982 and 1988, respectively) of ACOG's standards of care.

Other evidence, based on national health surveys and birth certificate data, has also helped clarify the role of gestational weight gain in the etiology of low birthweight and preterm birth. Outstanding among these contributions has been the work of Selma Taffel of the Division of Vital Statistics, National Center for Health Statistics. In addition to authoring several studies on low birthweight [54, 55], Taffel published an analysis of the gestational weight gain component of the 1980 National Natality Survey (NNS) and the 1980 National Fetal Mortality Survey (NFMS) [56]. These surveys included about 1 in 95 newborns weighing less than 2500 gm and about 1 in 400 newborns weighing more than 2500 gm, as well as 1 in 3 late fetal deaths (≥28 wk of gestation or ≥1000 gm) occurring in 1980.

Both surveys were weighted to provide estimates for all women for whom prenatal care information was available in 1980. Information was obtained from the birth certificate and, for married mothers, additional information was obtained through mailed questionnaires. Taffel reported that 23 percent of women giving birth in 1980 gained less than 21 lb, and 12 percent gained less than 16 lb [56]. Black mothers were 50 percent more likely to gain less than 21 lb and more than twice as likely as white mothers to gain less than 16 lb. A low weight gain during pregnancy was associated with a lower than average birthweight and a higher risk of LBW (≤2500 gm). For example, 29 percent of infants born to women weighing less than 100 lb and gaining less than 16 lb were low birthweight. The incidence of low birthweight declined sharply as weight gain increased, regardless of pregravid weight. The risk of fetal death was also lowered with added weight gain, up to 35 lb. For gestational periods of 32 to 40 weeks, the risk of fetal death dropped by about half as weight gain increased from less than 16 lb to 26 to 35 lb.

Despite the widely publicized results of the CPP in the late 1960s and the early 1970s and the integration of liberalized weight gain recommendations into standards of care by the mid to late 1970s, many practitioners continued to advise restricted weight gains. Data from the 1980 NNS indicated that 26.9 percent of married women giving birth in 1980 had been advised to limit their weight gain to less than 22 lb [57].

The findings of the CPP and the 1980 NNS, as well as the generally recognized need by the obstetric and nutritional professions for a reevaluation of previous recommendations, provided the impetus for the National Academy of Sciences' formulation of their latest report, *Nutrition During Pregnancy*, in 1990 [41]. This report, which critically reviews all available research on both gestational weight gain and nutrient supplements, recommends ranges of gain by pregravid weight-for-height categories. These recommendations include 28 to 40 lb for underweight women, 25 to 35 lb for normal-weight women, and 15 to 25 lb for overweight women. Research recommendations in this report include an evaluation of the effect of both total and rate of weight gain on preterm delivery, the relationship between high gestational weight gain and subsequent maternal obesity, and testing of recommended ranges of gestational weight gain against outcomes. From a historical perspective, this document not only represents the conclusion of a century of debate over the effect of maternal weight gain on birthweight, but also integrates the numerous points of view developed in the fields of obstetrics, pediatrics, and nutrition during this time. It is of interest that the research recommendations are multidisciplinary in nature and imply the use of large cohorts of women, whose pregnancy outcome should be examined using rigorous scientific standards. Parenthetically, it might be said that the Prochownick era has come to a close.

References

1. Gassner, UK: Ueber die Veranderungen des Korperewichtes bei Schwangeren, Gebarenden und Wochnerinnen. *Monatsschrift fur Geburtskunde Frauenkrankheiten* 19:1–68, 1862.
2. Guillot, N: Klinische bemerkungen uber Ammen und Sauglinge. *J. Kinderkr.* 19:113–125, 1852.
3. Shorter, E: *A History of Women's Bodies*. New York: Basic Books, 1982.
4. Smellie, W: *Treatise on the Theory and Practice of Midwifery*. London: D. Wilson, 1752 (facsimile printing by Scolar Press, London, 1974).
5. Williams, JW, and Sun, KC: A statistical study of the incidence and treatment of labor complicated by contracted pelvis in the obstetric service of the Johns Hopkins Hospital from 1896 to 1924. *Am. J. Obstet. Gynecol.* 11:735 755, 1926.

6. Findley, P: *Priests of Lucina.* Boston: Little, Brown, 1939.
7. DeLee, JB: *The Principles and Practice of Obstetrics.* Philadelphia: Saunders, 1913.
8. National Center for Health Statistics: NCHS Growth Charts, 1976. *Monthly Vital Statistics Report.* Vol. 25, No. 3, Suppl. (HRA) 76-1120, Rockville, MD, June 22, 1976.
9. Miller, HC, and Merritt, TA: *Fetal Growth in Humans.* Chicago: Year Book, 1979. P. 129.
10. LaFetra, LE: The hospital care of premature infants. *Trans. Am. Pediatr. Soc.* 28:90–105, 1916.
11. Prochownick, L: Ein Versuch zum Ersatze der kunstlichen Fruhgeburt. *Centralblatt Gynakologie* 33:577–581, 1889.
12. Klein, J: The relationship of maternal weight gain to the weight of the newborn infant. *Am. J. Obstet. Gynecol.* 52:574–580, 1946.
13. Prochownick, L: Ueber Ernahrungscuren in der Schwangerschaft. *Ther. Monatsh.* 15:446–463, 1901.
14. Davis, CH: Weight in pregnancy: Its value as a routine test. *Am. J. Obstet. Gynecol.* 6:575–581, 1923.
15. Hannah, CR: Weight during pregnancy with observations and statistics. *Am. J. Obstet. Gynecol.* 9:854–863, 1925.
16. Slemons, JM, and Fagan, RH: A study of the infant's birthweight and the mother's gain during pregnancy. *Am. J. Obstet. Gynecol.* 14:159–164, 1927.
17. Bingham, AW: The prevention of obstetric complications by diet and exercise. *Am. J. Obstet. Gynecol.* 23:38–44, 1932.
18. McIlroy, AL, and Rodway, HE: Weight—changes during and after pregnancy with special reference to the early diagnosis of toxemia. *J. Obstet. Gynecol. Br. Emp.* 44:221–244, 1937.
19. Robinson, HR, Guttmacher, AF, Harrison, EPH, and Spence, JM: Gain in weight during pregnancy. *Child Dev.* 14:131–141, 1943.
20. Browne, JC McC, and Dixon, G: *Browne's Antenatal Care* (10th ed.). Baltimore: Williams & Wilkins, 1970.
21. Williams, JW: *Obstetrics: A Textbook for the Use of Students and Practitioners.* New York: Appleton, 1903.
22. Paton, DN: The influence of diet in pregnancy on the weight of the offspring. *Lancet* 2:21–22, 1903.
23. Ehrenfest, H: Can labor be facilitated by a specific diet of the mother during pregnancy? *Trans. Am. Gynecol. Soc. Philadel.* 44:330–356, 1919.
24. Smith, GFD: Effects of the state of nutrition of the mother during pregnancy and labour on the condition of the child at birth and for the first few days of life. *Lancet* 2:54–56, 1916.
25. Kerwin, W: Weight estimates during pregnancy and the puerperium. *Am. J. Obstet. Gynecol.* 111:473–477, 1926.
26. Toombs, PW: The relationship between mother's gain during pregnancy and infant's birth weight. *Am. J. Obstet. Gynecol.* 22:851–856, 1931.

27. Chesley, LC: Weight changes and water balance in normal and toxic pregnancy. *Am. J. Obstet. Gynecol.*, 48:565–593, 1944.
28. Kerr, A: Weight gain in pregnancy and its relation to weight of infants and to length of labor. *Am. J. Obstet. Gynecol.* 45:950–960, 1943.
29. Randall, LM: The weight factor in pregnancy. *Am. J. Obstet. Gynecol.* 9:529–535, 1925.
30. Siddall, RS, and Mack, HC: Weight changes in the last four months of pregnancy. *Am. J. Obstet. Gynecol.* 26:244–249, 1933.
31. Cummings, HH: An interpretation of weight changes during pregnancy. *Am. J. Obstet. Gynecol.* 27:808–815, 1934.
32. Bray, PN: Weight changes in pregnancy. *Am. J. Obstet. Gynecol.* 35:802–809, 1938.
33. Stander, HJ, and Pastore, JB: Weight changes during pregnancy and puerperium. *Am. J. Obstet. Gynecol.* 39:928–937, 1940.
34. Waters, EG: Weight studies in pregnancy. *Am. J. Obstet. Gynecol.* 43:826–832, 1942.
35. Zangemeister, W: Ueber das Korpergewicht Schwangerer nebst Bemerkungen uber den Hydrops gravidarum. *Ztschr. Geburtsh Gynak.*, 78:325–365, 1916.
36. New York Academy of Medicine, Committee on Public Health Relations: Maternal Mortality in New York City: A study of all puerperal deaths, 1930–1932. New York: The Commonwealth Fund, 1933.
37. Eclampsia rare on war diet in Germany. *J.A.M.A.*, 68:732, 1917.
38. Rhoades, P: The significance of weight gain in pregnancy. *Lancet* 1:663–665, 1962.
39. Tompkins, WT, Wiehl, DG, and Mitchell, R McN: The underweight patient as an increased obstetric hazard. *Am. J. Obstet. Gynecol.* 69:114–123, 1955.
40. National Academy of Sciences: *Maternal Nutrition and the Course of Pregnancy*. Washington, DC: National Academy Press, 1970.
41. National Academy of Sciences: *Nutrition During Pregnancy*. Washington, DC: National Academy Press, 1990.
42. Beilly, JS, and Kurland, II: Relationship of maternal weight gain and weight of newborn infant. *Am. J. Obstet. Gynecol.* 50:202–206, 1945.
43. Humphreys, RC: An analysis of the maternal and foetal weight factors in normal pregnancy. *J. Obstet. Gynaecol. Br. Emp.* 61:764–771, 1954.
44. US Department of Health, Education, and Welfare, Public Health Service: *Vital Statistics of the United States, 1950*. Washington, DC: US Govert. Printing Office, 1954. Pp. 99–103.
45. Food and Nutrition Board, National Academy of Sciences: *Recommended Dietary Allowances*. Washington, DC: National Academy Press, 1943, 1945, 1948, 1953, 1958, 1964, 1968, 1974, 1980, 1989.
46. Niswander, KR, and Gordon, M: *The Women and Their Pregnancies*,

DHEW Pub. No. (NIH) 73-379. Washington, DC: US Govt. Printing Office, 1972.
47. Eastman, NJ, and Jackson, E: Weight relationships in pregnancy: The bearing of maternal weight gain and pre-pregnancy weight on birth weight in full term pregnancies. *Obstet. Gynecol. Survey* 23:1003–1025, 1968.
48. Niswander, KR, and Jackson, E: Physical characteristics of the gravida and their association with birth weight and perinatal death. *Am. J. Obstet. Gynecol.* 119:306–313, 1974.
49. Niswander, KR, Singer, J, Westphal, M, and Weiss, W: Weight gain during pregnancy and prepregnancy weight: Association with birth weight of term gestations. *Obstet. Gynecol.* 33:482–491, 1969.
50. Singer, JE, Westphal, M, and Niswander, KR: Relationship of weight gain during pregnancy to birth weight and infant growth and development in the first year of life. *Obstet. Gynecol.* 31:417–423, 1968.
51. Thomson, AM, and Billewicz, WZ: Clinical significance of weight trends during pregnancy. *Br. Med. J.* 1:243–247, 1957.
52. Hytten, FE, and Leitch, I: *The Physiology of Human Pregnancy* (2nd ed.). London: Blackwell Scientific Publications, 1971.
53. ACOG: *Manual of Standards in Obstetric–Gynecologic Practice.* Chicago: ACOG, 1959, 1965, 1974, 1982, 1985, 1988.
54. Taffel, S: Factors associated with low birth weight, United States, 1976. *Vital and Health Statistics,* Series 21, No. 37. Hyattsville, MD: National Center for Health Statistics, 1980.
55. Taffel, S: Trends in low birth weight, United States, 1975–85. *Vital and Health Statistics,* Series 21, No. 48. Hyattsville, MD: National Center for Health Statistics, 1989.
56. Taffel, S: Maternal weight gain and the outcome of pregnancy, United States, 1980. *Vital and Health Statistics,* Series 21, No. 44. Hyattsville, MD: National Center for Health Statistics, 1986.
57. Taffel, S, and Keppel, KG: Advice about weight gain during pregnancy and actual weight gain. *Am. J. Public Health* 76:1396–1399, 1986.

Frontispiece from the first edition of Williams' *Obstetrics*. Vertical mesial section through body of a woman dying in labor, with unruptured membranes protruding from vulva. (From J. Whitridge Williams. *Obstetrics: A Text-Book for the Use of Students and Practitioners*. New York: D. Appleton and Company, 1903.)

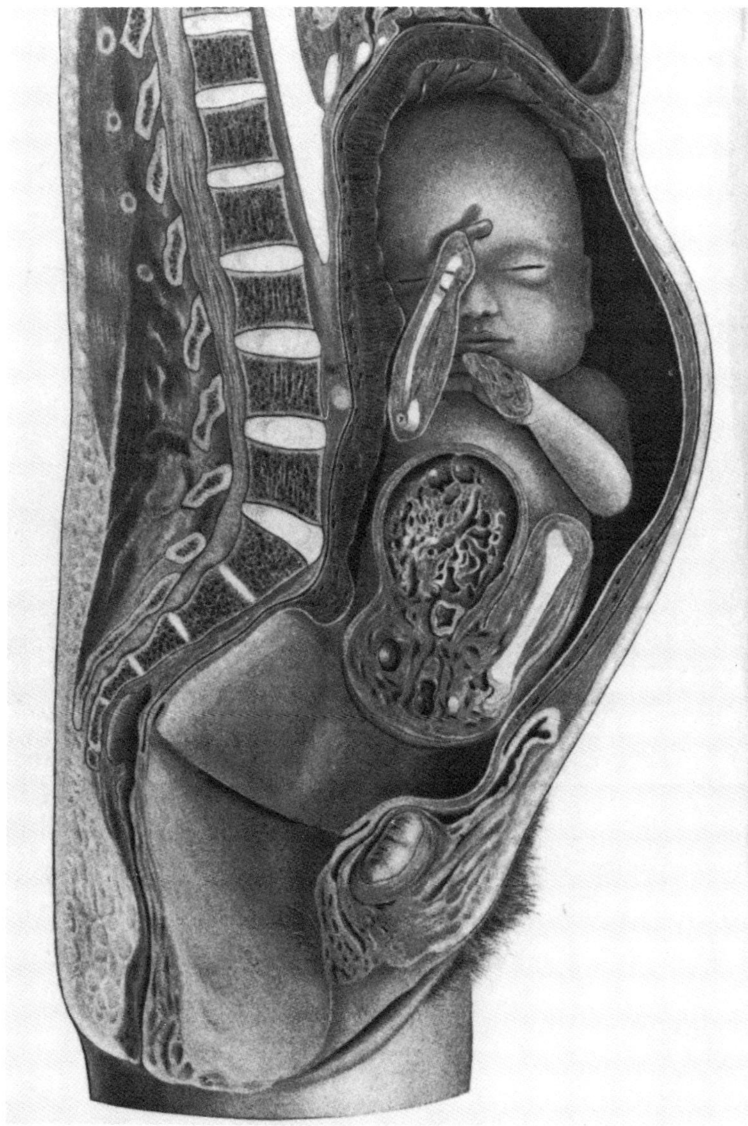

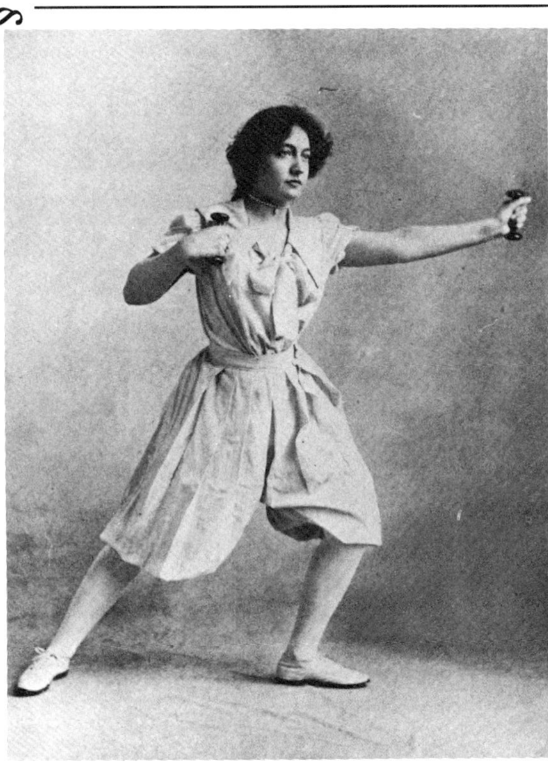

ARM EXERCISE WITH DUMB-BELLS

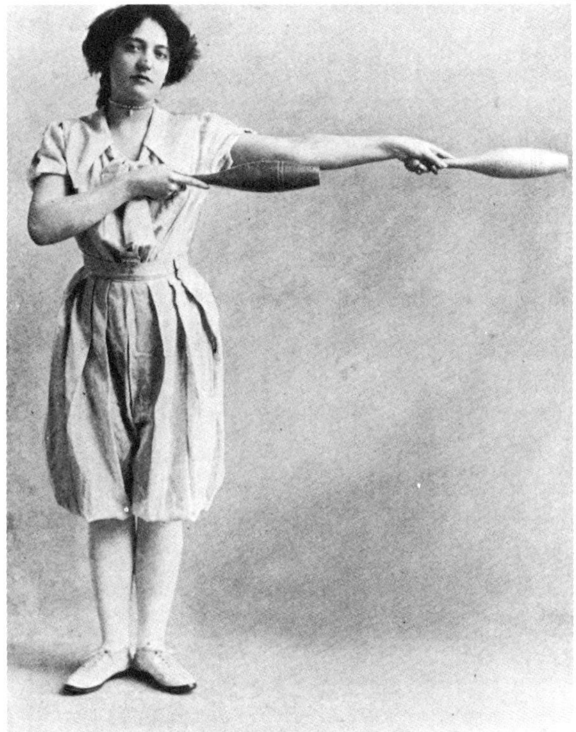

EXERCISE WITH INDIAN CLUBS.

Exercises for the modern woman. (From F. W. Pitcarin and E. J. Willard. *Woman's Guide to Health, Beauty, and Happiness.*)

2

Nutrition and Reproductive Health

This chapter presents the current evidence on the relationship between nutrition, particularly body composition, and reproductive health, including menarche, menstruation, and ovulation. The influence of physical training and weight loss on the menstrual cycle in women and reproductive health in men is discussed, including bone health and susceptibility to hormone-sensitive cancers. Dietary recommendations for optimal reproductive health are presented.

Menarche and Maturation

The maturation process resulting in menarche represents a complex interaction between hormonal and anthropometric factors [1]. The endogenous hormonal factors central to the maturation process cause height and weight changes, which are most likely the result of genetically controlled factors. Exogenous factors may modulate the timing of maturation events, particularly when these factors are extreme, but under normal circumstances genetic influences predominate. Other factors that influence growth and maturation have also been associated with menarche. For example, in obese girls menarche is accelerated, reflecting more rapid growth, whereas among girls living at high altitudes, menarche is delayed, reflecting slower growth [2].

Menarche itself does not reflect full reproductive maturity and does not imply initiation of regular hormonal or ovulatory cycles. Indeed, menarche is associated with a wide range of concurrent events, including the appearance of secondary sex characteristics [3, 4]; duration and amount of postmenarcheal growth in body weight [5–7], body fat [5, 8, 9], height [3, 5, 10], and lean body mass [8]; the completeness of pelvic growth [7, 11]; and the duration of postmenarcheal subfecundity [12].

Body Composition

Central to growth and development, menarche, and reproductive health is an appreciation of changes in body composition, in absolute and relative terms. Although some controversy surrounds the influence of body weight or body fat on reproductive health, body composition, particularly body fat, seems to play an important role in the reproductive process for both males and females.

Estimating Body Fat

Direct measurements of body fat are difficult to obtain. Instead, body fat estimates are usually derived from estimates or measurements of total body water (TBW). This derivation is based on the assumption that lean body mass (LBM) or fat-free mass has a water content of about 72 percent. Estimates of body fat can also be derived from measurements of specific gravity or relative density obtained from weighing individuals under water. These estimates are based on the principle that fat-free body mass has a fixed and high specific gravity (1.100 gm/cm^3) and adipose tissue has a fixed and low specific gravity (0.900 gm/cm^3).

Clinical studies typically utilize measurements of skinfold thickness to estimate body fat. Estimates using this method correlate well with simultaneous estimates using densitometry in adults [13] and body water in children [14], except in obese individuals. Two assumptions underlie the use of skinfold thickness to estimate body fat: (1) The thickness of the subcutaneous fat represents the total amount of body fat, and (2) the sites chosen for measurement, either singly or in combination, represent the average thickness of the subcutaneous fat [15].

Some investigators have estimated body fat indirectly [9]. Based on equations derived from deuterium oxide measurements, Mellits and Cheek [16] estimated TBW as:

$$TBW = -10.313 + 0.252 \text{ (weight in kg)} + 0.154 \text{ (height in cm)}$$

when height is greater than or equal to 110.8 cm (43.6 in.). Lean body mass (LBM) was then estimated as TBW/0.72. Next, body fat (BF) was estimated as:

$$BF = \text{body weight} - LBM$$

Each method has its advantages and drawbacks, and because there is no truly accurate technique for measuring or estimating body composition, including body fat, the theories regarding menarche that are based on body composition have been criticized [1, 17] (see later in text).

Changes During Childhood

About 50 years ago studies were conducted to evaluate growth patterns and physical changes during puberty at the Fels Research

Institute [8]; Berkeley, California [7, 18]; and the University of London [4]. These studies subsequently have become the standards on which to evaluate the numerous changes that occur during puberty and adolescence.

From birth, males and females differ in body composition, with males averaging greater length, weight, and muscle mass, and females more body fat (Table 2-1). These differences reflect the prenatal influences exerted by the fetal male and female sex hormones, respectively. During the last trimester, total body fat increases, so that by term a 3500-gm infant has about 12 percent body weight as fat. During the first postnatal year, body fat continues to increase, reaching a peak of about 20 percent by age 18 months. The relatively small gender differences in estimated body fat content in infants [19] and children [20, 21] increase dramatically at adolescence, although at any age or stage of growth body fat exhibits the most variability of any body component, reflecting caloric economy. Adipose tissue in adults functions as a labile energy reserve. The average man has about 12 percent body weight as fat compared to 25 percent in women.

Puberty refers to the collective morphologic and physiologic changes that occur in growing children as they enter the adult state. Puberty begins earlier for girls than boys and results in a greater gain of body fat. For boys, puberty begins 2 years later, on the average, and results in decreases in body fat and increases in stature and muscle mass.

Table 2-1
Body composition at different stages of growth

Gender and age	*Height*		*Body weight*		*% Body weight*	
	cm	*(in.)*	*kg*	*(lb)*	*Lean body mass*	*Fat body mass*
Newborn	50	(19.7)	3.5	(7.7)	20	12
Child, age 5	110	(43.3)	19.0	(41.9)	35	15
Child, age 10	140	(55.1)	31.0	(68.3)	37	15
Girl, age 13	160	(63.0)	45.0	(99.2)	39	18
Boy, age 14	160	(63.0)	50.0	(110.2)	42	12
Woman	162	(63.8)	55.0	(121.3)	35	25
Man	180	(70.9)	70.0	(154.3)	40	12

Source: Adapted from MA Holliday, Body Composition and Energy Needs During Growth. In F Falkner and JM Tanner (eds.), *Human Growth: A Comprehensive Treatise* (2nd ed.). Vol. 2, *Postnatal Growth and Neurobiology*. New York: Plenum, 1986. Pp. 101–117.

Because of their greater lean body mass, males have a greater basal metabolic rate than females. After adjusting for lean body mass, the energy metabolism of males and females is comparable. Peak height velocity, which usually precedes menarche in girls [4], is observed in girls at about age 12 compared to age 13.5 in boys. A moderately high correlation exists between age at menarche and skeletal maturity, with reduced variance in skeletal ages at the time of menarche [3, 22]. Skeletal maturation is influenced by gonadal and other hormones.

Several measures have been used to describe relative maturity around the time of puberty, including chronologic age, skeletal age, and gynecologic age (months after menarche). In addition, because the age at initiation of the adolescent growth spurt (and menarche in girls) varies, individuals are also categorized as early-, average-, or late-maturing. Among boys, those who mature early tend to be taller and heavier before age 15 compared to their late-maturing counterparts [7]. Among girls, those who mature early tend to be small for their skeletal age and have broader hips and narrower shoulders compared to those who mature later [7]. Between ages 7.5 and 12.5, early-maturing girls are taller and heavier, have greater muscle and body fat, and a lower rate of skeletal growth than do late-maturing girls [8].

Changes During Menarche

Menarche, or the onset of menses, is one of a series of maturational changes that occur around puberty, and is probably the most commonly used measure of relative reproductive maturity. The time interval from the first signs of puberty to complete maturity varies by as much as 1.5 to 6.0 years [4], with the onset of menarche occurring toward the beginning of puberty in early-maturing girls and toward the end in late-maturing girls. At menarche, most girls have attained 96 percent of their adult height and 80 percent of their adult weight [11].

Menarche is triggered by a series of endogenous maturational events regulated by developmental changes in the endocrine system. The rate at which these changes occur may be modified by exogenous events, including self-induced dieting or starvation, physical exercise or intense physical training, or psychological stress. Physical maturation and the ability to reproduce are linked to hormonal and compositional body changes. Over the past 200 years, there has been a secular trend toward earlier maturation. The average age at menarche has become earlier by 3 to 4 months per decade, paralleling an acceleration in achievement of height and weight of boys and girls during this same time period [23]. In developed countries, the average age of menarche in 1877 was 14.8 years, compared to 12.8 years today. Even within present-day studies, the range of age at which menarche occurs varies from 12.0 to 18.0 years (Table 2-2). Differences in nutrition and health status are primarily responsible for these secular changes and the contemporary variations in populations. Earlier age at menarche is associated with a variety of social and economic factors, particularly (1) improvement in the quality and accessibility of the food supply, with safe, fortified, and enriched food available all year; (2) eradication of the major infectious diseases and the availability of immunizations for most of those that are still prevalent; (3) the development and widespread use of antibiotics; and (4) the increased availability of endogenous vitamin D, secondary to changes in fashion with more exposure to sunlight. In

Table 2-2
Mean age at menarche in various populations

Country	*Year*	*Age (yr)*
New Guinea, highlands	1967	18.0
Nepal	1981	16.4
New Guinea, lowlands	1967	15.6
Egypt, Nubian	1966	15.2
Senegal, Dakar	1970	14.6
India, lower classes	1967	14.5
Mexico, rural	1976	14.3
Poland, rural	1976	13.4
Holland	1972	13.4
Denmark, Copenhagen	1964	13.2
France, urban	1966	13.0
USSR, Moscow	1970	13.0
Mexico, urban	1966	12.8
United States, white	1968	12.8
Poland, Warsaw	1976	12.7
Greece, middle class	1979	12.6
Egypt, upper class	1976	12.6
Chile, middle class	1970	12.6
United States, black	1968	12.5
Venezuela, middle class	1976	12.0

Source: Adapted from WA Marshall and JM Tanner, Puberty. In F Falkner and JM Tanner (eds.), *Human Growth: A Comprehensive Treatise* (2nd ed.). Vol. 2., *Postnatal Growth and Neurobiology*. New York: Plenum, 1986. Pp. 171–209.

general, better nutrition and health status have accelerated growth and development, including menarche, within a genetic range.

Hormonal Changes

The model of maturational events surrounding puberty in girls presented by Grumbach and associates [24] includes changes in the relationship between the hypothalamus, pituitary, and gonads, through the secretion of gonodatropin-releasing hormone (GnRH), gonodatropins, follicle-stimulating hormone (FSH), luteinizing hormone (LH), and estrogen. Through negative feedback exerted on the hypothalamus by estrogen, this system is maintained in a balanced state during childhood. Before puberty, the hypothalamus is highly sensitive to the gonadal steroids, and estrogen levels remain low as a result of this negative feedback system.

As part of the normal maturation process, the hypothalamus becomes increasingly less sensitive to the gonadal steroids, with GnRH, FSH, and LH levels slowly increasing. Estrogen levels, which had remained low during childhood, also increase, and trigger the changes of puberty and menarche. Changes in the ovarian follicles and central nervous system result in a positive feedback system, in which estrogen stimulates a surge of LH and the development of a pulsatile GnRH system. When this occurs, the reproductive system is mature and functions in a characteristic cyclic pattern.

In addition to changes in body fat, other alterations also occur in the perimenarcheal years, including changes in the lean body mass, pelvic breadth, metacarpal cortex thickness, and bone mass [15].

Skeletal Changes

As early-maturing girls approach maturity, their growth slows down and stops at an age when late-maturing girls are still growing fairly rapidly [7]. At the same skeletal age, early-maturing girls tend to be smaller than their late-maturing counterparts, and as adults these individuals remain shorter in stature. The skeletal age of early-maturing girls is significantly lower than that of late-maturing girls [7, 25].

Considerable pelvic growth continues after menarche [11]. More than 18 percent of the bispinous pelvic growth occurs after menarche, as well as 13 percent of the growth of the pelvic inlet and 14 percent of the inferior ischium. When early- versus late-maturing girls are compared, these differences are magnified (Table 2-3). At menarche, late-maturing girls have attained more linear and pelvic growth than early-maturing girls, and therefore have less growth to complete before maturity, including 2.8 versus 6.6 percent of stature, 15.6 versus 30.0 percent of weight, 8.5 versus 15.5 percent of the

Table 2-3
Percentage of growth remaining in years from menarche in early- versus late-maturing girls

Measurement	0 yr		1 yr		2 yr		Actual measures, adult (18 yr)	
	Early	Late	Early	Late	Early	Late	Early	Late
Body dimension								
Stature (cm)	6.6	2.8	3.1	1.2	2.2	0.2	163.3	167.0
Weight (kg)	30.0	15.6	20.8	10.5	15.3	5.7	60.6	56.3
Bicristal hip diameter (cm)	10.6	7.7	5.5	4.8	5.1	2.9	27.4	27.3
Pelvic diameters (cm)								
Inlet	15.5	8.5	8.5	3.1	6.2	2.3	12.9	13.0
Bispinous	20.2	12.7	9.1	6.9	7.1	4.9	9.9	10.2
Sacrum	16.1	10.3	9.3	6.0	5.9	2.6	11.8	11.7
Inferior ischium	25.5	16.7	17.3	11.8	9.2	4.9	9.8	10.2

Adapted from ML Moerman, Growth of the birth canal in adolescent girls. *Am. J. Obstet. Gynecol.* 143:528–532, 1982.

pelvic inlet, and 12.7 versus 20.2 percent of the bispinous diameter. Early-maturing girls have significantly smaller pelves at menarche compared to girls with late menarche. This pattern of pelvic growth has important implications for teenage pregnancies. Pregnancy in early-maturing girls of young chronologic age is associated with increased incidence of pelvic inlet contraction, cephalopelvic disproportion, forceps delivery, and cesarean section [26, 27].

Chemical Versus Compositional Maturity

For more than a century, it has been known that the chemical composition of young versus old tissues differs [28]. Young muscles contain less potassium, young bones less calcium, and young bodies less fat. The concept of "chemical maturity," as set forth by Moulton in 1923 [29], suggests that adult body composition is achieved at some point during growth. However, "maturity" is reached at different chronologic ages for various tissues. For example, ossification of the bones is not complete until after puberty, although skeletal muscle attains adult values for potassium, chloride, and water by age six [30].

Critical Weight and/or Fat Theory of Menarche

Frisch and McArthur [31] hypothesized that menarche is triggered by the attainment of a critical lean body weight : fat ratio, represented by about 17 percent body weight as fat at menarche (about 47 kg or 103.6 lb) and 22 percent body weight as fat (57 kg or 125.7 lb) at the completion of growth at age 18. Based on estimates of body composition using the equations of Mellits and Cheek [16], Frisch and McArthur estimated that, in both early- and late-maturing girls, body fat increased about 120 percent (from 5 kg to 11 kg), compared to a 44 percent increase in lean body mass. This represented a change in the ratio of lean body weight to fat from 5 : 1 at the initiation of the adolescent growth spurt to 3 : 1 at menarche [9]. These investigators reported that menarche is associated with the attainment of 22 percent of body weight as fat and a ratio of lean body weight to fat of 3 : 1. Because body fat increases at a slower rate in late-maturing compared to early-maturing girls, this proportion and ratio are attained later in late-maturing girls. Because fat can convert androgens to estrogens [32], the relative proportion of fatness can be directly related to the amount of circulating estrogen. In addition, the biologic effectiveness of estrogen is also related to body weight [33, 34]. Frisch [35] later hypothesized that the rate of gain of fat is the mechanism relating rate of growth, nutrition, and physical activity to the energy requirements for reproduction.

Using the percentage of body weight as total body water as an index of fatness, Frisch and McArthur [31] estimated the minimal weight-for-height necessary for menarche (Fig. 2-1) and for resumption of menstruation when the amenorrhea is secondary to undernutrition or intense physical training, or both (Fig. 2-2). These investigators found that 56.1 percent total body water/body weight (equivalent to 22% body fat) was the minimal weight-for-height necessary for the restoration and maintenance of menstrual cycles. The weights at which menstrual cycles ceased or resumed in postmenarcheal girls aged 16 years or older were about 10 percent heavier than the minimal weights for the same height observed at menarche. Both early- and late-maturing girls gain an average of 4.5 kg fat from menarche to age 18, with most of this gain achieved by age 16.

Frisch and associates [9] have shown that early-maturers have a different body composition than late-maturers at both the initiation of the adolescent growth spurt and at menarche. As shown in Table 2-4, when girls at the extremes of age at the initiation of the adolescent growth spurt are compared, early-maturers have significantly more body fat and less lean body mass, total body water, and percentage of body weight as total body water than late-maturers. At menarche, this same pattern remains, with early-maturers having more weight as body fat and less weight as total body water (Table 2-5).

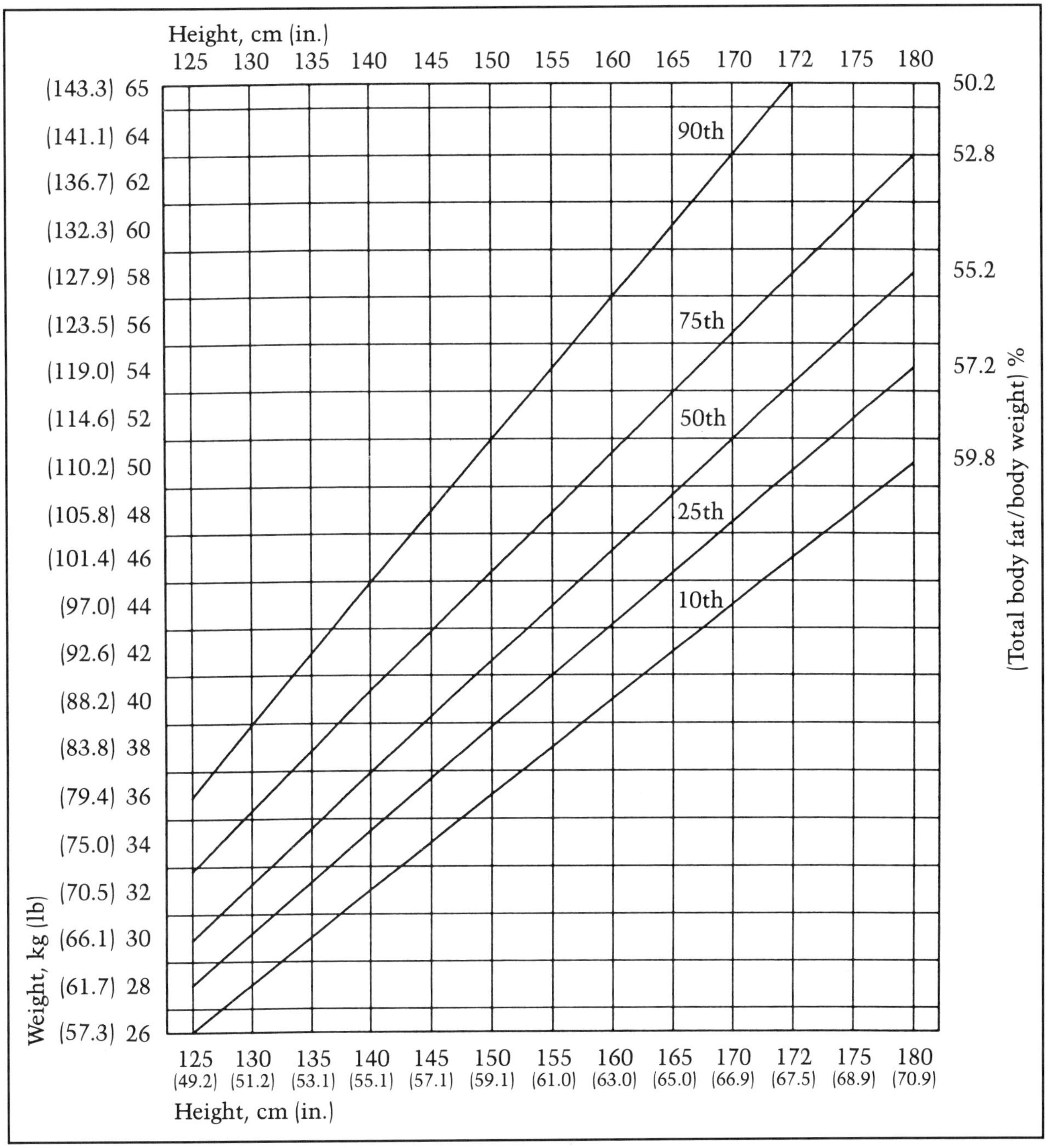

Fig. 2-1
Minimal weight-for-height for onset of menarche. TBW, total body water; BWT, body weight. (Adapted from RE Frisch, Body fat, menarche, fitness and fertility. In RE Frisch (ed.), *Adipose Tissue and Reproduction*. Vol. 14, *Progress in Reproductive Biology and Medicine*. Basel, Switzerland: Karger, 1990. Pp. 1–26.)

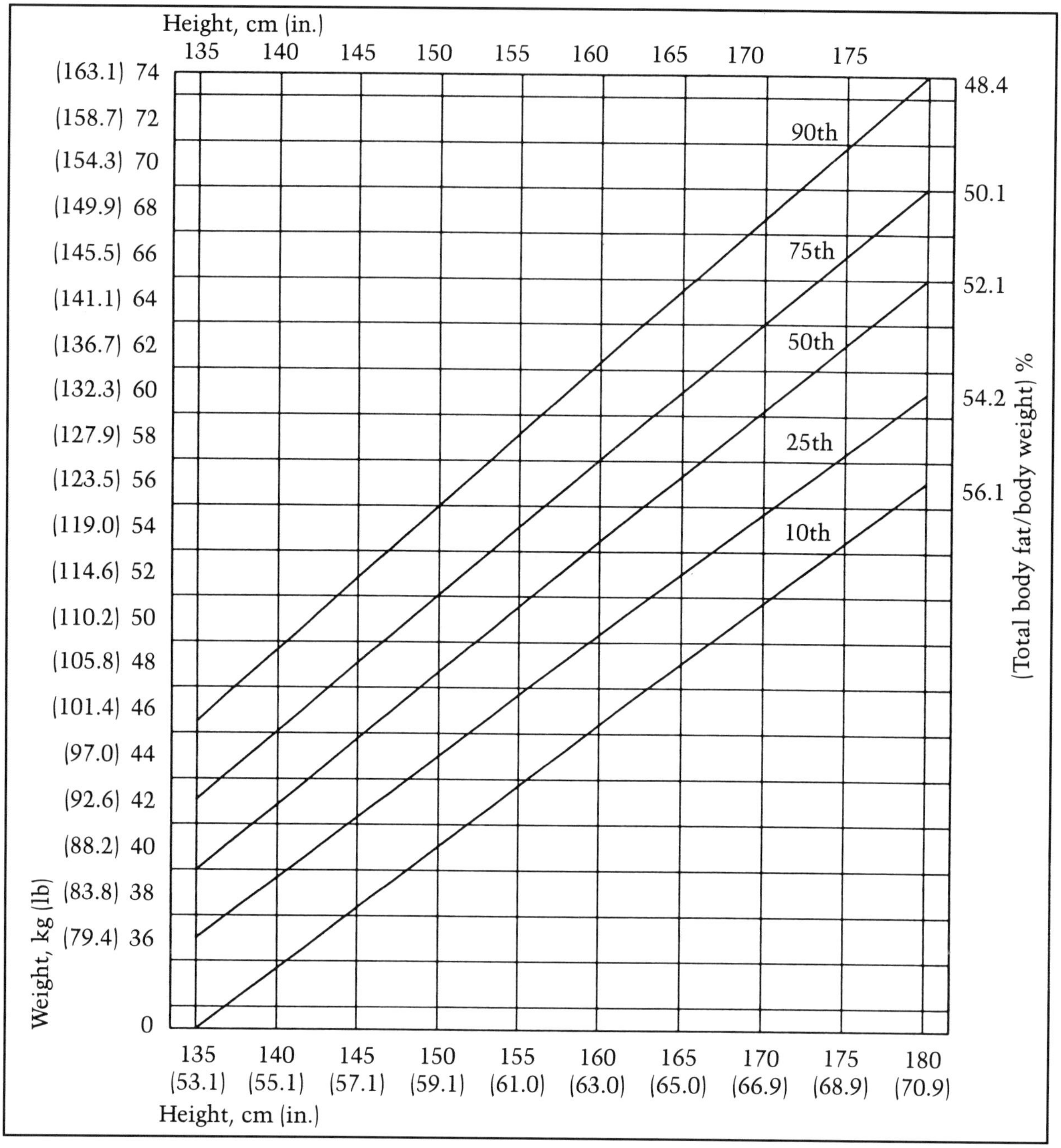

Fig. 2-2
Minimal weight-for-height for restoration of menstrual cycles. TBW, total body water; BWT, body weight. (Adapted from RE Frisch, Body fat, menarche, fitness and fertility. In RE Frisch (ed.), *Adipose Tissue and Reproduction*. Vol. 14, *Progress in Reproductive Biology and Medicine*. Basel, Switzerland: Karger, 1990. Pp. 1–26.)

Table 2-4
Estimated body composition at the initiation of the adolescent growth spurt in girls

		Age at initiation of growth spurt (yr)			
		≤8.5	9.0–9.5	10.0–10.5	≥11.0
Mean age at initiation of growth spurt	(yr)	7.9	9.0	10.0	11.3
Mean total body water	(kg)	17.4*	18.4	18.4	19.3
	(lb)	(38.4)	(40.6)	(40.6)	(42.5)
Percent body weight as water	(%)	58.8*	59.5	61.3	61.8*
Mean lean body mass	(kg)	24.2*	25.5	25.6	26.8*
	(lb)	(53.4)	(56.2)	(56.4)	(59.1)
Mean body fat	(kg)	5.7*	5.6	4.6	4.5*
	(lb)	(12.6)	(12.3)	(10.1)	(9.9)

*Difference significant at $p < .02$.

Source: Adapted from RE Frisch, R Revelle, and S Cook, Components of weight at menarche and the initiation of the adolescent growth spurt in girls: Estimated total water, lean body weight, and fat. *Hum. Biol.* 45:469–483, 1973.

Table 2-5
Estimated changes in body composition by age at menarche

		Age at menarche (yr)			
		≤11.9	12.0–12.9	13.0–13.9	≥14.0
Mean age at menarche	(yr)	11.4	12.4	13.4	14.5
Mean weight	(kg)	47.9	48.7	47.2	47.2
	(lb)	(105.6)	(107.4)	(104.0)	(104.0)
Mean body fat	(kg)	12.0	12.2	10.9	10.6
	(lb)	(26.5)	(26.9)	(24.0)	(23.4)
Percent body weight as fat at menarche	(%)	24.6	24.4	22.7	21.9
Mean lean body mass	(kg)	35.9	36.5	36.2	36.6
	(lb)	(79.1)	(80.5)	(79.8)	(80.7)
Mean total body water	(kg)	26.8	27.1	26.7	26.6
	(lb)	(59.1)	(59.7)	(58.9)	(58.6)
Percent body weight as water at menarche	(%)	54.3*	54.4	55.8	56.2*

*Difference significant at $p < .02$.

Source: Adapted from RE Frisch, R Revelle, and S Cook, Components of weight at menarche and the initiation of the adolescent growth spurt in girls: Estimated total water, lean body weight, and fat. *Hum. Biol.*, 45:469–483, 1973.

Frisch [35] suggests that there are at least four mechanisms by which body fat may directly affect ovulation, menstruation, and fertility. First, body fat acts as a significant extragonadal source of estrogen, accounting for a third of the circulating estrogen of premenopausal women. Second, body weight (and therefore body fat) influences the direction of estrogen metabolism to more potent or less potent forms, with very thin women having an increase in the relatively inactive 2-hydroxylated form of estrogen and heavier women having an increase in the more potent 16-hydroxylated form. Third, overweight women and young girls who are fatter have a diminished capacity for estrogen to bind to serum sex hormone–binding globulin (SHBG), resulting in an elevated percentage of free serum estradiol. Through changes in the proportion of body fat, SHBG regulates the availability of estradiol to the brain and other target tissues, influencing reproductive performance. Fourth, because body fat stores steroid hormones, changes in the proportion of body fat affect reproductive ability indirectly through hypothalamic regulation of body temperature, energy balance, and response to luteinizing hormone–releasing hormone.

Structural Maturity Theory

Ellison [36] has suggested that menarche is more closely related to the attainment of "structural maturity" (as measured by height), than to "compositional" or "chemical maturity" (as measured by weight or body fat). Skeletal maturity is more closely related to menarche than weight or body fat [37]. Several investigators have shown that of all variables measured, height has the least variability around menarche, suggesting it as a critical variable [36, 38, 39]. Individuals who mature early have advanced skeletal age for their chonologic age [5, 7, 25].

Estrogen, a key hormone in the maturation process, is also related to bone growth. Estrogen levels are correlated with the fusion of long-bone epiphyses in girls. Exogenous administration of estrogen to premenarcheal girls triggers menstruation and causes a cessation of linear growth [40]. Prolonged hypoestrogenism in premenarcheal girls delays epiphyseal closure and in postmenarcheal women accelerates demineralization [41]. In a study of 75 female professional ballet dancers, Warren and associates [42] reported a 24 percent prevalence of scoliosis, with highest prevalence among dancers who had delayed menarche (83%). Scoliosis was also associated with a higher prevalence and duration of secondary amenorrhea. Sixty-one percent of the dancers experienced fractures, and the proportion rose with increasing age at menarche. Sixty-nine percent of all fractures occurred nontraumatically (stress fractures). The incidence of secondary amenorrhea was twice as high and its duration longer among dancers with stress fractures.

Effects of Exercise and Physical Training

Regular physical training results in an increase in lean body mass and a decrease in body fat in children, adolescents, and adults [43]. In addition, physical training raises the lean : fat ratio, resulting in delayed menarche in athletes who begin training before menarche [44, 45], with a delay of 5 months for each year of premenarcheal training. In a study of 38 college swimmers and runners, Frisch and associates [44] reported that the mean age of menarche was significantly older for athletes than for the general population (13.9 vs. 12.8 years). In addition, the mean age of menarche for athletes who began training before menarche was 15.1 years, compared to 12.8 years for those who began training after menarche.

Amenorrhea has long been associated with intense physical training. The estimated incidence of amenorrhea in the general population is 1 to 5 percent [46–50]. Among top athletes the incidence is far higher. For example, among female Olympic athletes the incidence increased from 26 percent in 1968 to 68 percent in 1978 [51, 52]. Exercise-associated amenorrhea is particularly prevalent among runners, although an increased incidence has been reported among all female athletes. Among the athletes studied by Frisch and associates [44], 83 percent of those who began training before menarche were either amenorrheic or had irregular cycles, compared to 40 percent of the athletes who began training after menarche. Other investigators have reported an increased incidence of exercise-induced amenorrhea in women under age 25 [53, 54], and in nulliparas compared to multiparas [55]. The percentage of body fat is strongly implicated in exercise-induced amenorrhea, with mature nonathletic women having 25 to 28 percent body fat compared to 15 percent in recreational joggers and 7 to 8 percent in marathon runners [54].

Sanborn and associates [56] surveyed swimmers and runners from the United States National Collegiate championships and world-class competitive cyclists. These investigators reported the incidence of amenorrhea to be 25.7 percent among runners, 12.3 percent among swimmers, and 12.1 percent among cyclists. The prevalence of amenorrhea correlated with an index of body fat in all athletes.

Among runners, the prevalence increased with decreasing body weight and paralleled increasing miles run per week.

The amount of weight lost while training is also associated with exercise-induced amenorrhea. Among runners who lost more than 9 kg (19.8 lb), the incidence of amenorrhea was 17.5 percent [54]. In their survey of 1841 women who participated in the 1979 New York Marathon, Shangold and Levine [57] reported that the pretraining menstrual pattern was the best predictor of the menstrual pattern during training, but that thinness was associated with amenorrhea regardless of intensity of training.

Intense training may be accompanied by luteal phase irregularities, suggestive of anovulatory cycles [58, 59]. This induced estrogen deficit may lead to bone demineralization [60–62]. In contrast, other studies show that bone density increases in physically active individuals [63–65].

Drinkwater and associates [66] matched amenorrheic athletes to eumenorrheic athletes for age, height, weight, sport, and training regimens. These investigators reported a significant decrease in vertebral mineral density (1.12 gm/cm^2 vs. 1.30 gm/cm^2), estradiol concentrations (38.58 pg/ml vs. 106.99 pg/ml), and lower progesterone peak (1.25 ng/ml vs. 12.75 ng/ml). They concluded that amenorrhea observed in female athletes may be accompanied by a decrease in mineral density of the lumbar vertebrae.

Jones and associates [67] compared four groups of women: amenorrheic athletes, those with weight-loss–associated amenorrhea, those with premature menopause, and menstruating control subjects. Bone density was significantly decreased in patients with weight-loss amenorrhea and menopause compared to controls. Linear regression demonstrated a significant correlation between months of amenorrhea and bone density. These authors concluded that weight-bearing athletes and menstruating women may have better bone health than women with weight-loss amenorrhea.

Reproductive changes also occur among male athletes. Male marathon runners have decreased hypothalamic GnRH secretion [68] and serum testosterone and prolactin levels [69]. Weight loss in wrestlers is associated with changes in serum testosterone levels [70].

There is no agreement regarding the association between body fat or body weight and menstrual dysfunction in athletes. Studies have shown no differences in body composition between athletes with or without amenorrhea, and when training is interrupted, return of menses may occur without changes in body weight or the lean : fat ratio [44, 71, 72]. Stress may be an important factor in exercise amenorrhea, and may operate within the predisposing genetic and phenotypic make-up of the individual [73]. Delayed menarche and amenorrhea may be associated with a genetic and physical tendency toward athleticism. It has been proposed that the body build of late-maturing girls (long legs and narrow hips) offers a physical advantage in sports [74]. In contrast, early-maturing girls may be socialized away from participation in physical activity [74].

In summary, the factors that predispose a female athlete to menstrual irregularities are: (1) prior menstrual dysfunction in the pretraining period, (2) nulliparity, (3) weight loss of 10 to 15 percent of normal weight during training, and (4) a decrease in percentage of body fat below 22 percent [75].

The long-term implications of delayed menarche and altered hormonal and menstrual cycles among athletes have been reported in several studies [76–80]. In a 10-year follow-up study of former female athletes, Eriksson and associates [76] reported normal reproductive capability. Frisch and colleagues [77] compared the lifetime occurrence of breast cancer and cancers of the reproductive system of former college athletes to nonathletes in a study of college alumnae. Former athletes had significantly lower occurrence of cancer than nonathletes, even after controlling for such confounding factors as age, age at menarche, age at first birth, smoking, and family history of cancer. The relative risk for nonathletes versus athletes for cancers of the reproductive system was 2.53; for breast cancer it was 1.86. In every age group compared, the former college athletes were leaner than the nonathletes. Frisch suggests that the most likely explanation is that the former athletes, because they remained significantly leaner even beyond college, had lower levels of estrogen, and more of the estrogen was metabolized to the nonpotent catechol estrogens [77, 78]. In addition, former athletes had lower lifetime occurrence of benign tumors of the breast and reproductive system [79] and a lower incidence of diabetes after age 40 [80].

Effects of Weight Loss

Secondary amenorrhea (cessation of menses after menarche) occurs in dieting women at weights of 85 to 90 percent normal weight-for-height [31, 81]. This weight loss is equivalent to the loss of about one third of body fat [31, 82]. Primary amenorrhea (absence of menarche at age 16 or older) also occurs with excessive leanness and dieting, and among highly trained athletes [41, 44, 55, 71], as discussed previously. Excessive fatness is also associated with infertility [83, 84], and weight loss to achieve a body weight within normal range restores fertility in many of these women [84].

The amenorrhea observed in anorexia nervosa results in endocrine changes similar to those associated with simple weight-loss (dieting) amenorrhea and protein–calorie malnutrition. In addition, the hypothalamic and endocrine state of weight-loss amenorrhea, regardless of cause, is very similar to the prepubescent state [75]. Most consistent findings are that the plasma LH and FSH levels are low to normal and endogenous production of estrogen is decreased in the prepubescent girl, and in women suffering from anorexia nervosa, dietary amenorrhea, or protein–calorie malnutrition [85–87]. Levels of these hormones become normal when body weight is regained in most, but not all, individuals [88].

Rigotti and associates [89] studied women who were anorexic or bulimic, had been amenorrheic for at least one year, and had not received any estrogen or progesterone therapy. Significant reductions were noted in levels of gonadotropins and estradiol, as well as bone density, all of which correlated with age, relative weight, and duration of the eating disorder. Two patients who had decreased bone mass also had multiple, nontraumatic vertebral compression fractures, resulting in a loss of height at ages 19 and 24, after 5 years of low body weight and amenorrhea. Those anorectic women who were more physically active had significantly greater mean bone density than did less active anorectic women.

The long-term effect of anorexia nervosa on linear growth was investigated by Pfeiffer and associates [90]. Despite weight losses of up to 45 percent of body weight before age 16, by adulthood, most patients had grown to expected norms.

Conclusions and Recommendations

The attainment of reproductive maturity is associated with changes in body composition, particularly the relative and absolute amounts of body fat. Differences in the rate of growth between early- and late-maturing girls may influence the proportion of body fat and skeletal maturity attained at menarche. Early-maturing girls have attained less of their adult growth by the time they reach menarche compared to late-maturing girls, and this difference has clinical implications for adolescent pregnancy. The attainment of 22 percent body weight as fat and a ratio of lean body weight to fat of 3 : 1 is associated with the onset of menarche.

Intense physical training and weight loss of 10 to 15 percent of normal body weight is associated with endocrine changes resulting in amenorrhea. Restoration of menses and normal hormonal levels is achieved with weight gain. Studies indicate no significant adverse long-term effects of amenorrhea and menstrual irregularities on reproductive capability, and the incidence of hormone-sensitive cancers and adult-onset diabetes is lower among physically active women with low levels of body fat. Chronic estrogen deficiency, secondary to low body fat and menstrual irregularities, may have a detrimental effect on bone health, leading to delay in epiphyseal closure and accelerated demineralization. Women with low body fat from whatever cause should have ample calcium intakes through dietary and supplemental sources with good bioavailability.

References

1. Scott, EC, and Johnston, FE: Critical fat, menarche, and the maintenance of menstrual cycles: A critical review. *J. Adoles. Health Care* 2:249–260, 1982.
2. Frisch, RE, and Revelle, R: Height and weight at menarche and a hypothesis of menarche. *Arch. Dis. Child.* 46:695–701, 1971.
3. Tanner, JM: *Growth at Adolescence* (2nd ed.). London: Blackwell Scientific, 1962.
4. Marshall, WA, and Tanner, JM: Variations in pattern of pubertal changes in girls. *Arch. Dis. Child.*, 44:291–303, 1969.
5. Simmons, K, and Greulich, WW: Menarcheal age and the height, weight, and skeletal age of girls age 7 to 17 years. *J. Pediatr.* 22:518–548, 1943.
6. Roche, AF, and Davila, GH: Late adolescent growth in stature. *Pediatrics* 50:874–880, 1972.
7. Bayley, N: Size and body build of adolescents in relation to rate of skeletal maturing. *Child. Dev.* 14:47–90, 1943.
8. Reynolds, EL: Sexual maturation and the growth of fat, muscle, and bone in girls. *Child Dev.* 17:121–144,1946.
9. Frisch, RE, Revelle, R, and Cook, S: Components of weight at menarche and the initiation of the adolescent growth spurt in girls: Estimated total water, lean body weight and fat. *Hum. Biol.*, 45:469–483, 1973.
10. Deming, J: Application of the Compertz curve to the observed pat-

tern of growth in length of 48 individual boys and girls during the adolescent growth cycle. *Hum. Biol.* 29:85–122, 1957.
11. Moerman, ML: Growth of the birth canal in adolescent girls. *Am. J. Obstet. Gynecol.* 143:528–532, 1982.
12. Baanders-Van Halewijn, EA, and DeWaard, F: Menstrual cycles shortly after menarche in European and Bantu girls. *Hum. Biol.* 40:314–330,1968.
13. Durnin, JVGA, and Rahaman, MM: The assessment of the amount of fat in the human body from measurement of skin fold thickness. *Br. J. Nutr.* 21:681–689, 1967.
14. Brook, CGD: Determination of body composition of children from skin fold measurements. *Arch. Dis. Child.* 46:182–184, 1971.
15. Forbes, GB: Body Composition in Adolescence. In F Falkner and JM Tanner (eds.), *Human Growth: A Comprehensive Treatise.* Vol. 2. *Postnatal Growth and Neurobiology* (2nd ed.). New York: Plenum, 1986. Pp. 119–145.
16. Mellits, ED, and Cheek, DB: Growth and Body Water. In DB Cheek, *Human Growth.* Philadelphia: Lea & Febiger, 1968. P. 135.
17. Billewicz, WZ, Fellowes, HM, and Hytten, CA: Comments on the critical metabolic mass and the age of menarche. *Ann. Hum. Biol.,* 3:51–59, 1976.
18. Nicolson, AB, and Hanley, C: Indices of physiological maturity: Derivation and interrelationships. *Child Dev.* 24:1–38, 1953.
19. Owen, GM, Jensen, RL, and Fomon, SJ: Sex-related difference in total body water and exchangeable chloride during infancy. *J. Pediatr.* 60:858–868, 1962.
20. Novak, LP: Total body water and solids in six to seven-year-old children: Differences between the sexes. *Pediatrics* 38:483–489, 1966.
21. Flynn, MA, Murthy, Y, Clark, J, et al: Body composition of Negro and white children. *Arch. Environ. Health* 20:604–607, 1970.
22. Malina, RM: Adolescent growth and maturation: Selected aspects of current research. *Yearbook Phys. Anthropol.* 21:63–94, 1978.
23. Wyshak, G, and Frisch, RE: Evidence for a secular trend in age of menarche. *N. Engl. J. Med.* 306:1033–1035, 1982.
24. Grumbach, M, Grave, GD, and Mayer, F (eds.): *Control of the Onset of Puberty.* New York: Wiley, 1974.
25. Stevens-Simon, C, Forbes, GB, Kreipe, RE, and McAnarney, ER: A comparison of chronologic age and gynecologic age as indices of biologic maturity. *Am. J. Dis. Child.* 140:702–705, 1986.
26. Duenhoelter, JH, Jimenez, JM, and Baumann, G: Pregnancy performance of patients under fifteen years of age. *Obstet. Gynecol.,* 46:49–52, 1975.
27. Graham, D: The obstetric and neonatal consequences of adolescent pregnancy. *Birth Defects: Original Article Series,* Vol. XVII, No. 3, 1981. Pp. 49–67.
28. Bezold, A von: Untersuchungen uber die Vertheilung von Wasser,

organischer Materie und anorganische Verbindungen im Thierreiche. *Z. Wiss. Zool.* 8:486, 1857. In [15].
29. Moulton, CR: Age and chemical development in mammals. *J. Biol. Chem.* 57:79–97, 1923.
30. Nichols, BL, Hazelwood, CF, and Barnes, DJ: Percutaneous needle biopsy of quadriceps muscle: Potassium analysis in normal children. *J. Pediatr.* 72:840–852, 1968.
31. Frisch, RE, and McArthur, JW: Menstrual cycles: Fatness as a determinant of minimum weight for height necessary for their maintenance or onset. *Science* 185:949–951, 1974.
32. Siiteri, PK, and MacDonald, PC: Role of Extraglandular Estrogen In Human Endocrinology. In SR Geiger, EG Astwood, and RO Greep (eds.), *Handbook of Physiology*. New York: American Physiology Society, 1973. Pp. 615–629.
33. Fishman, J, Boyar, RM, and Hellman, L: Influence of body weight on estradiol metabolism in young women. *J. Clin. Endocrinol. Metab.* 41:989–991, 1975.
34. Schneider, J, Bradlow, HL, Strain, G, et al: Effects of obesity on estradiol metabolism: Decreased formation of nonuterotropic metabolites. *J. Clin. Endocrinol. Metab.* 56:973–978, 1983.
35. Frisch, RE: Body Fat, Menarche, Fitness and Fertility. In RE Frisch (ed.), *Adipose Tissue and Reproduction. Prog. Reprod. Biol. Med.* 14:1–26, 1990.
36. Ellison, PT: Physical growth and reproductive maturity in humans (abstract). *Am. J. Phys. Anthropol.* 54:216, 1981.
37. Marshall, WA, and De Limongi, Y: Skeletal maturity and the prediction of age at menarche. *Ann. Hum. Biol.* 3:235–243, 1976.
38. Ellison, PT: Prediction of age at menarche from annual height increments. *Am. J. Phys. Anthropol.* 56:71–75, 1981.
39. Anderson, M, Hwang, SC, and Green, WT: Growth of the normal trunk in boys and girls during the second decade of life related to age, maturity and ossification of the iliac epiphyses. *J. Bone Joint Surg.* 47A:1534–1564, 1966.
40. Whitelaw, MJ: Experiences in treating excessive height in girls with cyclic oestradiol valerate. *Acta Endocrinol.* 54:473–484, 1967.
41. Warren, MP: The effects of exercise on pubertal progression and reproductive function in girls. *J. Clin. Endocrinol. Metab.* 51:1150–1157, 1980.
42. Warren, WP, Brooks-Gunn, J, Hamilton, LH, et al: Scoliosis and fractures in young ballet dancers. *N. Engl. J. Med.* 314:1348–1353, 1986.
43. Bailey, DA, Malina, RM, and Mirwald, RL: Physical Activity and Growth of the Child. In F Falkner and JM Tanner (eds.), *Human Growth: A Comprehensive Treatise* (2nd ed.). Vol. 2, *Postnatal Growth and Neurobiology*. New York: Plenum, 1986. Pp. 147–170.
44. Frisch, RE, von Gotz-Welbergen, A, McArthur, JW, et al: Delayed menarche and amenorrhea of college athletes in relation to age of onset of training. *J.A.M.A.* 246:1559–1563, 1981.

45. Malina, RM: Menarche in athletes: A synthesis and hypothesis. *Ann. Hum. Biol.*, 10:1–24, 1983.
46. Treloar, AE, Boynton, RE, Behn, BG, et al: Variation of the human menstrual cycle through reproductive life. *Int. J. Fertil.* 12:77–126, 1967.
47. Singh, KB: Menstrual disorders in college students. *Am. J. Obstet. Gynecol.* 140:299–302, 1981.
48. Pettersson, F, Fries, H, and Nillius, SJ: Epidemiology of secondary amenorrhea. I. Incidence and prevalence rates. *Am. J. Obstet. Gynecol.* 117:80–86, 1973.
49. Fries, H, Nillius, SJ, and Pettersson, F: Epidemiology of secondary amenorrhea. II. A retrospective evaluation of etiology with special regard to psychogenic factors and weight loss. *Am. J. Obstet. Gynecol.* 118:473–479, 1974.
50. Bachmann, GA, and Kemmann, E: Prevalence of oligomenorrhea and amenorrhea in a college population. *Am. J. Obstet. Gynecol.* 144:98–102, 1982.
51. Zaharieva, E: Survey of sportswomen at the Tokyo Olympics. *J. Sports Med.* 5:215–219, 1965.
52. Webb, WL, Millan, DL, and Stolz, CJ: Gynecologic survey of American female athletes competing at the Montreal Olympic games. *J. Sports Med.* 19:405–412, 1979.
53. Baker, E: Menstrual dysfunction and hormonal status in athletic women: A review. *Fertil. Steril.* 36:691–696, 1974.
54. Speroff, L, and Redwine, DB: Exercise and menstrual function. *Phys. Sports Med.* 8:41–47, 1980.
55. Dale, E, Gerlach, DH, and Wilhite, AL: Menstrual dysfunction in distance runners. *Obstet. Gynecol.* 54:47–53, 1979.
56. Sanborn, CF, Martin, BJ, and Wagner, WW: Is athletic amenorrhea specific to runners? *Am. J. Obstet. Gynecol.* 143:859–861, 1982.
57. Shangold, MM, and Levine, HS: The effect of marathon training upon menstrual function. *Am. J. Obstet. Gynecol.* 143:862–869, 1982.
58. Shangold, M, Freeman, R, Thysen, B, and Gatz, M: The relationship between long distance running, plasma progesterone, and luteal phase length. *Fertil. Steril.* 31:130–133, 1979.
59. Prior, JC, Cameron, K, Yuen, BG, and Thomas, J: Menstrual cycle changes with marathon training: Anovulation and short luteal phase. *Can. J. Appl. Sports Sci.*, 7:173–177, 1982.
60. Cann, CE: Hypothalamic amenorrhea in premenopausal women associated with bone loss. *Calcif. Tissue Int.* 35:A49, 1984.
61. Gonzalez, ER: Premature bone loss found in some nonmenstruating sportswomen. *J.A.M.A.*, 248:513–514, 1982.
62. Jacobs, HS: Amenorrhea in athletes. *Br. J. Obstet. Gynaecol.* 89:498–499, 1982.
63. Dalen, N, and Olsson, KE: Bone mineral content and physical activity. *Acta Orthop. Scand.* 45:170–174, 1974.

64. Cumming, DC, Strich, G, Brunsting, LA, et al: Acute exercise related endocrine changes in women runners and nonrunners. *Fertil. Steril.* 36:421–422, 1981.
65. Jones, HH, Priest, JD, Hayes, WC, et al: Humeral hypertrophy in response to exercise. *J. Bone Joint Surg.* 59A:204–208, 1977.
66. Drinkwater, BL, Nilson, K, Chesnut, CH, et al: Bone mineral content of amenorrheic and eumenorrheic athletes. *N. Engl. J. Med.* 311:277–281, 1984.
67. Jones, KP, Ravnikar, VA, Tulchinsky, D, and Schiff, I: Comparison of bone density in amenorrheic women due to athletics, weight loss, and premature menopause. *Obstet. Gynecol.* 66:5–7, 1985.
68. MacConnie, SE, Barkan, A, Lampman, RM, et al: Decreased hypothalamic gonadotropin-releasing hormone secretion in male marathon runners. *N. Engl. J. Med.* 315:411–417, 1986.
69. Wheeler, GD, Wall, SR, Belcastro, AN, et al: Reduced serum testosterone and prolactin levels in male distance runners. *J.A.M.A.* 252:514–516, 1984.
70. Strauss, RH, Lanese, RR, and Malarkey, WB: Weight loss in amateur wrestlers and its effect on serum testosterone levels. *J.A.M.A.* 254:3337–3338, 1985.
71. Frisch, RE, Wyshak, G, and Vincent, L: Delayed menarche and amenorrhea in ballet dancers. *N. Engl. J. Med.* 303:17–19, 1980.
72. Abraham, SF, Beumont, PJV, Fraser, IS, and Llewellyn-Jones, D: Body weight, exercise and menstrual status among ballet dancers in training. *Br. J. Obstet. Gynaecol.* 89:507–510, 1982.
73. Editorial: Running, jumping, and . . . amenorrhea. *Lancet*, 2:638–640, 1982.
74. Malina, RM, Spirduso, WW, Tate, C, and Baylor, AM: Age at menarche and selected menstrual characteristics in athletes at different competitive levels and in different sports. *Med. Sci. Sports* 10:218–222, 1978.
75. Garner, PR: The effect of body weight on menstrual function. *Curr. Probl. Obstet. Gynecol.* 7:4–37, 1984.
76. Eriksson, BO, Engstrom, L, Karlberg, P, et al: Long-term effect of previous swim training in girls: A 10-year follow-up on the "girl swimmers." *Acta Paediatr. Scand.* 67:285–292, 1978.
77. Frisch, RE, Wyshak, G, Albright, NL, et al: Lower prevalence of breast cancer and cancers of the reproductive system among former college athletes compared to nonathletes. *Br. J. Cancer* 52:885–891, 1985.
78. Hershcopf, RJ, and Bradlow, HL: Obesity, diet, endogenous estrogens, and their risk of hormone-sensitive cancer. *Am. J. Clin. Nutr.* 45:283–289, 1987.
79. Wyshak, G, Frisch, RE, Albright, NL, et al: Lower prevalence of benign diseases of the breast and benign tumors of the reproductive system among former college athletes compared to nonathletes. *Br. J. Cancer* 54:841–845, 1986.

80. Frisch, RE, Wyshak, G, Albright, TE, et al: Lower prevalence of diabetes in female former college athletes compared with nonathletes. *Diabetes* 35:1101–1105, 1986.
81. Vigersky, RA, Andersen, AE, Thompson, RH, et al: Hypothalamic dysfunction in secondary amenorrhea associated with simple weight loss. *N. Engl. J. Med.* 297:1141–1145, 1977.
82. Wentz, AC: Body weight and amenorrhea. *Obstet. Gynecol.* 56:482–487, 1980.
83. Hartz, AJ, Barboriak, PN, Wong, A, et al: The association of obesity with infertility and related menstrual abnormalities in women. *Int. J. Obes.* 3:57–73, 1979.
84. Pasquali, R, Antenucci, D, Casimirri, F, et al: Clinical and hormonal characteristics of obese amenorrheic hyperandrogenic women before and after weight loss. *J. Clin. Endocrinol. Metab.* 68:173–179, 1989.
85. Lev-Ran, A: Secondary amenorrhea resulting from uncontrolled weight-reducing diets. *Fertil. Steril.* 25:459–462, 1974.
86. McArthur, JW, O'Loughlin, KM, Johnson, L, et al: Endocrine studies during the refeeding of young women with nutritional amenorrhea and infertility. *Mayo Clin. Proc.* 51:607–616, 1976.
87. Pimstone, B: Endocrine function in protein–calorie malnutrition. *Clin. Endocrinol.* 5:79–95, 1976.
88. Nakamura, Y, Yoshimura, Y, Oda, T, et al: Clinical and endocrine studies on patients with amenorrhea associated with weight loss. *Clin. Endocrinol.* 23:643–651, 1985.
89. Rigotti, NA, Nussbaum, SR, Herzog, DB, and Neer, RM: Osteoporosis in women with anorexia nervosa. *N. Engl. J. Med.* 311:1601–1606, 1984.
90. Pfeiffer, RJ, Lucas, AR, and Ilstrup, DM: Effect of anorexia nervosa on linear growth. *Clin. Pediatr.* 25:7–12, 1986.

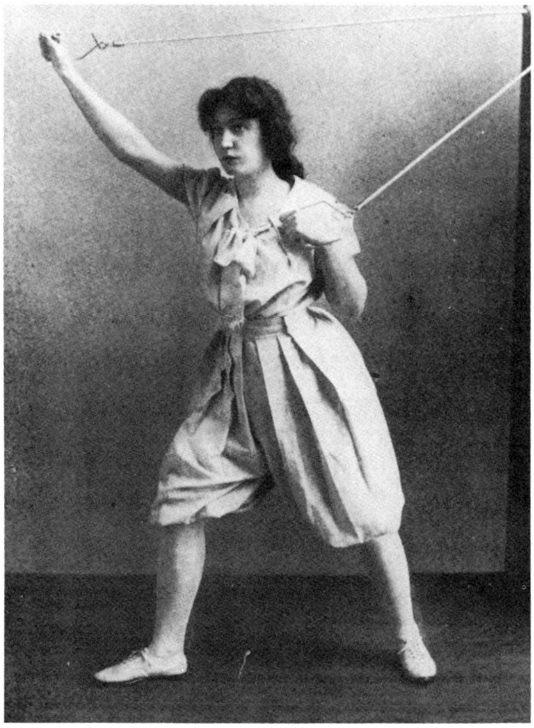

DEVELOPING A GOOD FIGURE.

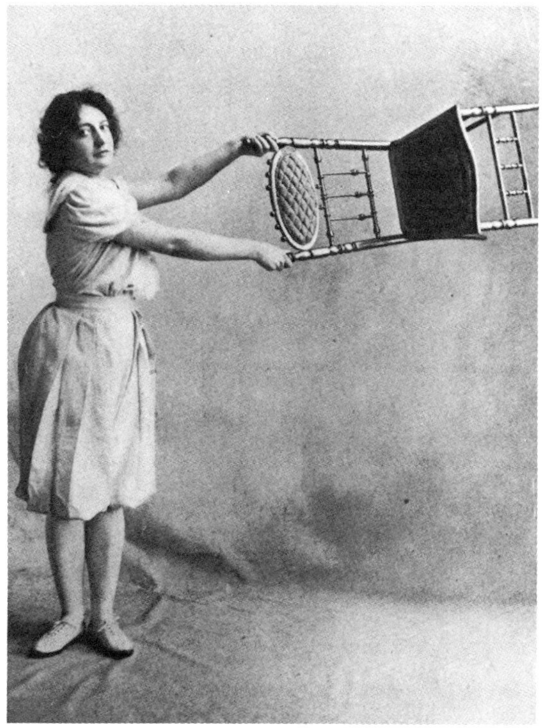

GYMNASTICS WITH HOME APPARATUS.

Exercises for the modern woman. (From F. W. Pitcarin and E. J. Willard. *Woman's Guide to Health, Beauty, and Happiness.*)

Fourteenth-century maternity dress. (From G. J. Witowski. *Anecdotes & Curiosites historiques sur les Accouchements*. Paris: G. Steinheil, 1892.)

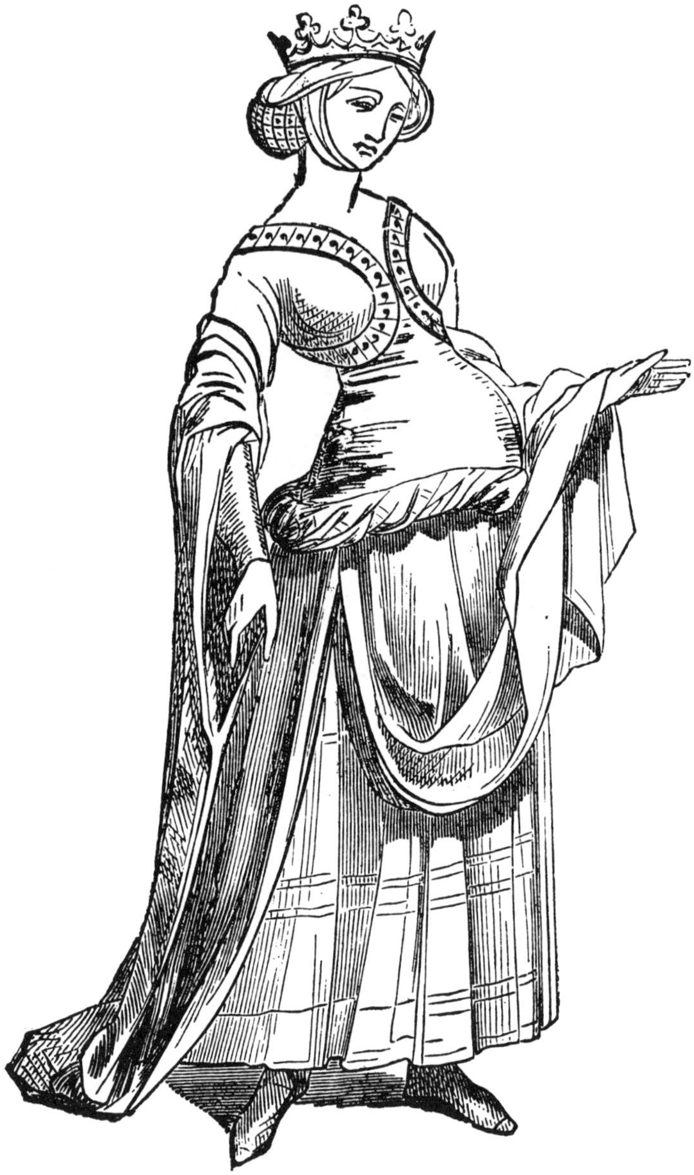

3

Maternal Anthropometric Characteristics: Height, Pregravid Weight, and Weight Gain

The three major anthropometric components associated with pregnancy outcome – maternal height, pregravid weight, and gestational weight gain – represent a combination of genetic and environmental factors. Although each factor independently influences birthweight and length of gestation, the effects are neither equal nor additive. This chapter reviews the literature on the association between each of these anthropometric factors, singly and in combination, with pregnancy outcome. Measures and techniques for evaluation of these anthropometric factors are also presented, as well as recommendations for the use of anthropometric data in the clinical setting.

Maternal Height

The ability to reproduce is closely correlated with physical growth and development. Specifically, the onset and maintenance of menstrual cycles are associated with the attainment of a minimum weight-for-height, representing a critical fat store [1] (see Chap. 2). At menarche, most girls are in the deceleration phase of growth and have attained all but 2 in. of their adult height [2]. Maternal height at puberty results from the combined influences of genetic inheritance and pre- and postnatal environment, including nutrition. Of the biosocial factors before puberty associated with attainment of adult height, low socioeconomic status, large family size, malnutrition, chronic disease, and emotional and psychological stress have all been significantly correlated with shorter stature [3]. The effect of these adverse factors, manifesting as short stature, frequently becomes intergenerational, passing on from mother to child. For example, women who were growth retarded at birth tend to have growth-retarded infants [4]. Ounsted and Ounsted [4] hypothesize that "it seems possible that the degree to which the maternal regulator constrains intra-uterine growth is a function of the degree of growth constraint imposed on the mother when she herself was a foetus." There is a strong tendency for this cycle to repeat unless it is reversed through preventive measures, such as nutritional interventions, including higher prenatal weight gain or an enriched childhood diet, thereby allowing a fuller expression of the genetic potential for physical development.

The strong association between maternal height and low birthweight was demonstrated by Sir Dugald Baird based on all births in Aberdeen, Scotland, between 1951 and 1959 [5]. As shown in Table 3-1, short maternal stature secondary to an adverse environment (low socioeconomic class) rather than genetics (high socioeconomic

Table 3-1
Low birthweight (LBW) rate and attributable risk of LBW due to short stature by maternal height and husband's social class

	Maternal height			*Attributable risk*	
*Husband's social class**	*Short, <61 in.*	*Average, 61–64 in.*	*Tall, >64 in.*	*Short vs. average*	*Short vs. tall*
I and II	8.2	5.8	4.1	2.4	4.1
III	10.8	6.4	4.2	4.4	6.6
IV and V	15.6	10.5	6.3	5.1	9.3
All classes	12.0	7.2	4.6	4.8	7.4

*Classes I and II include professionals and managers, class III includes clerical and skilled manual workers, and classes IV and V include semi-skilled and unskilled workers.

Source: Adapted from D Baird, Environmental and obstetrical factors in prematurity, with special reference to experience in Aberdeen. *Bull. W.H.O.* 26:291–295, 1962.

class) magnifies the risk of low birthweight. Compared to women of average height, the increased risk of having a low-birthweight infant attributable to short stature was 2.4 among the higher class, 4.4 among the middle class, and 5.1 among the lower class. These risks were magnified further when the rates of low birthweight were compared for tall versus short women: 4.1 among the upper class, 6.6 among the middle class, and 9.3 among the lower class. When evaluated by gestational age, the relationship between maternal height and low birthweight persisted, as shown in Fig. 3-1. Although other factors, including higher pregravid weight associated with taller stature, may also play an important role, this early study provides an interesting insight into the association between maternal height and birthweight.

Of note, women with heights of more than 64 in. were considered tall in this Aberdeen study 30 years ago [5]. In the United States, the average height of adult women has been increasing and the percentage of women of short stature has been decreasing. Between 1960 and 1980, three large national health surveys documented this trend: (1) the National Health Examination Survey, Cycle I (HES, 1960–1962) [6]; (2) the first National Health and Nutrition Examination Survey (NHANES I, 1971–1974) [7]; and (3) the second National Health and Nutrition Examination Survey (NHANES II, 1976–1980) [8]. Data from these surveys show that the mean height of women aged 18 to 24 years increased 1.8 cm (0.7 in.) between 1960 and 1962 and 1976 and 1980. During this 20-year period changes in the proportion of women of short stature have been more dramatic. In the 1960 to 1962 survey, 40.1 percent of women were less than 63 in. in height and 24.6

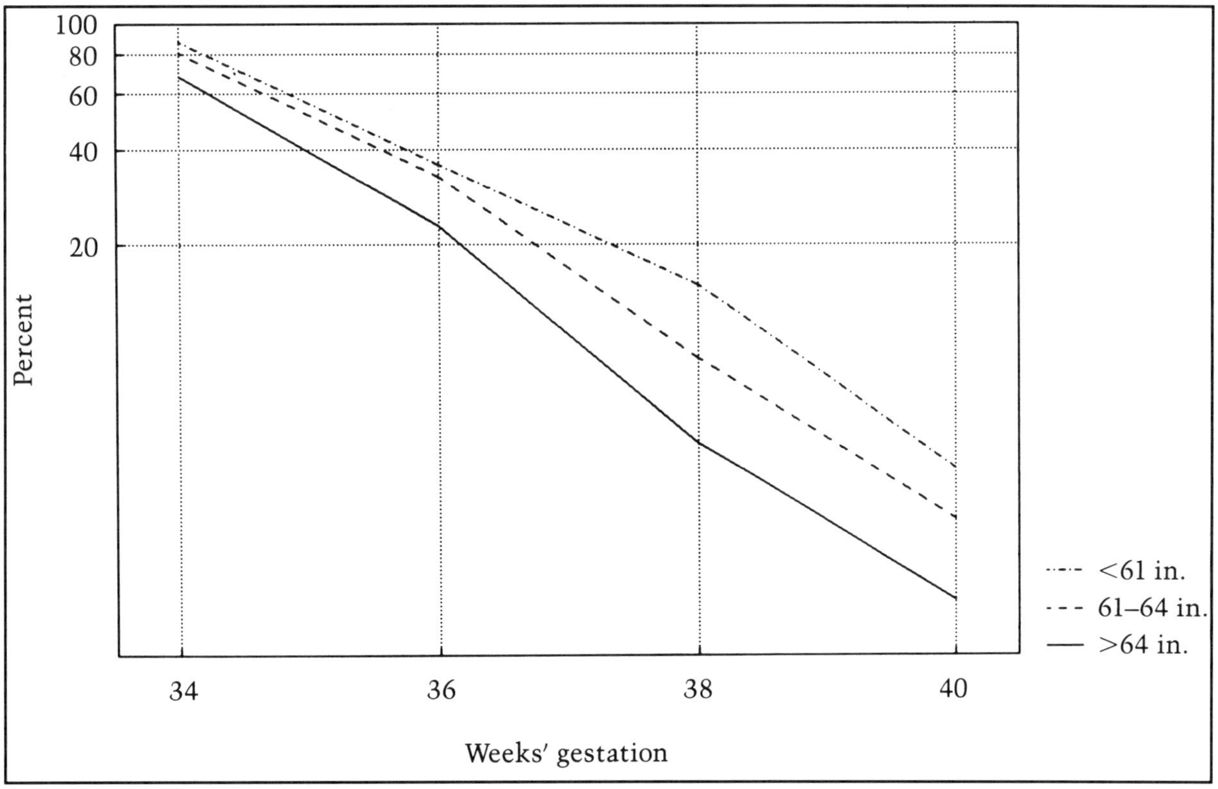

Fig. 3-1
Percent low birthweight by length of gestation and maternal height, Aberdeen primiparas, singleton births, 1951–1959. (Adapted from D Baird, Environmental and obstetrical factors in prematurity, special reference to experience in Aberdeen. *Bull. W.H.O.* 26:291–295, 1962.)

percent were less than 62 in., compared to 29.1 and 17.8 percent, respectively, in the 1976 to 1980 survey.

Few studies have evaluated the effect of maternal height on reproductive performance. Some of the earliest work in this area was published by Cawley, McKeown, and Record in a series of classic papers in the 1950s [9, 10]. These investigators reported that birthweight increased regularly as the height of the mother increased, and that the association between birthweight and the height of the father was less marked and less consistent [9]. They also found that birthweight correlated more closely with the height of the mother than the height of the father, even after the height of the other parent was held constant. The association between maternal height and infant birthweight was also stronger for first than subsequent pregnancies [10]. These investigators also evaluated the weight of the infant at 6, 9, 12, and 24 months after birth. At every interval, infant weight was more highly correlated with the height of the mother than the father, and the correlations did not differ significantly from those at birth. These correlations remained even after controlling for duration of gestation, birth rank, and maternal age.

Among malnourished women, the lower birthweights associated with short maternal stature are also significantly correlated with higher infant mortality [11–13]. Seidman and associates [14], in a study of more than 14,000 singleton term births, reported that maternal height was positively correlated with infant birthweight, by 12.6 gm/cm. These authors also found maternal body mass index (weight/[height]^2) to be positively correlated with birthweight, with 26.6 gm/(kg/cm^2). Witter and Luke [15] compared birthweight and birthlength of infants born to short women (59–62 in.) versus infants born to tall women (66–69 in.) (Fig. 3-2). Statistically significant differences between the infants of the two groups of women were evident for birthweight and birthlength at 35 weeks of gestation. The mean difference between the two groups from 35 and 42 weeks was 211 gm in birthweight and 1.1 cm in birthlength. The infants of the shorter women were symmetrically smaller than the infants of the taller women, as there were no significant differences between their ponderal indexes [(birthweight/birthlength)^3].

Luke and associates [16] reported that the incidence of both severe and moderate intrauterine growth retardation was inversely proportional to increasing delivery weight among women of short and average stature. These investigators found that adequate pregravid weight and liberal weight gains augmented optimal intrauterine growth for infants of all women, but were of particular benefit to the infant of the short woman.

Winikoff and Debrovner [17] demonstrated that among singleton term births, the anthropometric factor most correlated with birthweight varied by maternal weight-for-height status. For example, in women of low weight-for-height, weight gain was most significantly associated with birthweight. In women of intermediate weight-for-height, pregravid weight was the most significant factor, and in women with high weight-for-height birthweight was most significantly correlated with maternal height. These findings suggest that the relative value of genetic and environmental factors may differ depending on maternal body type.

Other studies that considered height concluded that taller women have heavier infants by virtue of their higher pregravid weight [18–20]. Love

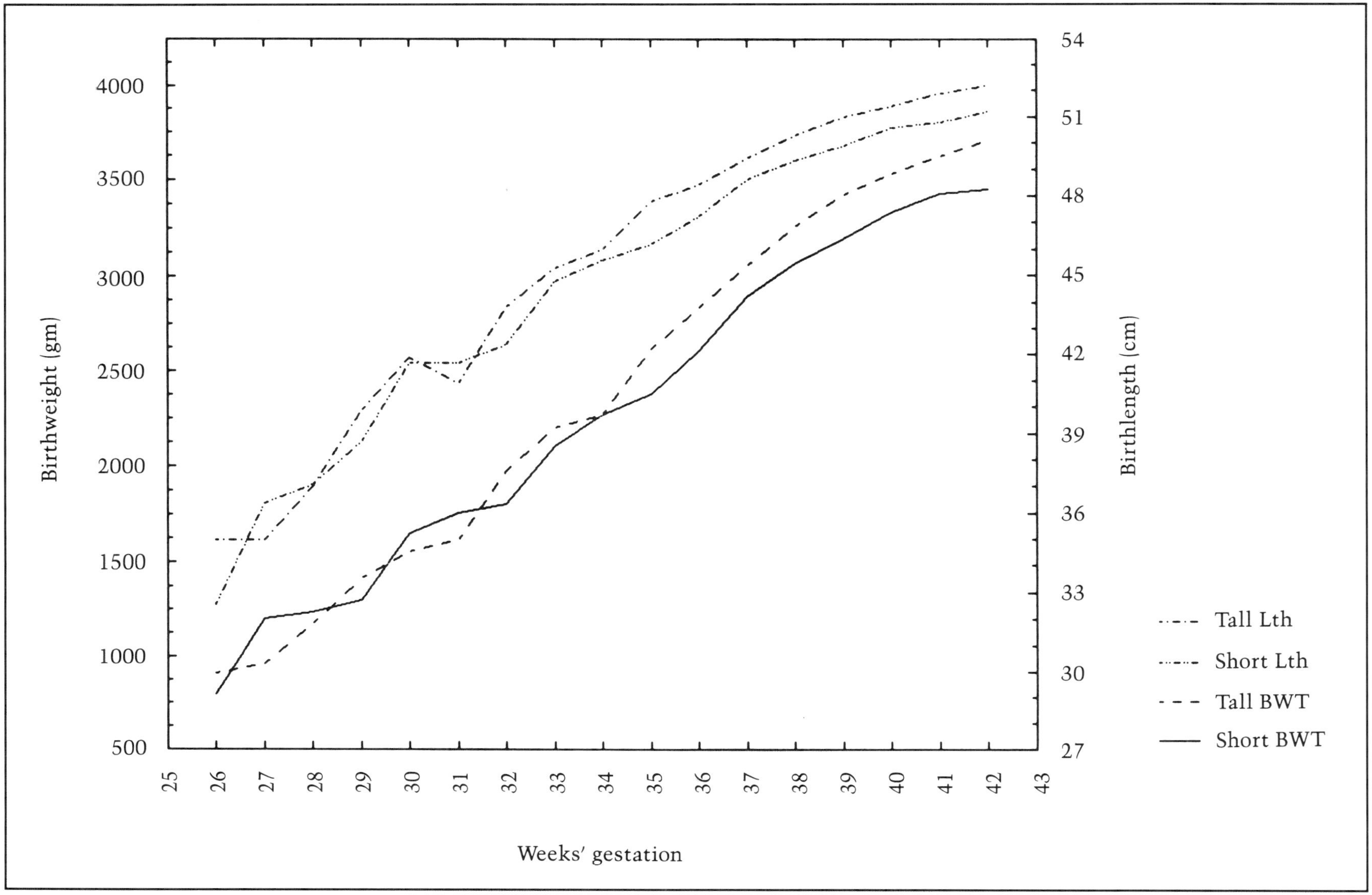

Fig. 3-2
Comparison of mean birthweight (BWT) and mean birthlength (Lth) for short women (59–62 in.) versus tall women (66–69 in.). (Adapted from FR Witter and B Luke, The effect of maternal height on birth weight and birth length. *Early Hum. Dev.* 25:181–186, 1991.)

and Kinch [18] reported that taller women have heavier infants because of higher body weight. They found that the correlation between maternal height and birthweight was less than that between maternal weight and birthweight, and that when corrected by the maternal weight, its influence was insignificant. However, they also found that taller women tended to gain more weight and therefore have larger infants.

Based on data from the Collaborative Perinatal Project (CPP), Eastman and Jackson concluded that "matenal height per se plays a very minor role in determining birth weight since any apparent relationship is through the medium of weight; the same is true of maternal age and parity" [19]. Low weight-for-height and short stature have both been shown to be risk factors for low birthweight (LBW) and preterm delivery. Data from the CPP demonstrated a positive association between increasing maternal heights and higher mean birthweights [20]. Among white gravidas, the incidence of LBW at term decreased from 128.8 per 1000 live births for women less than 58 in. tall to 57.3 per 1000 live births for women over 66 in. tall. Among black gravidas, the incidence of LBW at term also decreased with increasing maternal height, from 174 per 1000 live births for those under 58 in. in height to 105 per 1000 live births for those taller than 66 in. [20]. Across the range of maternal height groups studied in the CPP, a twofold reduction was seen in the rate of LBW for women of both races, as well as an increase in mean birthweight as maternal height increased (Fig. 3-3).

Other authors, in particular Bergner and Susser [21], interpret the association between maternal height and birthweight as being more indirect:

> Mother's height is best considered as an indirect index of her weight, for the effect of height on birthweight disappears when the mother's weight is controlled. While the fixed character of height gives its associations with birth weight the semblance of predetermination, adult weight is not fixed and its sensitivity to current influences in pregnancy is reflected in birthweight.

Maternal Weight-for-Height

Anthropometric indices that incorporate more than one measure may more accurately reflect nutritional status [22]. These measures include body mass index and percent ideal weight-for-height. Body mass index (BMI), also known as Quetelet's index, is the ratio of weight to the square of height. When evaluated in studies of body composition and skinfold thickness, BMI showed a high correlation with body fat, and therefore the degree of obesity [23, 24]. For this reason, the National

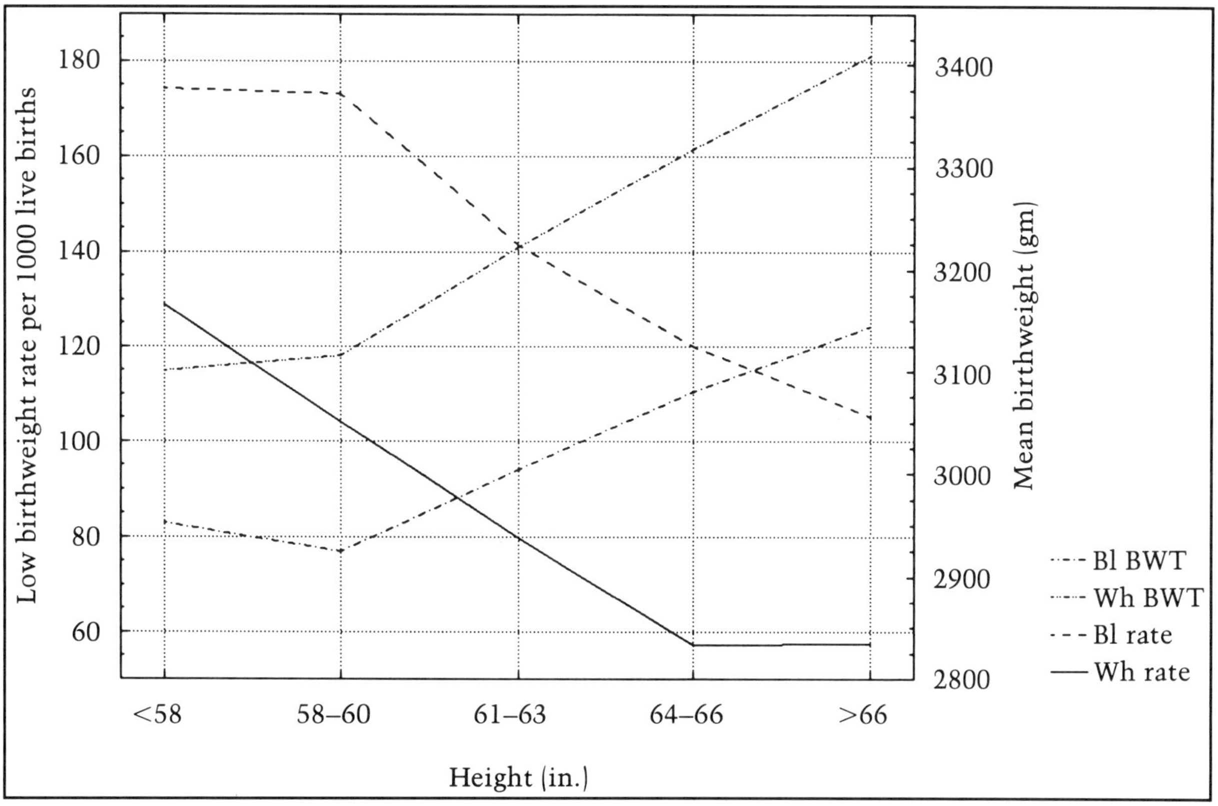

Fig. 3-3
Low birthweight (BWT) rate per 1000 live births and mean birthweight by maternal height and race. Wh, white; Bl, black. (Adapted from KR Niswander and M Gordon, *The Women and Their Pregnancies, the Collaborative Perinatal Study of the National Institute of Neurological Diseases and Stroke*. DHEW Pub. No. (NIH) 73-379. Washington: U.S. GPO, 1972. Pp. 80–93.)

Academy of Sciences has recently recommended its use in the clinical setting [22]. Regardless, not all studies have reported an advantage in using body mass index over absolute weight in predicting birthweight, antepartum complications, or adverse pregnancy outcomes [25, 26]. Some investigators have argued that the BMI is unduly influenced by body proportions, with shorter-legged individuals having higher BMIs, and by both lean and fat components of the body [27].

A traditional and more widely used measure is the determination of weight as a percentage of an ideal weight-for-height. The most commonly used references for ideal weight-for-height are the Metropolitan Life Insurance Company tabular data, which are specific for both gender and body build [28, 29]. These tables, which indicate the weights at which mortality is lowest and longevity highest, are based on extensive mortality studies of thousands of insured adults conducted by the Society of Actuaries and the Association of Life Insurance Medical Directors of America. The two most commonly used tables were published in 1959 and 1983, respectively (Table 3-2). The weight values for the more recent study are higher than in 1959, but are still far below average weights. The designations of body build as small, medium, and large were developed from NHANES I, 1971 to 1974 [7], with 50 percent of the population having a medium frame and 25 percent each having small and large frames. The range and midpoint of ideal weight-for-height by small, medium, and large frame for 1959 and 1983 are presented in Table 3-2.

Absolute height, absolute weight, percent ideal weight-for-height, and **weight/(height)^2 (BMI)** have all been used in studies of maternal nutrition. As noted above, most studies of the association between **absolute maternal height** and pregnancy outcome were published in the 1950s and 1960s [5, 9–11], with only a few appearing in the 1980s and 1990s [3, 13, 15, 16]. Most studies evaluating **absolute maternal weight** and pregnancy outcome are also older, having been published in the 1970s and 1980s [30–37]. The vast majority of studies of maternal nutrition, dating from the 1950s to the 1990s, has used **percent ideal weight-for-height,** based on the Metropolitan Life Insurance Company tables [16, 17, 38–55] or the British equivalent [56, 57]. Since 1986, an increasing number of studies have used **BMI** [14, 58–64]. Several established investigators, including Abrams [59, 61], Hediger [60, 62], and Luke [64] have recently changed from percent ideal weight-for-height to BMI, or are using both measures. Because the standards, as well as their cutoff points and ranges, have varied, it is difficult to evaluate published studies that have examined associations between maternal anthropometric characteristics and pregnancy outcome using different anthropometric measures.

To facilitate comparisons between absolute height, absolute weight, percent ideal weight-for-height, and BMI, values comparable to the traditional ranges of 90 percent or lower (underweight), 91 to 119 percent (normal weight), 120 to 134 percent (overweight), and 135 percent or above (obese) are given in absolute weight (lb and kg) and BMI (in English and metric units) for heights of 57 to 70 in. in Table 3-3.

Pregravid Weight

Clinical Studies

Numerous studies have demonstrated that birthweight parallels increases in maternal pregravid weight or pregravid body mass. Pregravid weight and gestational weight gain act together in their

Table 3-2
Metropolitan Life Insurance Company height and weight tables for adult women

Height (in.)	Small frame (lb)		Medium frame (lb)		Large frame (lb)	
	1959	1983	1959	1983	1959	1983
57						
Midpoint	93.5	103.5	100	112	110	121.5
Range	90–97	99–108	94–106	106–118	102–118	115–128
58						
Midpoint	94	105	103	114	113	124
Range	92–100	100–110	97–109	108–120	105–121	117–131
59						
Midpoint	99	106.5	106	117.5	116	126.5
Range	95–103	101–112	100–112	110–123	108–124	119–134
60						
Midpoint	102	109	109	119	119	129.5
Range	98–106	103–115	103–115	112–126	111–127	122–137
61						
Midpoint	105	111.5	112	122	122	132.5
Range	101–109	105–118	106–118	115–129	114–130	125–140
62						
Midpoint	108	114.5	115.5	125	125.5	136
Range	104–112	108–121	109–122	118–132	117–134	128–144
63						
Midpoint	111	117.5	119	128	129.5	139.5
Range	107–115	111–124	112–126	121–135	121–138	131–148
64						
Midpoint	114.5	120.5	123.5	131	133.5	143
Range	110–119	114–127	116–131	124–138	125–142	134–152
65						
Midpoint	118.5	123.5	127.5	134	137.5	146.5
Range	114–123	117–130	120–135	127–141	129–146	137–156
66						
Midpoint	122.5	126.5	131.5	137	141.5	150
Range	118–127	120–133	124–139	130–144	133–150	140–160
67						
Midpoint	126.5	129.5	135.5	140	145.5	153.5
Range	122–131	123–136	128–143	133–147	137–154	143–164
68						
Midpoint	131	132.5	139.5	143	150	156.5
Range	126–136	126–139	132–147	136–150	141–159	146–167
69						
Midpoint	135	135.5	143.5	146	154.5	159.5
Range	130–140	129–142	136–151	139–153	145–164	149–170
70						
Midpoint	139	138.5	147.5	149	159	162.5
Range	134–144	132–145	140–155	142–156	149–169	152–173

Source: Adapted from *Statistical Bulletin of the Metropolitan Life Insurance Company* 40:1–4, 1959 and 64:2–9, 1983.

Table 3-3
*Reference weight-for-height (wt-ht)**

	Underweight ≤90% wt-ht		*Normal weight 91–119% wt-ht*		*Overweight 120–134% wt-ht*		*Obese ≥135% wt-ht*	
Height	*Weight*	*BMI**	*Weight*	*BMI*	*Weight*	*BMI*	*Weight*	*BMI*
57	101	3.11	102–133	3.14–4.09	134–150	4.12–4.62	151	4.65
[1.45	45.8	21.8	46.3–60.3	22.0–28.6	60.8–68.0	28.8–32.3	68.5	32.5]
58	103	3.06	104–136	3.09–4.04	137–153	4.07–4.55	154	4.58
[1.47	46.7	21.4	47.2–61.7	21.6–28.3	62.1–69.4	28.5–31.9	69.9	32.1]
59	106	3.05	107–140	3.07–4.02	141–157	4.05–4.51	158	4.54
[1.49	48.1	21.4	48.5–63.5	21.5–28.1	64.0–71.2	28.4–31.6	71.7	31.8]
60	107	2.97	108–142	3.00–3.94	143–159	3.97–4.42	160	4.44
[1.52	48.5	20.8	49.0–64.4	21.0–27.6	64.9–72.1	27.8–30.9	72.6	31.1]
61	110	2.96	111–145	2.98–3.90	146–164	3.92–4.41	165	4.43
[1.55	49.9	20.7	50.3–65.8	20.9–27.3	66.2–74.4	27.4–30.9	74.8	31.0]
62	113	2.94	114–149	2.97–3.88	150–168	3.90–4.37	169	4.40
[1.57	51.3	20.6	51.7–67.6	20.8–27.2	68.0–76.2	27.3–30.6	76.7	30.8]
63	115	2.90	116–152	2.92–3.83	153–172	3.85–4.33	173	4.36
[1.60	52.2	20.3	52.6–68.9	20.4–26.8	69.4–78.0	27.0–30.3	78.5	30.2]
64	118	2.88	119–156	2.91–3.81	157–176	3.83–4.30	177	4.32
[1.62	53.5	20.2	54.0–70.8	20.4–26.7	71.2–79.8	26.8–30.1	80.3	30.2]
65	121	2.86	122–160	2.89–3.79	161–180	3.81–4.26	181	4.28
[1.65	54.9	20.0	55.3–72.6	20.2–26.5	73.0–81.6	26.7–29.8	82.1	30.0]
66	123	2.82	124–163	2.85–3.74	164–184	3.76–4.22	185	4.25
[1.67	55.8	19.7	56.2–73.9	20.0–26.2	74.4–83.5	26.3–29.5	83.9	29.8]
67	126	2.81	127–167	2.83–3.72	168–188	3.74–4.19	189	4.21
[1.70	57.2	19.7	57.6–75.7	19.8–26.0	76.2–85.3	26.2–29.3	85.7	29.5]
68	129	2.79	130–170	2.81–3.68	171–192	3.70–4.15	193	4.17
[1.73	58.5	19.5	59.0–77.1	19.7–25.8	77.6–87.0	25.9–29.1	87.5	29.2]
69	132	2.77	133–174	2.79–3.65	175–196	3.68–4.12	197	4.14
[1.75	59.9	19.4	60.3–78.9	19.5–25.6	79.4–88.9	25.8–28.8	89.4	29.0]
70	134	2.73	135–178	2.76–3.36	179–200	3.65–4.08	201	4.10
[1.78	60.8	19.1	61.2–80.7	19.3–25.4	81.2–90.7	25.6–28.6	91.2	28.7]

*Unbracketed heights and weights are in English and standard units (in. and lb, respectively); bracketed values are in metric units (meters for height and kg for weight). BMI values are based on English units as [weight/(height)^2] × 100 or metric units as weight/(height)^2.

Source: Based on the midpoint of the medium frame ideal weight-for-height of the 1983 Metropolitan Life Height and Weight tables (*Statistical Bulletin of the Metropolitan Life Insurance Company* 64:2–9, 1983).

effect on birthweight, although this effect varies across the spectrum of pregravid weights. Data on live births from the 1980 National Natality Survey illustrate this association, as shown in Table 3-4 and Fig. 3-4 [58]. **The percentage of low birthweight is highest among women with the lowest pregravid weights and lowest gestational weight gains; with gains of 26 lb or more, the differences between maternal pregravid weight categories no longer exist.** When differences in maternal age and education, infant gender, and gestational age were accounted for, women gaining less than 21 lb were 2.3 times as likely to have a low-birthweight infant as women with higher weight gains.

As shown in Table 3-4, within each category of gestational weight gain, mean birthweights increased with BMI from underweight to overweight. The difference in mean birthweights of infants born to underweight versus overweight women was 203 gm, or about 6 percent. When stratified by weight gain categories, the difference in mean birthweights of infants born to underweight versus over-

Table 3-4
Mean birthweights (gm) of term live births by maternal pregravid BMI and gestational weight gain of nonsmoking women, United States, 1980 National Natality Survey

	Weight gain						*Birthweight difference <16 vs. ≥36 lb weight gain*	
BMI[a]	*<16 lb*	*16–20 lb*	*21–25 lb*	*26–35 lb*	*≥36 lb*	*All*	*Grams*	*Percent*
Underweight	2927	3100	3276	3374	3483	3323	556	19.0
Normal weight	3097	3231	3428	3471	3606	3453	509	16.4
Overweight	3330	3458	3526	3581	3665	3526	335	10.0
All BMIs	3189	3266	3411	3467	3592	3440	403	12.6
Birthweight difference[b]								
Grams	403	358	250	207	182	203		
Percent	13.8	11.5	7.6	6.1	5.2	6.1		

[a]BMI categories divided as: underweight, equal to the first quartile of the study population; normal weight, the second and third quartiles; and overweight, the fourth quartile.
[b]Difference between under- vs. overweight.

Source: Adapted from S Taffel, Maternal weight gain and the outcome of pregnancy, United States, 1980. *Vital and Health Statistics*, Series 21, No. 44. DHHS Pub. No. (PHS) 86-1922. Public Health Service. Washington, DC: US Govt. Printing Office, 1986.

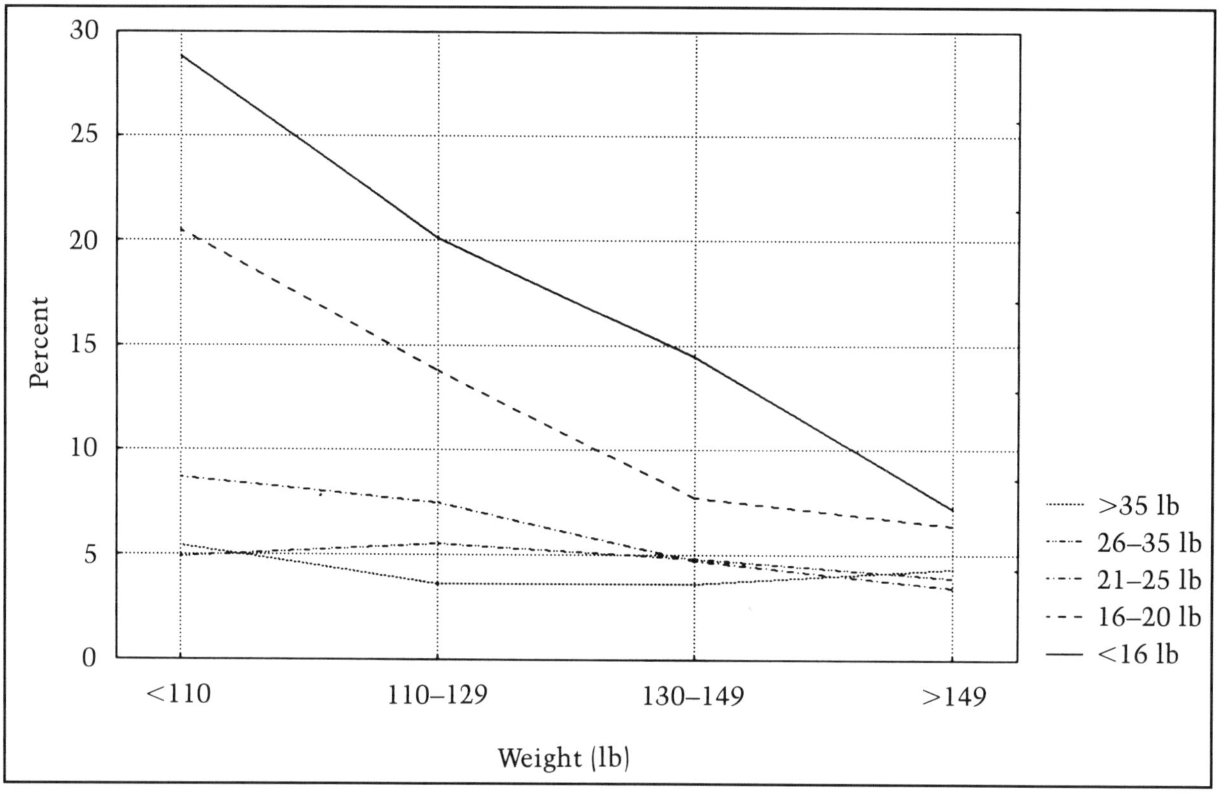

Fig. 3-4
Percent of low-birthweight infants by maternal pregravid weight and weight gain, United States, 1980 National Natality Survey. (Adapted from S Taffel, Maternal weight gain and the outcome of pregnancy, United States, 1980. *Vital and Health Statistics*, Series 21, No. 44. DHHS Pub. No. (PHS) 86-1922. Public Health Service. Washington, DC: US Govt. Printing Office, 1986.)

weight women was greatest with gains of 16 lb or less (403 gm, 13.8%), and decreased with gains of 36 lb or more (182 gm, 5.2%). **Higher gestational weight gains exert the greatest effect on the birthweights of underweight women; such women must gain more than their normal-weight counterparts for their newborns to achieve comparable birthweights.** As is also shown in Table 3-4, mean birthweights increased across the range of gestational weight gain from 16 lb or less to 36 lb or greater by 556 gm, or 19 percent, for infants of underweight women, to 509 gm, or 16.4 percent for normal-weight women, and 335 gm, or 10 percent, for infants of overweight women. **Among term births, mean birthweight of about 3400 gm was achieved with weight gains of 36 lb or more in underweight women, compared to 21 to 25 lb in normal-weight women, and 16 to 20 lb in overweight women.**

Other investigators have also shown that underweight women must gain more than their normal-weight or overweight counterparts to achieve comparable birthweights. Mitchell and Lerner [53] reported that each kilogram increase in maternal weight gain was associated with a 12.85-gm increase in birthweight in the infants of underweight women, compared to an 8.59-gm increase in the birthweight of normal-weight women. Abrams and Laros [59] found that each kilogram increase in maternal weight gain was associated with an increase in birthweight of 25.9 gm among infants of underweight women, 28.3 gm among infants of normal-weight women, and 17.8 gm among infants of moderately overweight women. In a study of postpartum weight-for-height, Luke and Petrie [41] reported that each 10 percent increase in body weight was associated with a 214-gm increase in birthweight for underweight women, a 41.9-gm increase for normal-weight women, and a 29.8-gm decrease in overweight women.

Because of the strong evidence from clinical studies, current weight gain recommendations suggest taking maternal pregravid weight into account. The 1990 recommendations from the National Academy of Sciences' Food and Nutrition Board [22] suggest that for normal-weight women (BMI 19.8–26.0, or 91–119% ideal weight-for-height), total weight gain should be 25 to 35 lb; for underweight women (BMI <19.8, or 10% or more below ideal weight-for-height), 28 to 40 lb; and for overweight women (BMI >26.0, or 20% or more above ideal weight-for-height), 15 to 25 lb. The recommended weight gain in the overweight and obese woman has been a matter of controversy for many years. In two recent studies [51, 59], weight gain was not significantly correlated with birthweight for women more than 135 percent above ideal weight-for-height, although a third study [43] found that massively obese women (>150% ideal weight-for-height) needed to gain more than 12 lb to achieve infant birthweights greater than 3000 gm.

Rate of Weight Gain

The traditional studies of weight gain in pregnancy were conducted by Hytten [65], and provided the basis of clinical recommendations for decades (see Chap. 1). These studies, based on weight gains of 486 healthy primiparas in Aberdeen, Scotland, between 1950 and 1955, suggested that the rate of gain, when plotted, is generally sigmoid in shape, with the steepest slope, corresponding to a maximum rate of gain, at or before midgestation. During the first trimester, weight accumulation was minimal and almost all in the maternal compartment. The rate of gain increased to about 0.3 kg (0.66 lb) per week in the second trimester, of which 50 percent was in the maternal compartment. The rate remained about the same during the third trimester, except that approximately 90 percent was in the fetal compartment. Hytten estimated that from the 13th to the 18th week of gestation, the rate of weight gain was about 0.36 kg (0.8 lb) per week, increasing to 0.45 kg (1.0 lb) per week during midgestation, then slowing to 0.36 to 0.41 kg (0.8–0.9 lb) per week to term.

The National Academy of Sciences' 1990 recommendations suggest a rate of gain for underweight women of 5 lb during the first trimester, followed by slightly more than 1 lb per week for the second and third trimesters [22]. For normal-weight women, the suggested rate is 3.5 lb during the first trimester, and 1 lb per week during the second and third trimesters. For overweight women, gain in the first trimester is suggested to be about 2 lb, with a rate of gain of 0.66 lb per week for the second and third trimesters.

The actual rates of weight gain associated with good pregnancy outcomes (birthweights of ≥3000 gm at term) are much higher than those of Hytten's Aberdeen primiparas [65] or the recommendations of the National Academy of Sciences [22]. A recent American study by Petitti and associates [66] of low-risk women delivered of infants with birthweights of 3000 gm or greater at term reported a rate of gain of 0.66 lb per week from the 8th to 20th weeks and 1.06 lb per week from the 20th week to term. A comparison of net weight gain to 10, 20, 30, and 40 weeks of gestation as recommended by Hytten [67] and the National Academy of Sciences [22] and as reported by Pettiti and colleagues [66] is shown in Table 3-5. The data from Petitti suggest a higher rate of gain during the second half of pregnancy, from 20 weeks of gestation to term. This higher net weight gain may represent the accretion of fat stores earlier than observed by Hytten.

Maternal pregravid weight and the rate of gestational weight gain are each independently associated with birthweight and length of gesta-

Table 3-5
Net weight gain (lb)

	Week of gestation			
Source	*10*	*20*	*30*	*40*
Hytten and Leitch (1971) [67]	1.5	9.0	19	27.5
NAS (1990) [22]	2.7	10.5	20.5	30.5
Petitti (1991) [66]	5.3	10.5	24.2	35.1

tion. Inadequate early rate of gain (<4.3 kg [9.5 lb] by 24 weeks of gestation) is associated with an increased risk of small-for-gestational-age (SGA) birthweight, whereas inadequate late rate of gain (<0.4 kg [0.9 lb]/week after 24 weeks of gestation) or an overall low rate of gain (<0.27 kg [0.6 lb]/week) is associated with a significant increase in preterm delivery [54, 60].

Role of Maternal Body Fat

The effects of maternal weight gain, both as the rate and net gain to various gestational ages, are mediated through maternal body weight. As noted earlier, the effects of weight gain on birthweight are stronger among underweight women and weaker among normal-weight and overweight women. Maternal pregravid weight, alone or in combination with gestational weight gain, may exert its effect on birthweight through the presence (or absence) of maternal nutrient reserves, in particular body fat. According to Frisch [68], there are at least four mechanisms by which maternal body fat may directly affect ovulation, menstruation, fertility, and gestation. First, body fat acts as a significant extragonadal source of estrogen, accounting for a third of the circulating estrogen of premenopausal women. Second, body weight (and therefore body fat) influences the direction of estrogen metabolism to more or less potent forms. Very thin women have an increase in the relatively inactive 2-hydroxylated form of estrogen, whereas heavier women have an increase in the more potent 16-hydroxylated form. Third, overweight women and young girls who are fatter have a diminished capacity for estrogen to bind serum sex hormone–binding globulin (SHBG), resulting in an elevated percentage of free serum estradiol. Through changes in the proportion of body fat, SHBG regulates the availability of estradiol to the brain and other target tissues, influencing reproductive performance. Lastly, because maternal body fat stores steroid hormones, changes in the proportion of body fat affect reproductive ability indirectly through hypothalamic regulation of body temperature, energy balance, and response to luteinizing hormone–releasing hormone.

As a buffer against environmental stresses and fluctuations in dietary intake, maternal body fat may also play an important role in the hormonal and biochemical aspects of gestation. In addition to paralleling longer length of gestation [45], increasing maternal body weight (an indirect measure of body fat) as pregravid weight or weight attained at various points in gestation is associated with better intrauterine growth [30–33, 37–42, 44, 45, 49–55, 58–62, 66].

The interrelationship of body fat and birthweight was demonstrated most dramatically in the studies of the Dutch famine during World

War II [32, 33]. Famine conditions existed in the Netherlands from October 1944 until May 1945 (8 months). The most severe conditions occurred between December 1944 and May 1945. A graphic presentation of the changes in infant birthweight, birthlength, placental weight, maternal body weight (postpartum), length of gestation, and caloric rations per day during the 20-month period around the famine is presented in Fig. 3-5. Infant birthweight, birthlength, placental weight, maternal body weight (postpartum), and length of gestation are given in Z-scores (standard deviations from a norm), and caloric rations are given in absolute calories. The Dutch women had been well nourished before the famine. However, as food rations fell below 1500 kcal per day, maternal body weight was adversely affected, followed by infant birthweight. Birthlength was much less affected, and length of gestation was affected least of all indices studied. Maternal body weight absorbed the first impacts of the famine, preceding a decline in placental weight and newborn measures. Only after a lower threshold limit of maternal body weight was reached, representing a depletion of maternal body fat, did nutritional deprivation have a significant direct effect on the products of conception (first the placenta, followed by birthweight). With the provision of additional food after the liberation of the Netherlands in May 1945, the metabolic needs of the mother and the placenta took priority; maternal body weight and placental weight were quicker to recover, with birthweight increasing only after a time lag.

Research on **skinfold changes during pregnancy**, estimating the accretion and utilization of body fat during gestation, reflects this concept of optimal maternal nutrient reserves associated with better pregnancy outcome (as longer gestation and higher birthweight) [69–72]. In studies of healthy women with term pregnancies, total maternal body fat increased during pregnancy, reaching a peak between 24 and 28 weeks, and followed by a decrease during the remaining 12 weeks [69, 70]. By 6 to 8 weeks postpartum, total body fat was similar to the amount present at 10 weeks of gestation. Increases in total body fat were less for multiparas than for primiparas and for overweight women compared to normal-weight or underweight women [69].

In a series of studies comparing anthropometric changes during pregnancy in Asian and European mothers who had small-for-gestational-age (SGA) versus appropriate-for-gestational-age (AGA) infants, Bissenden and associates [71, 72] demonstrated the effect of the accretion of body fat on length of gestation and birthweight. Asian

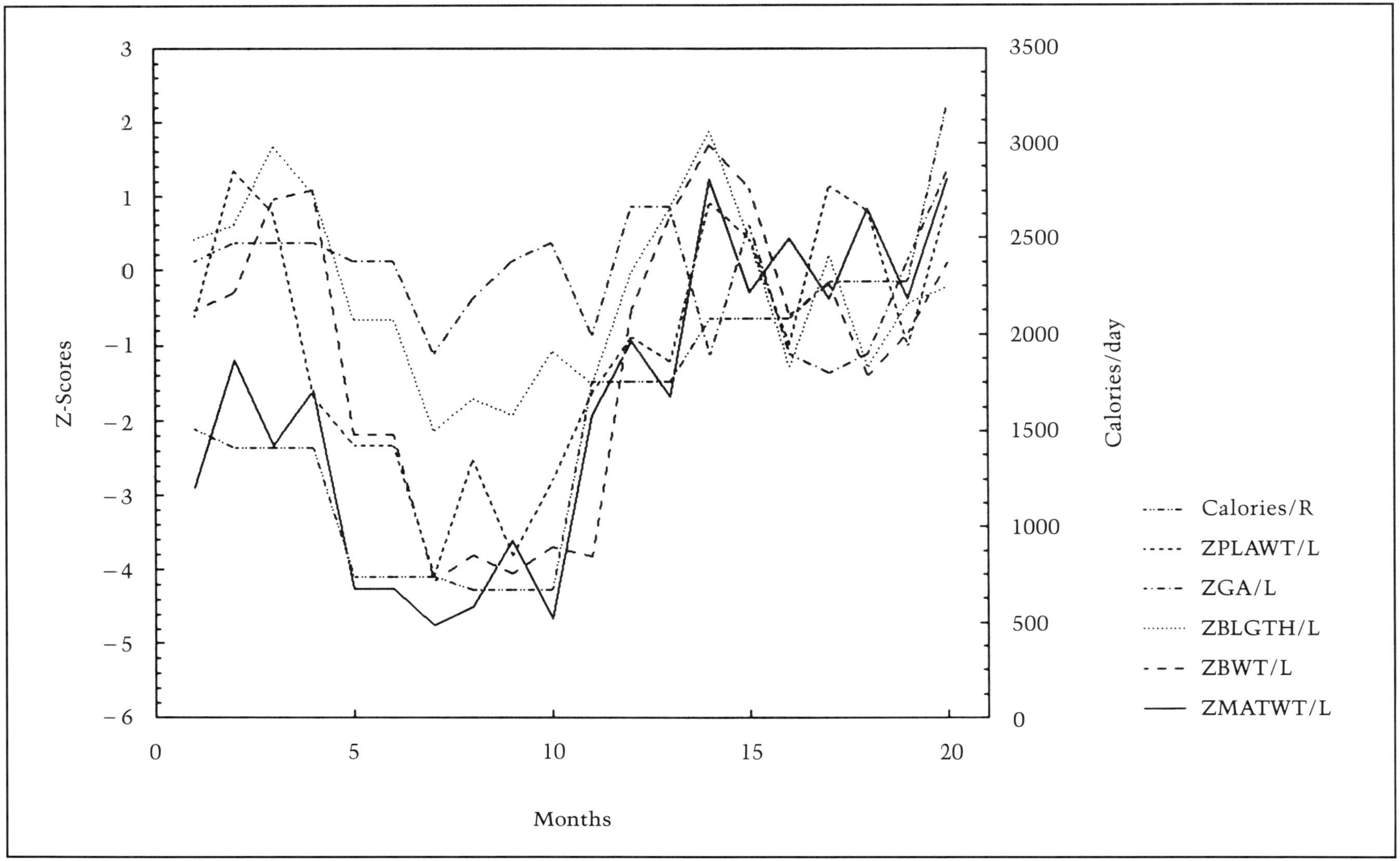

Fig. 3-5
Mean caloric intake and Z-scores of mean maternal weight (ZMATWT), infant birthweight (ZBWT), birthlength (ZBLGTH), length of gestation (ZGA), and placental weight (ZPLAWT) in Rotterdam, the Netherlands from August 1944 through March 1946. (Adapted from Z Stein and M Susser, The Dutch famine, 1944–45, and the reproductive process. II. Interrelations of caloric rations and six indices at birth. *Pediatr. Res.* 9:76–83, 1975.)

women with SGA infants had gained less weight and fat during the second trimester, and had pregnancies that averaged 1.6 weeks shorter than those of European women with SGA infants [71]. Asian women with AGA infants had comparable length of gestation and weight gains, but double the increase in body fat compared to European women with AGA infants [72].

Other ethnic and racial differences may account for differing effects of weight gain, body weight, and body fat on birthweight. In addition to the acknowledged differences between blacks and whites in birthweights for comparable pregravid weight, weight gain, and length of gestation [58, 73], new evidence suggests that metabolic differences may exist between racial groups as well [63]. Green and associates [63] reported that despite significantly lower maternal pregravid weight, Chinese women had significantly higher mean serum glucose levels than white, Hispanic, or black women. As a result, mean birthweights for Chinese infants were comparable to those of the other racial groups. These findings suggest that racial and ethnic differences in metabolism may mediate the known relationships between maternal pregravid weight, weight gain, body fat, and birthweight.

Maternal Weight Gain

Components of Weight Gain

In *The Physiology of Human Pregnancy*, Hytten and Leitch [67] presented their classic studies of the components of pregnancy. Although average weight gains have increased (see Table 3-5) from the 27.5 lb on which these authors based their evaluations in 1950 to 1955, their descriptions of the distribution of gain are probably still relevant today.

Table 3-6 gives the components of weight gain by week of gestation as originally described by Hytten and Leitch [67]. Both placental and maternal components of weight gain, including accumulation of body fat, precede peak fetal growth. Until the 30th week of gestation, maternal body fat accounts for the largest percentage of total gain; by 40 weeks, fetal weight accounts for the largest percentage. By the 10th week of gestation, the fetus has attained less than 1 percent of its final weight, compared to 3 percent for the placenta and 9 percent for maternal body fat. Between 10 and 20 weeks of gestation, maternal body fat increases most rapidly, at about 5.2 percent (175 gm) per week, compared to 2.3 percent per week for the placenta and other maternal tissues, and less than 1 percent per week for the fetus.

Table 3-6
Components of gestational weight gain

Site	*10*		*20*		*30*		*40*
	Week of gestation						
Fetus							
Weight (gm)	5		300		1500		3400
% of total growth	<1		<10		44		100
Rate/wk as % of total growth		<1		3.4		5.6	
Placenta							
Weight (gm)	20		170		430		650
% of total growth	3		26		66		100
Rate/wk as % of total growth		2.3		4.0		4.4	
Maternal fat							
Weight (gm)	310		2050		3480		3345
% of total growth	9		61		104		100
Rate/wk as % of total growth		5.2		4.3		−0.4	
*Other maternal tissues**							
Weight (gm)	315		1480		3090		5105
% of total growth	6		29		61		100
Rate/wk as % of total growth		2.3		3.2		3.9	

*Includes amniotic fluid, uterus, mammary glands, blood, and extracellular fluid.

Source: Adapted from FE Hytten and I Leitch, *The Physiology of Human Pregnancy* (2nd ed.). London: Blackwell Scientific, 1971.

Between the 20th and 30th weeks, the increase in placental, maternal, and fetal compartments is approximately equal, averaging about 3.2 to 4.3 percent per week. Between the 30th and 40th weeks, fetal growth is most rapid, with an average increase of 5.6 percent per week, and a peak rate of about 250 gm per week at the 33rd week [74]. During these last 10 weeks of a normal, term pregnancy, placental growth slows to about 4.4 percent per week, and maternal body fat is utilized at a rate of about 14 gm per week.

Consequences of Inadequate Maternal Nutrition

Short-Term. The two most common short-term consequences of inadequate maternal nutrition, as low pregravid weight and poor weight gain, are increased morbidity and mortality of the newborn. Although the severity of the intrauterine growth deficit and prognosis may be related to the pattern of maternal weight gain [76], children who are born growth retarded are at increased risk for neonatal or infant mortality [74, 75, 77, 78]. Studies of the relative effects of birthweight and gestational age on infant mortality indicate that birthweight is the predominant factor, although maturity, as reflected by gestational age, may have a more important role in long-term development [75, 77]. **The lowest mortality is among term infants with birthweights of 3000 to 3500 gm** [75]. **With birthweights below 2500 gm, mortality increases exponentially with decreasing birthweight. Compared to infants of normal birthweight, those with low birthweights (<2500 gm) are 40 times more likely to die during the neonatal period; for infants with birthweights of 1500 gm or less, the relative risk of neonatal death is nearly 200 times greater** [79]. Data from the National Infant Mortality Surveillance project (NIMS), which evaluated the 1980 birth cohort, indicated that low-birthweight infants accounted for fewer than 6 percent of all newborns in 1980, but these infants were responsible for 57 percent of all infant deaths, including 73 percent of all neonatal deaths and 27 percent of all postneonatal deaths [80].

Anatomic studies of growth-retarded infants indicate that, in addition to reduced birthweight and birthlength, individual organs, including the thymus, spleen, liver, adrenals, heart, and kidneys, are also adversely affected [81–83]. The implications of such organ cell deficits among surviving growth-retarded infants is unknown, although they may contribute to the higher incidence of chronic illness and poor postnatal development frequently observed in these children.

Long-Term. Among survivors, children who were low birthweight have three times the risk of adverse neurologic sequelae [84]. Data from both the Collaborative Perinatal Project [85] and the Child Health and Development Studies [86] indicate that inadequate gestational weight gain is associated with poor mental and motor development of surviving infants at 1 year of age [85] and 5 years of age [86]. As shown in Table 3-7, higher maternal weight gains were associated with better childhood growth and development.

Other studies have evaluated growth-retarded infants at birth at 1 year [87, 88], 2 years [89], and 7 years [90, 91]. Nearly all studies report that these children fall behind their normal-birthweight counterparts in growth and development, while exhibiting an increase in the rate of behavioral problems [91]. In addition, children who were low birthweight have more chronic health conditions and more hospitalizations, and lose more school days due to illness, than children who had normal birthweights [92].

Table 3-7
Percentage of infants with abnormal growth and performance by maternal weight gain

	Infant measures				
Weight gain (lb)	*Mental*	*Motor*	*Height*	*Weight*	*Neurologic*
0–15	12.5	11.3	10.1	15.8	8.8
16–25	9.3	8.0	7.5	11.2	7.5
26–35	8.3	6.8	6.5	8.4	7.9
≥36	7.5	5.2	7.3	6.2	7.1

Source: Adapted from JE Singer, M Westphal, and K Niswander, Relationship of weight gain during pregnancy to birth weight and infant growth and development in the first year of life. *Obstet. Gynecol.* 31:417–422, 1968.

Conclusions and Recommendations

Maternal anthropometric indices—height, pregravid weight, and gestational weight gain—have well-established direct effects on intrauterine growth. In addition, pregravid weight has a direct effect on length of gestation [93]. As such, these factors can profoundly influence birthweight and subsequent infant morbidity and mortality, as well as future growth and development. Few factors have such long-reaching effects on the health and well-being of generations, and because of their strong influence, deserve a central role in the provision of adequate preconceptional and prenatal care [94].

Of primary importance is adequate maternal pregravid weight-for-height. If a woman is planning to become pregnant, correction of a pregravid weight deficit (or, of less importance, reduction of excess weight) should be achieved through appropriate dietary interventions. As discussed in other chapters, attention to all aspects of nutrition, including iron and calcium status, and particularly the intake of folic acid, is important during the preconceptional period. **Once conception has occurred, weight loss should be discouraged, since it may have adverse effects on pregnancy outcome.**

During the prenatal period, weight gain is of prime concern, particularly the adequate deposition of fat stores by midgestation. Because it is not possible to predict the duration of gestation, a liberal rate of early weight gain should be encouraged, depending on maternal pregravid weight. All women, regardless of pregravid weight status, should gain during pregnancy to maximize optimal birthweight and neonatal vitality. Dietary intake to achieve this gain should be through nutrient-rich foods, particularly those high in protein; vitamins A, C, and B_{12}; folate; calcium; and trace minerals (i.e., zinc and magnesium), as well as in carbohydrates and calories. Higher weight gains are associated with better short- and long-term outcomes. The anthropometric factors of pregravid weight and gestational weight gain are particularly important in primiparas because there is a strong tendency to repeat gestational ages and birthweights in subsequent pregnancies [95]. Nutrition plays an important role in pregnancy outcome for all populations, and is a powerful, although often unrecognized, mechanism by which to augment intrauterine growth and enhance duration of gestation.

References

1. Frisch, RE: Population, food intake, and fertility. *Science* 199:22–30, 1978.
2. National Academy of Sciences, Food and Nutrition Board, Committee on Maternal Nutrition: Relation of Nutrition to Pregnancy in Adolescence. In *Maternal Nutrition and the Course of Pregnancy*. Washington, DC: National Academy Press 1970. Pp. 139–162.
3. Mascie-Taylor, CG: Biosocial influences on stature: A review. *J. Biosoc. Sci.* 23:113–128, 1991.
4. Ounsted, M, and Ounsted, C: Maternal regulation of intra-uterine growth. *Nature* 212:995–997, 1966.
5. Baird, D: Environmental and obstetrical factors in prematurity, with special reference to experience in Aberdeen. *Bulletin W.H.O.* 26:291–295, 1962.
6. National Center for Health Statistics: *Weight, Height, and Selected Body Dimensions of Adults, United States 1960–62. Vital and Health Statistics*, Series 11, No. 8 Pub. No. (PHS) 1000. Hyattsville, MD: US Dept. of Health and Human Services, 1965.
7. Abraham, S, Johnson, CL, and Najjar, MF: *Weight and Height of Adults 18–74 Years of Age, United States, 1971–74. Vital and Health Statistics*, Series 11, No. 211 Pub. No. (PHS) 79-1659. Hyattsville, MD: US Dept. of Health and Human Services, 1979.
8. Najjar, MF and Rowland, M: *Anthropometric Reference Data and Prevalence of Overweight, United States, 1976–80. Vital and Health Statistics*, Series No. 11, No. 238 Pub. No. (PHS) 87-1688. Hyattsville, MD: US Dept. of Health and Human Services, 1987.
9. Cawley, RH, McKeown, T, and Record, RG: Parental stature and birth weight. *Am. J. Hum. Genet.* 6:448–456, 1954.
10. McKeown, T, and Record, RG: Influence of pre-natal environment on correlation between birth weight and parental height. *Am. J. Hum. Genet.* 6:457–463, 1954.
11. Furusho, T: Relationship between the stature of parents and the mortality of their children. *Jap. J. Hum. Genet.* 9:18–34, 1964.

12. Lechtig, A, Delgado, H, Yarbrough, C, et al: A simple assessment of the risk of low birth weight to select women for nutritional intervention. *Am. J. Obstet. Gynecol.* 125:25–34, 1976.
13. Martorell, R, Delgado, HL, Valverde, V, and Klein, RE: Maternal stature, fertility and infant mortality. *Hum. Biol.* 53:303–312, 1981.
14. Seidman, DS, Ever-Hadani, P, and Gale, R: The effect of maternal weight gain in pregnancy on birth weight. *Obstet. Gynecol.* 74:240–246, 1989.
15. Witter, FR, and Luke, B: The effect of maternal height on birth weight and birth length. *Early Hum. Dev.* 25:181–186, 1991.
16. Luke, B, Jonaitis, MA, and Petrie, RH: A consideration of height as a function of prepregnancy nutritional background and its potential influence on birth weight. *J. Am. Dietet. Assoc.* 84:176–181, 1984.
17. Winikoff, B, and Debrovner, CH: Anthropometric determinants of birth weight. *Obstet. Gynecol.* 58:678–684, 1981.
18. Love, EJ, and Kinch, RAH: Factors influencing the birth weight in normal pregnancy. *Am. J. Obstet. Gynecol.* 91:342–348, 1965.
19. Eastman, NJ, and Jackson, E: Weight relationships in pregnancy. *Obstet. Gynecol. Surv.* 23:1003–1025, 1968.
20. Niswander, KR, and Gordon, M: *The Women and Their Pregnancies, the Collaborative Perinatal Study of the National Institute of Neurological Diseases and Stroke.* DHEW Pub. No. (NIH) 73-379. Washington, DC: US Govt. Printing Office, 1972. Pp. 80–93.
21. Bergner, L, and Susser, MW: Low birth weight and prenatal nutrition: An interpretative review. *Pediatrics* 46:946–952, 1970.
22. National Academy of Sciences: *Nutrition During Pregnancy: Weight Gain and Nutrient Supplements.* Washington, DC: National Academy Press, 1990.
23. Garrow, JS, and Webster, J: Quetelet's index (W/H^2) as a measure of fatness. *Int. J. Obes.* 9:147–153, 1985.
24. Frisancho, AR, and Flegel, PN: Relative merits of old and new indices of body mass with reference to skinfold thickness. *Am. J. Clin. Nutr.* 36:697–699, 1982.
25. Garn, SM, and Pesick, SD: Relationship between various maternal body mass measures and size of the newborn. *Am. J. Clin. Nutr.* 36:664–668, 1982.
26. Wolfe, HM, Zador, IE, Gross, TL, et al: The clinical utility of maternal body mass index in pregnancy. *Am. J. Obstet. Gynecol.* 164:1306–1310, 1991.
27. Garn, SM, Leonard, WR, and Hawthorne, VM: Three limitations of the body mass index. *Am. J. Clin. Nutr.* 44:996–997, 1986.
28. New weight standards for men and women. *Statistical Bulletin of the Metropolitan Life Insurance Company* 40:1–4, 1959.
29. 1983 Metropolitan height and weight tables. *Statistical Bulletin of the Metropolitan Life Insurance Company* 64:2–9, 1983.
30. Niswander, K, and Jackson, EC: Physical characteristics of the grav-

ida and their association with birth weight and perinatal death. *Am. J. Obstet. Gynecol.* 119:306–313, 1974.

31. Simpson, JW, Lawless, RW, and Mitchell, AC: Responsibility of the obstetrician to the fetus. II. Influence of prepregnancy weight and pregnancy weight gain on birthweight. *Obstet. Gynecol.* 45:481–487, 1975.
32. Stein, Z, and Susser, M: The Dutch famine, 1944–1945, and the reproductive process. I. Effects on six indices at birth. *Pediatr. Res.* 9:70–76, 1975.
33. Stein, Z, and Susser, M: The Dutch famine, 1944–1945, and the reproductive process. II. Interrelations of caloric rations and six indices at birth. *Pediatr. Res.* 9:76–83, 1975.
34. Fedrick, J, and Anderson, ABM: Factors associated with spontaneous pre-term birth. *Br. J. Obstet. Gynaecol.* 83:342–350, 1976.
35. Berkowitz, GS: An epidemiologic study of preterm delivery. *Am. J. Epidemiol.* 113:81–92, 1981.
36. Calandra, C, Abell, DA, and Beischer, NA: Maternal obesity in pregnancy. *Obstet. Gynecol.* 57:8–12, 1981.
37. Anderson, GD, Blidner, IN, McClemont, S, and Sinclair, JC: Determinants of size at birth in a Canadian population. *Am. J. Obstet. Gynecol.* 150:236–244, 1984.
38. Tompkins, WT, Wiehl, DG, and Mitchell, R McN: The underweight patient as an increased obstetric hazard. *Am. J. Obstet. Gynecol.* 69:114–123, 1955.
39. Peckham, CH, and Christianson, RE: The relationship between prepregnancy weight and certain obstetric factors. *Am. J. Obstet. Gynecol.* 111:1–7, 1971.
40. Edwards, SE, Alton, JR, Barrada, I, and Hakanson, JKY: Pregnancy in the underweight woman. *Am. J. Obstet. Gynecol.* 135:297–302, 1979.
41. Luke, B, and Petrie, RH: Intrauterine growth: Correlation of infant birthweight and maternal postpartum weight. *Am. J. Clin. Nutr.* 33:2311–2317, 1980.
42. Gormican, A, Valentine, J, and Satter, E: Relationships of maternal weight gain, prepregnancy weight, and infant birthweight. *J. Am. Diet. Assoc.* 77:662–667, 1980.
43. Harrison, GG, Udall, JN, and Morrow, G: Maternal obesity, weight gain in pregnancy, and infant birthweight. *Am. J. Obstet. Gynecol.* 136:411–412, 1980.
44. Luke, B, Dickinson, C, and Petrie, RH: Intrauterine growth: Correlations of maternal nutritional status and rate of gestational weight gain. *Eur. J. Obstet. Gynecol. Reprod. Biol.* 12:113–121, 1981.
45. Brown, JE, Jacobson, HN, Askue, LH, and Peick, MG: Influence of pregnancy weight gain on the size of infants born to underweight women. *Obstet. Gynecol.* 57:13–17, 1981.
46. George, NN, Kim, SK, and Duhring, JL: Prepregnancy weights and weight gains related to birth weights of infants born to overweight women. *J. Am. Diet. Assoc.* 84:450–452, 1984.

47. Garbaciak, JA, Richter, M, Miller, S, and Barton, JJ: Maternal weight and pregnancy complications. *Am. J. Obstet. Gynecol.* 152:238–245, 1985.
48. Loris, P, Dewey, KG, and Poirier-Brode, K: Weight gain and dietary intake of pregnant teenagers. *J. Am. Diet. Assoc.* 85:1296–1305, 1985.
49. Brown, JE, Berdan, KW, Splett, P, and Robinson, M: Prenatal weight gains related to the birth of healthy-sized infants to low-income women. *J. Am. Diet. Assoc.* 86:1679–1683, 1986.
50. Mitchell, MC, and Lerner, E: Factors that influence the outcome of pregnancy in middle-class women. *J. Am. Diet. Assoc.* 87:731–735, 1987.
51. Frentzen, BH, Dimperio, DL, and Cruz, AC: Maternal weight gain: Effect on infant birth weight among overweight and average-weight low-income women. *Am. J. Obstet. Gynecol.* 159:1114–1117, 1988.
52. Scholl, TO, Salmon, RW, Miller, LK, et al: Weight gain during adolescent pregnancy. *J. Adolesc. Health Care* 9:286–290, 1988.
53. Mitchell, MC, and Lerner, E: Weight gain and pregnancy outcome in underweight and normal weight women. *J. Am. Diet. Assoc.* 89:634–641, 1989.
54. Abrams, B, Newman, V, Key, T, and Parker, J: Maternal weight gain and preterm delivery. *Obstet. Gynecol.* 74:577–583, 1989.
55. Abrams, B, and Newman, V: Small-for-gestational age birth: Maternal predictors and comparison with risk factors of spontaneous preterm delivery in the same cohort. *Am. J. Obstet. Gynecol.* 164:785–790, 1991.
56. Kerr, MG: The problem of the overweight patient in pregnancy. *J. Obstet. Gynaecol. Br. Commwlth.* 69:988–995, 1962.
57. Billewicz, WZ, and Thomson, AM: Body weight in parous women. *Br. J. Prev. Soc. Med.* 24:97–104, 1970.
58. Taffel, S: Maternal weight gain and the outcome of pregnancy, United States, 1980. *Vital and Health Statistics*, Series 21, No. 44. DHHS Pub. No. (PHS) 86-1922. Public Health Service. Washington, DC: US Govt. Printing Office, 1986.
59. Abrams, BF, and Laros, RK: Prepregnancy weight, weight gain, and birth weight. *Am. J. Obstet. Gynecol.* 154:503–509, 1986.
60. Hediger, ML, Scholl, TO, Belsky, DH, et al: Patterns of weight gain in adolescent pregnancy: Effects on birth weight and preterm delivery. *Obstet. Gynecol.* 74:6–12, 1989.
61. Abrams, B, and Parker, JD: Maternal weight gain in women with good pregnancy outcome. *Obstet. Gynecol.* 76:1–7, 1990.
62. Hediger, ML, Scholl, TO, Ances, IG, et al: Rate and amount of weight gain during adolescent pregnancy: Associations with maternal weight-for-height and birth weight. *Am. J. Clin. Nutr.* 52:793–799, 1990.
63. Green, JR, Schumacher, LB, Pawson, IG, et al: Influence of maternal body habitus and glucose tolerance on birth weight. *Obstet. Gynecol.* 78:235–240, 1991.

64. Luke, B, Minogue, J, Abbey, H, et al: The association between maternal weight gain and the birthweight of twins. *J. Maternal-Fetal Medicine* 1:267–276, 1992.
65. Hytten, FE: Weight Gain in Pregnancy. In FE Hytten and G Chamberlain (eds.), *Clinical Physiology in Obstetrics* (2nd ed.). London: Blackwell Scientific, 1991. Pp. 173–203.
66. Petitti, DB, Croughan-Minihane, MS, and Hiatt, RA: Weight gain by gestational age in both black and white women delivered of normal birthweight and low birthweight infants. *Am. J. Obstet. Gynecol.* 164:801–805, 1991.
67. Hytten, FE, and Leitch, I: *The Physiology of Human Pregnancy* (2nd ed.). London: Blackwell Scientific, 1971.
68. Frisch, RE (ed.): *Adipose Tissue and Reproduction*. Basel: Karger, 1990.
69. Pipe, NGJ, Smith, T, Halliday, D, et al: Changes in fat, fat-free mass, and body water in human normal pregnancy. *Br. J. Obstet. Gynaecol.* 86:929–940, 1979.
70. Taggart, NR, Holliday, RM, Billewicz, WZ, et al: Changes in skinfolds during pregnancy. *Br. J. Nutr.* 21:439–451, 1967.
71. Bissenden, JG, Scott, PH, King, J, et al: Anthropometric and biochemical changes during pregnancy in Asian and European mothers having light for gestational age babies. *Br. J. Obstet. Gynaecol.* 88:999–1008, 1981.
72. Bissenden, JG, Scott, PH, Hallum, J, et al: Anthropometric and biochemical changes during pregnancy in Asian and European mothers having well grown babies. *Br. J. Obstet. Gynaecol.* 88:992–998, 1981.
73. Kleinman, JC, and Kessel, SS: Racial differences in low birth weight. *N. Engl. J. Med.* 317:749–753, 1987.
74. Susser, M, Marolla, FA, and Fleiss, J: Birth weight, fetal age, and perinatal mortality. *Am. J. Epidemiol.* 96:197–204, 1972.
75. Williams, RL, Creasy, RK, Cunningham, GC, et al: Fetal growth and perinatal viability in California. *Obstet. Gynecol.* 59:624–632, 1982.
76. Villar, J, and Belizan, JM: The timing factor in the pathophysiology of the intrauterine growth retardation syndrome. *Obstet. Gynecol. Surv.* 37:499–506, 1982.
77. Koops, BL, Morgan, LJ, and Battaglia, FC: Neonatal mortality risk in relation to birth weight and gestational age: Update. *J. Pediatr.* 101:969–977, 1982.
78. Myers, SA, and Ferguson, R: A population study of the relationship between fetal death and altered fetal growth. *Obstet. Gynecol.* 74:325–331, 1989.
79. Shapiro, S, McCormick, MC, Starfield, BH, et al: Relevance of correlates of infant deaths for significant morbidity at 1 year of age. *Am. J. Obstet. Gynecol.* 136:363–373, 1980.
80. National Infant Mortality Surveillance (NIMS) 1980. *MMWR/CDC Surveillance Summaries*. Vol. 38, No. SS-3, 1989.
81. Naeye, RL, Diener, MM, and Dellinger, WS: Urban poverty: Effects on prenatal nutrition. *Science* 166:1026–1027, 1969.

82. Naeye, RL: Malnutrition: Probable cause of fetal growth retardation. *Arch. Pathol.* 79:284–291, 1965.
83. Cassady, G: Body composition in intrauterine growth retardation. *Pediatr. Clin. North Am.* 17:79–99, 1970.
84. Papile, L-A, Munsick-Bruno, G, and Schaefer, A: Relationship of cerebral intraventricular hemorrhage and early childhood neurologic handicaps. *J. Pediatr.* 103:273–277, 1983.
85. Singer, JE, Westphal, M, and Niswander, K: Relationship of weight gain during pregnancy to birthweight and infant growth and development in the first year of life: A report from the Collaborative Study of Cerebral Palsy. *Obstet. Gynecol.* 31:417–422, 1968.
86. Tavris, DR, and Read, JA: Effect of maternal weight gain on fetal, infant, and childhood death and on cognitive development. *Obstet. Gynecol.* 60:689–694, 1982.
87. Low, JA, Galbraith, RS, Muir, D, et al: Intrauterine growth retardation: A study of long-term morbidity. *Am. J. Obstet. Gynecol.* 142:670–677, 1982.
88. Ounsted, M, Moar, VA, and Scott, A: Neurological development of small-for-gestational age babies during the first year of life. *Early Hum. Dev.* 16:163–172, 1988.
89. Fitzhardinge, PM, and Inwood, S: Long-term growth in small-for-date children. *Acta Paediatr. Scand.* 349 (Suppl.):27–33, 1989.
90. Ounsted, M, Moar, VA, and Scott, A: Children of deviant birthweight at the age of seven years: Health, handicap, size and developmental status. *Early Human Dev.* 9:323–340, 1984.
91. Walther, FJ: Growth and development of term disproportionate small-for-gestational age infants at the age of 7 years. *Early Hum. Dev.* 18:1–11, 1988.
92. Overpeck, MD, Moss, AJ, Hoffman, HJ, and Hendershot, GE: A comparison of the childhood health status of normal birth weight and low birth weight infants. *Public Health Rep.* 104:58–70, 1989.
93. Kramer, MS: Intrauterine growth and gestational duration determinants. *Pediatrics* 80:502–511, 1987.
94. Brown, JE: Improving pregnancy outcomes in the United States: The importance of preventive nutrition services. *J. Am. Diet. Assoc.* 89:631–633, 1989.
95. Bakketeig, LS, Hoffman, HJ, and Harley, EE: The tendency to repeat gestational age and birth weight in successive births. *Am. J. Obstet. Gynecol.* 135:1086–1103, 1979.

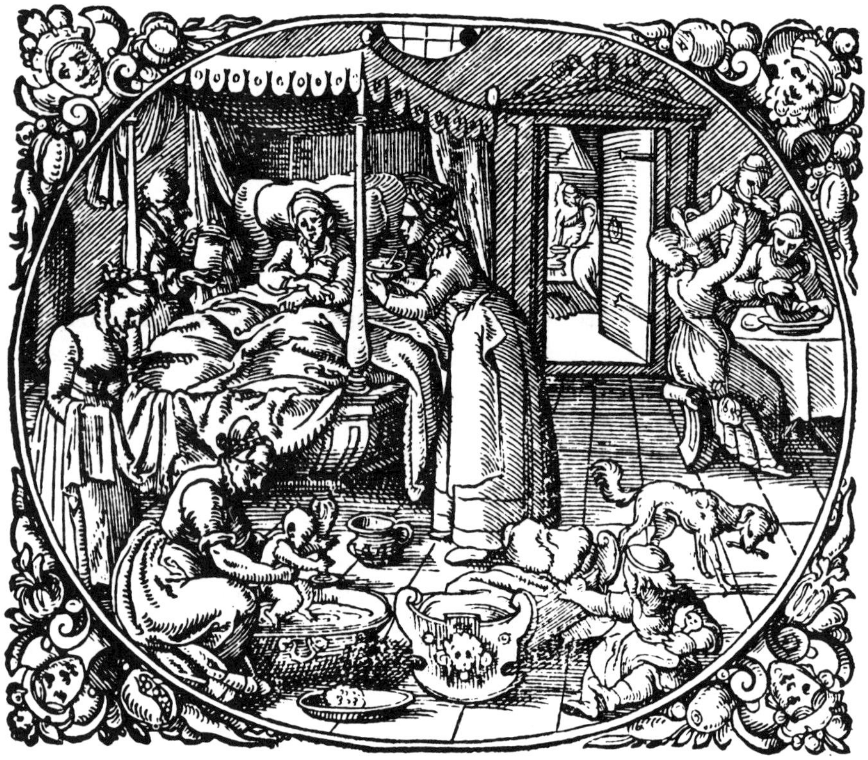

Childbirth in 1580. (From Jacobus Rueff. *De Conceptu.*
Frankfurt: S. Feyerabendt, 1580.)

4

Maternal Sociodemographic Characteristics

Age, race, and socioeconomic status are among the most frequently cited factors associated with low birthweight and preterm delivery. Next to low pregravid weight and inadequate gestational weight gain, young maternal age, black race, and low socioeconomic status are most often associated with adverse pregnancy outcomes [1–5].

In addition, these three major factors are surrogates for a host of biologic, behavioral, environmental, and medical factors that potentiate the risk of poor reproductive performance. Once a woman has a history of an adverse pregnancy outcome, the pattern has a strong tendency to repeat itself [6, 7]. Therefore, minimizing the untoward effects of each major and associated factor benefits not only the current pregnancy, but subsequent pregnancies as well. This chapter presents a review of the literature on the effects of age, race, and socioeconomic status, singly, and in combination with associated factors, on pregnancy outcome. Factor-specific recommendations are made to minimize adverse effects on pregnancy outcome.

Age

Extremes of maternal age have traditionally been associated with adverse pregnancy outcomes, including increased risks of stillbirths, perinatal mortality, low birthweight and intrauterine growth retardation, preterm delivery, and congenital anomalies. However, the precise ages associated with these increased risks is not clear. Some risk scoring systems use ≤15 years and ≥35 years [8–10]; others use <20 years and a >40 years [11–13], and still others suggest ≤20 years and ≥40 years [14].

Adolescent Pregnancy

Although the rates of first births (Fig. 4-1) and all births (Fig. 4-2) to adolescents has declined since 1970, they are still much higher than for other age groups. Between 1970 and 1986, the rate of first births and all births to adolescents aged 15 to 19 decreased by 27 and 18 percent, respectively [15]. Despite these declines, in 1988, nearly half a million births, or more than 12 percent of all births, were to adolescents [15].

As discussed in Chap. 2, both gynecologic age (years after menarche) and chronologic age influence biologic maturity. Although a girl may conceive soon after menarche, her own physical growth may not yet be complete. Between the ages of 10 and 17, height increases 15 percent, weight 69 percent, and body mass index 26 percent (Table 4-1). Numerous studies have documented continued adolescent growth during pregnancy and between successive pregnancies [11–20]. In an

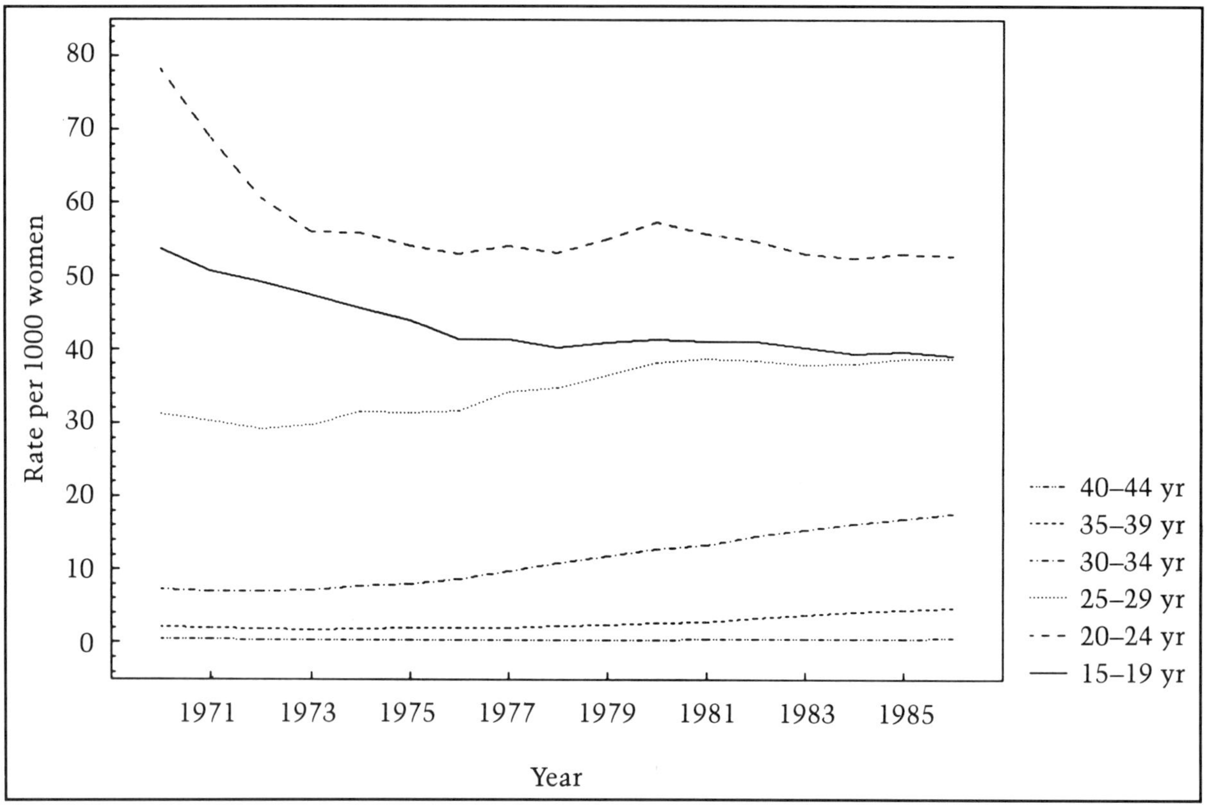

Fig. 4-1
Rate of first births by age of mother, United States, 1970 to 1986. (Adapted from SJ Ventura, Trends and Variations in first births to older women, 1970–86. *Vital and Health Statistics*, Series 21, No. 47. National Center for Health Statistics, 1989.)

American study of adolescents 16 years of age or younger, mean pregravid weight increased 2.2 kg (4.9 lb) and mean height increased 0.79 cm (0.03 in.) between first and second pregnancies [17]. In Zaria, Nigeria, increases in maternal height of as much as 16 cm (6.3 in.) were documented in primigravidas aged 16 and younger [18, 19]. Greater growth was observed among adolescent mothers taking antimalarial drugs, iron, and folic acid supplements compared to those not taking these preventive measures. Evaluations of linear growth during adolescent pregnancy have also been conducted with serial measurements of the lower leg [20]. Primigravidas aged 12 to 15 grew the most during pregnancy, followed by multigravidas aged 15 to 18; mature control subjects aged 18 to 29 grew the least.

The amount of growth during adolescence is influenced by the chronologic age at menarche. Among late-maturing girls, menarche occurs toward the end of the adolescent growth spurt, whereas for

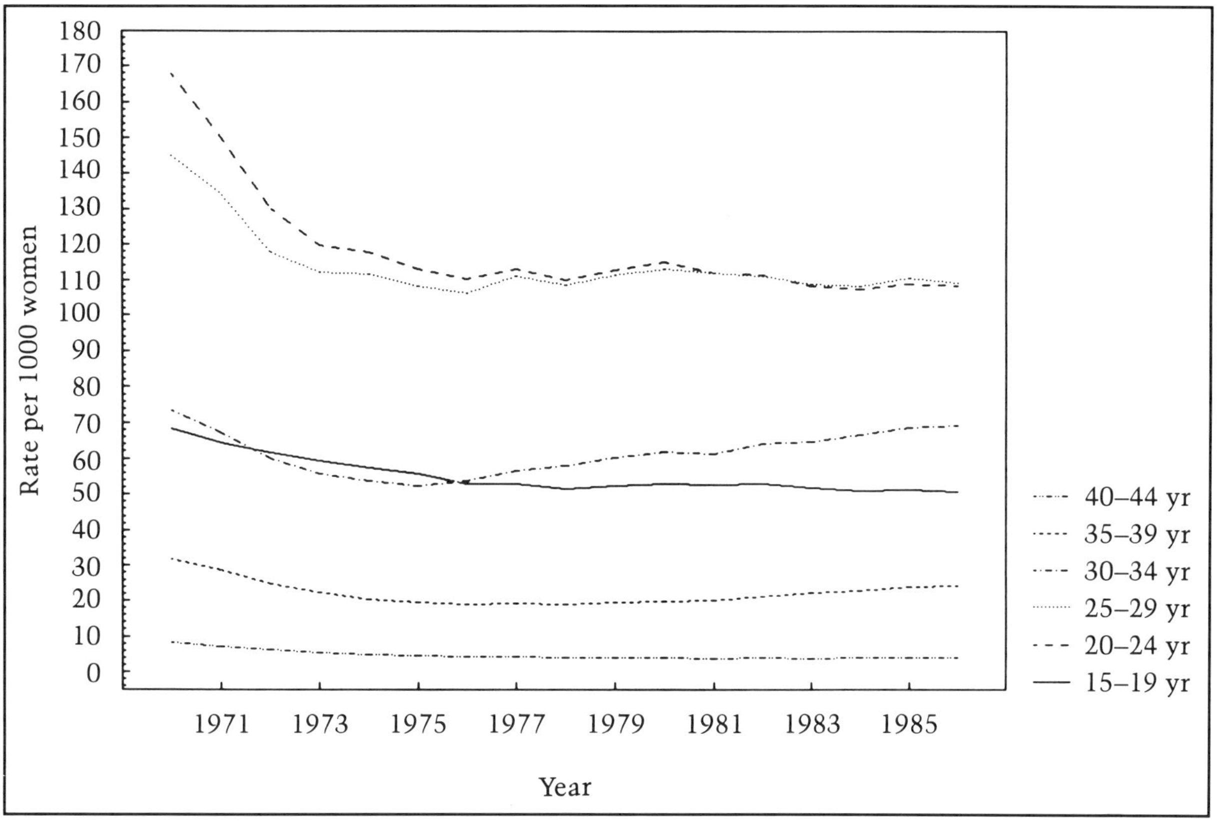

Fig. 4-2
Rate of all births by age of mother, United States, 1970 to 1986. (Adapted from SJ Ventura, Trends and variations in first births to older women, 1970–86. *Vital and Health Statistics*, Series 21, No. 47. National Center for Health Statistics, 1989.)

early-maturing girls it occurs toward the beginning. Early-maturing girls, therefore, have about twice as much growth, including skeletal growth, remaining before they achieve physical maturity compared to late-maturing girls. At the same chronologic age, early-maturing girls have much younger bone age and have completed less pelvic growth than late-maturing girls. This difference has important consequences for adolescent pregnancy [21–23]. Data from the Collaborative Perinatal Project [24] showed that in successive pregnancies, early-maturing girls grew substantially more both in height and weight than late-maturing girls.

Adverse Pregnancy Outcomes

The competition between the growing mother and her growing fetus for available nutrients is associated with less favorable reproductive outcomes [17, 20, 25–30]. The risk of low birthweight is increased among adolescents, as shown in Fig. 4-3. In evaluating all live births in the United States in 1988, the birthweight distributions shift to

Table 4-1
Comparison of anthropometric parameters (50th percentile) of females by age (NHANES II)

Age (yr)	Height (in.)	Weight (lb)	Body mass index	Skinfold measurements (mm) Triceps	Skinfold measurements (mm) Subscapular	Mid–upper arm circumference
Adolescents						
10	55.7	76.1	17.0	13.5	8.0	21.7
11	58.2	89.0	18.1	14.0	8.0	22.5
12	61.0	100.1	18.8	13.5	9.0	23.6
13	62.6	108.1	19.3	15.0	9.5	24.2
14	63.3	117.1	20.4	17.0	10.5	25.3
15	64.2	117.6	19.9	16.5	10.5	25.1
16	64.3	122.6	21.0	18.0	12.0	26.4
17	64.2	128.8	21.4	20.0	13.0	27.1
% increase 10–17 yr	15	69	26	48	63	25
Adult						
18–24	64.5	128.0	21.6	19.0	13.0	27.1
25–34	64.2	134.3	22.6	22.0	16.0	28.3
35–44	64.0	139.8	23.8	25.0	19.0	29.6
% increase 18–44 yr	None	9	10	32	46	9

NHANES II, National Nutrition and Health Examination Survey, 1976–1980.

Source: Adapted from MF Najjar and M Rowland, Anthropometric reference data and prevalence of overweight, United States, 1976–80. *Vital and Health Statistics*, Series 11, No. 238. DHHS Pub. No. (PHS) 87-1688. Public Health Service. Washington, DC: US Govt. Printing Office, 1987.

the right (heavier categories) with increasing maternal age. In 1988, adolescents 15 years of age or younger had the highest low birthweight rate (13.6%) (Table 4-2).

The risk of low birthweight is increased by young chronologic age and young gynecologic age, and is magnified in the presence of both factors. In a study of pregnancy outcomes among gravidas aged 17 years or younger, Zlatnik and Burmeister [26] showed that the proportion of low-birthweight infants was higher among girls with chronologic ages <16 versus ≥16 (12 vs. 7%), and gynecologic ages <3 years versus ≥3 (13 vs. 7%). The incidence of low birthweight was nearly 2.5 times higher among gravidas with chronologic ages <15 and gynecologic ages <2 than for gravidas ≥15 years with gynecologic ages ≥2 (16 vs. 6.6%). Among only 15-year-olds, the incidence of low birthweight was nearly double among gravidas with gynecologic age of ≤2 compared to those greater >2 (17 vs. 9%).

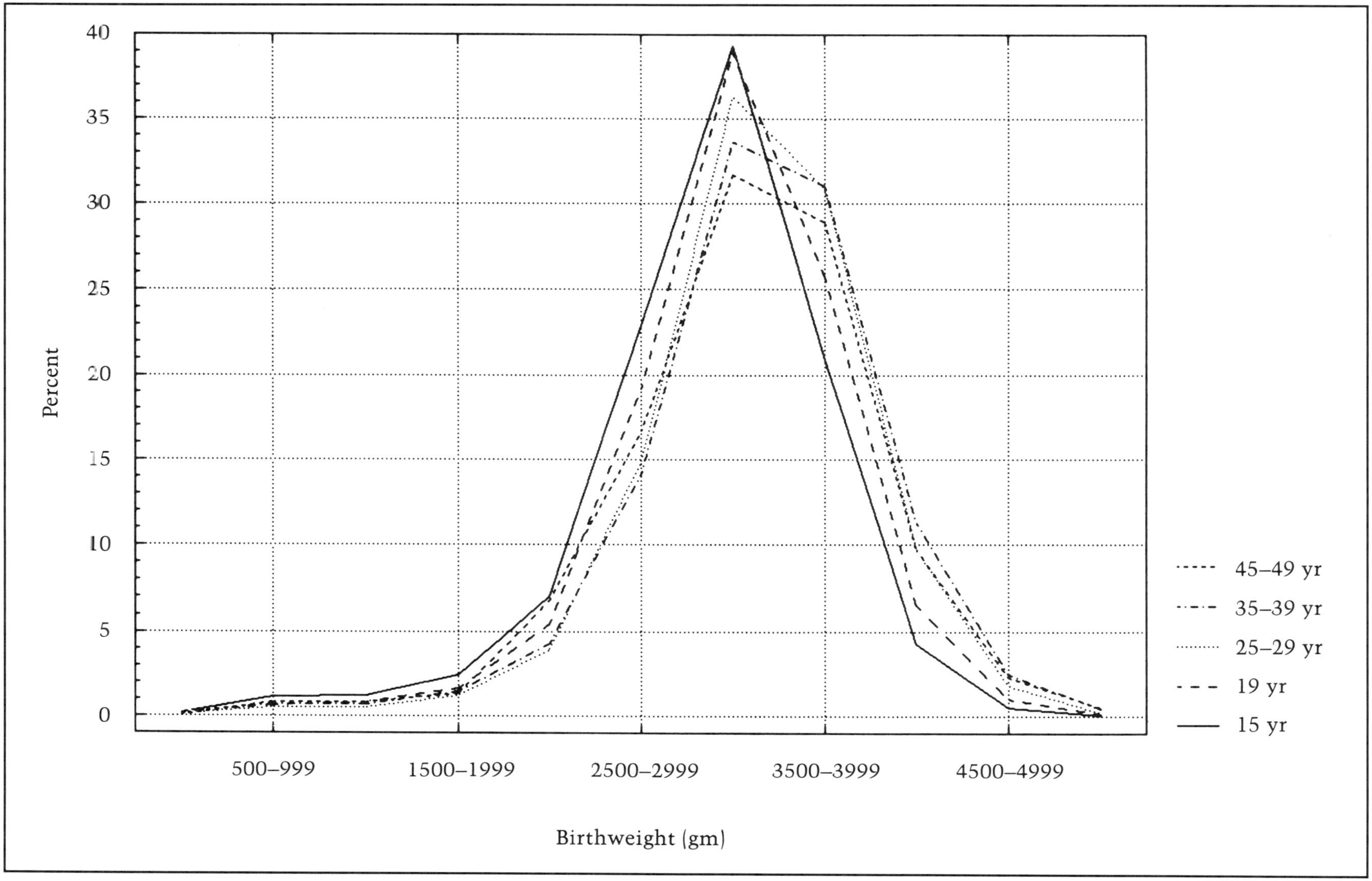

Fig. 4-3
Percent distribution of live births by birthweight and maternal age, United States, 1988. (Adapted from National Center for Health Statistics: Vital Statistics of the United States, 1988. Vol. 1, *Natality. Public Health Service.* Washington, DC: Government Printing Office, 1990. P. 241.)

Table 4-2
Percentage of all live births with low birthweight (<2500 gm), by mother's age and race, United States, 1988

Age (yr)	Race		
	All	*White*	*Black*
All ages	6.9	5.6	11.5
<15	13.6	11.0	15.2
15–19	9.9	7.5	12.6
20–24	7.2	5.8	11.3
25–29	6.1	5.0	11.0
30–34	6.3	5.2	11.0
35–39	7.1	6.1	11.3
40–44	8.2	7.1	12.1
45–49	9.8	9.3	11.1

Source: Adapted from Advance report of final natality statistics. *Monthly Vital Statistics Report*, Vol. 39, No. 4, Supplement, August 15, 1990.

In a study in which girls with gynecologic ages of 2.6 years or less were matched to girls with gynecologic ages of 4.1 years or greater, Sukanich and associates [17] reported that despite similar weight gains (28 lb), the younger gynecologic age group had a significantly shorter length of gestation (38 vs. 39.9 wk), and lighter birthweight (2967 vs. 3092 gm). In addition, rates of cesarean section and abruptio placentae were significantly higher among the younger group (11.5 vs. 3.7% and 3.8 vs. 0%, respectively), as were incidences of low birthweight (18.3 vs. 11.1%), stillbirth (2.9 vs. 0.9%), and neonatal death (2.9 vs. 0.9%).

Other investigators reported similar adverse outcomes associated with young chronologic and gynecologic age. In comparing pregnancy outcomes of girls 15 years of age or younger versus those 19 to 24 years old, Duenhoelter and associates [25] reported shorter gestations among younger gravidas. The percentage of gestations of less than 35 weeks was nearly twice that of the older gravidas (10.5 vs. 5.4%). In addition, these investigators reported significantly more pelvic inlet contractions and reduced pelvic midplane diameters among younger gravidas (7.4 vs. 2.8% and 3.0 vs. 1.7%, respectively), resulting in higher rates of midforceps and cesarean delivery (4.2 vs. 2.1% and 10.4 vs. 7%, respectively). Other studies of adolescent pregnancies have also reported higher cesarean section and forceps delivery rates [27]. In a study of all adolescent pregnancies at Johns Hopkins Medical Institutions in 1979, more than 46 percent of the indications for cesarean delivery were for cephalopelvic disproportion.

Influence of Nutrition

Unlike its effect on infants of mature gravidas, parity does not exert a positive effect on birthweight in successive pregnancies in adolescents [17, 20, 28, 29], particularly among girls who are still growing. The lack of a positive effect of parity in successive pregnancies during adolescence may represent depletion of maternal nutritional stores compounded by competition with the fetus for available nutrients [28]. Among mature gravidas, birthweight increases 150 to 200 gm in subsequent pregnancies. No similar increase occurs among adolescents [20]. Using Collaborative Perinatal Project data, Naeye [28] showed that among younger primiparas (10–16 yr), those who were normal weight or underweight before conception had a significantly higher proportion of growth-retarded infants than those who were overweight.

Even when matched for nutritional status, infants of adolescent mothers are lighter compared to those of their older counterparts. With the same level of gestational weight gain, infants of young adolescent (13–15 yr) mothers were both lighter and thinner than infants born to older mothers [17, 30].

The lower mean birthweight of infants of adolescents, compared to older gravidas, is in large part due to differences in anthropometric parameters, reflecting inadequate body fat, as indicated by increasing skinfold measurements. As shown in Table 4-1, body fat increases throughout adolescence and even during adulthood. From age 15 to young adulthood (ages 18–24 yr), skinfold measurements of subcutaneous fat increase at the triceps by 15 percent, at the subscapular area by 24 percent, and at the mid–upper arm circumference by 8 percent. Comparisons to older age categories (25–34 and 35–44 yr) are even more dramatic. In normal-weight, mature women, total maternal body fat increases during pregnancy, reaching a peak between 24 and 28 weeks, and is followed by a decrease during the remaining 12 weeks [31, 32]. Bissenden and associates [33, 34] reported that to achieve infants of comparable birthweight for gestational age, mature women of smaller body habitus (Asian) had to increase body fat by twice as much as women of average body habitus (European). Inadequate increases in skinfold thickness in mature gravidas during the second trimester, particularly triceps measurements, were significant predictors of poor fetal growth [35].

Underweight or normal-weight adolescents may still be lighter and have lower body fat than mature women. In addition, the normal accretion of body fat that accompanies gestation may be diverted to provide energy for maternal growth, particularly in early-maturers and adolescents of young chronologic age. Maso and associates [36] demonstrated different patterns of anthropometric changes in adolescents who had low-birthweight infants compared to those who had normal-birthweight infants. In particular, increases in mid-arm circumferences were significantly less among adolescents who had low-birthweight versus normal-birthweight infants (0.05 vs. 0.80 mm/wk).

Higher pregravid weight among adolescents may lessen the difference in birthweight outcomes compared to older gravidas. When pregnancy occurs before completion of the adolescent growth spurt, the mother's metabolic needs compete with those of her fetus for available nutrients [28]. Changes in maternal nutritional status, as reflected by the deposition and utilization of body fat, may partially mediate birthweight outcome in adolescent pregnancies.

Adolescents may particularly benefit from higher gestational weight gains and dietary supplementation. Horon and associates [37] reported that among mature gravidas race and gender of the infant were more important predictors of birthweight, whereas among adolescents maternal weight gain was more important. Although they would benefit most from higher weight gains, younger adolescents tend to gain less weight during pregnancy [38, 39]. Pregnancy weight gains among adolescents are significantly associated with the trimester the adolescent enrolls in the Supplemental Food Program for Women, Infants, and Children (WIC) [39], which provides additional foods to high-risk gravidas, including adolescents [40, 41]. Scholl and colleagues reported that among adolescents, birthweight was significantly associated with total maternal weight gain independent of pregravid weight [42] and the pattern of maternal weight gain [43]. Inadequate early weight gain (<4.3 kg, or 9.5 lb, by 24 wk) is associated with a significant risk of intrauterine growth retardation [43].

Frisancho and associates [30] suggest that the average weight gain of 3 kg (6.6 lb) per year due to normal growth in nonpregnant adolescents be added to the weight gain in pregnancy to help optimize gestational outcome. Guidelines from the American Dietetic Association on the nutritional management of adolescent pregnancy [44] suggest that weight gain be calculated based on (1) the expected weight increase as a result of nonpregnant growth during the 9 months of pregnancy, (2) a weight increase to support pregnancy, and (3) if underweight, a weight increase to achieve an average weight-for-height.

Few studies have evaluated the prenatal diet of adolescents. Some report adequate dietary intakes (2800 kcal and 110 gm protein), with levels of all nutrients, except iron, exceeding the Recommended Dietary Allowances (RDAs) [45]; others report inadequate intakes of protein, calcium, iron, and vitamins A and C [27]. Because adolescents, particularly those of young chronologic or gynecologic age, are still actively growing, they may benefit from dietary supplementation during pregnancy, either through the WIC program to augment foods in the home [39] or with a balanced nutrient supplement [46]. Paige and associates [46] reported significant increases in birthweight among infants of adolescents who received a daily dietary supplement of 240 kcal, 14.5 gm protein, with vitamins and minerals over an average period of 15 weeks. Infants of adolescents who received the supplement averaged 157 gm heavier than those who had not; the birthweights of infants of younger adolescents (<16 yr) and smokers particularly benefited from dietary supplementation.

In summary, pregnancy before physical maturation results in substantially compromised outcome, including shorter gestation, lighter birthweight, increased surgical delivery due to pelvic immaturity, and increased complications of preterm birth. Therapeutic measures to reduce the risk of adverse outcomes include higher maternal weight gain, particularly earlier than 24 weeks of gestation, based on the adolescent's pregravid weight, gynecologic and chronologic ages, and the estimated needs for pregnancy. Anthropometric monitoring of the triceps skinfold measurement or mid–upper arm circumference, or both, to evaluate the increase in body fat may be a useful indicator of nutritional status and progress in meeting the needs of both growing mother and her fetus.

Associated Factors for the Younger Gravida

Beyond the biologic constraints of adolescent pregnancy, associated physiologic factors, such as maternal smoking, potentiate adverse outcomes (see Chap. 12). The 1990 national school-based Youth Risk Behavior Survey of the Centers for Disease Control [47] reported that more than one third of all students in grades 9 through 12 used tobacco. The prevalence of tobacco use was significantly greater among male students (40.4%) than among female students (31.7%), and among white students (41.2%) than among Hispanic (32.0%) or black (16.8%) students. Tobacco use increased by the grade of students, from 32.1 percent of 9th graders to 41.2 percent of 12th graders.

Once pregnant, younger gravidas are more likely to quit smoking than are older gravidas. Data from the 1985 National Health Survey [48] indicate that younger women, across all education and income levels, are more likely to stop smoking during pregnancy (Table 4-3). In addition, the adverse effect of smoking on fetal growth and

Table 4-3
Percentage of women aged 18 to 44 years who quit smoking once pregnant, by age, race, education, income, and marital and employment status (1985 National Health Interview Survey)

	Age (yr)				
Characteristic	*18–24*	*25–29*	*30–34*	*35–44*	*Total*
All women	21.1	23.6	18.9	16.7	21.2
Race					
White	21.5	24.6	19.1	16.6	21.7
Black	17.3	17.5	19.2	19.0	17.9
Hispanic	28.8	45.0	40.0	31.6	38.9
Education (yr)					
<12	17.7	13.7	6.6	10.8	14.8
12	29.3	35.8	24.0	22.8	29.4
13–15	29.3	35.8	24.0	22.8	29.4
≥16	85.7	34.5	37.0	34.6	37.5
Income					
<$10,000	16.8	17.6	15.9	11.1	16.4
10,000–19,999	24.3	25.7	13.0	19.7	22.8
20,000–34,999	19.2	24.2	19.3	13.0	20.8
35,000–49,999	27.4	26.3	22.0	25.8	25.1
≥50,000	14.3	39.2	28.9	15.1	26.9
Marital status					
Married	21.8	26.6	19.3	16.7	22.5
Single	19.9	16.3	26.1	–	19.2
Employment status					
Employed	24.8	26.3	17.4	14.3	22.7
Unemployed	27.3	25.5	39.6	16.7	28.1

Source: Adapted from CA Schoenborn, Health promotion and disease prevention: United States, 1985. *Vital and Health Statistics*, Series 10, No. 163. DHHS Pub. No. (PHS) 88-1591. Public Health Service. Washington, DC: US Govt. Printing Office, 1988. P. 55.

gestational age is significantly greater as maternal age advances [49]. Wen and associates [49] reported a fivefold increased risk of growth retardation in women 35 years of age or older, but less than a twofold increased risk in women under 17 years of age. These investigators also reported that smoking reduced birthweight by 134 gm in young women compared to 301 gm in women over 35.

Social disadvantages represent the overwhelming associated factor with adolescent pregnancy [50]. The 1987 National Academy of Sciences' report, *Risking the Future* [50], summarized the current situation in the United States:

> Teenage families with children are disproportionately fatherless, and most are poor. Teenage marriages, when they occur, are characterized by a high degree of instability. In addition, teenage parents, both male and female, suffer the negative impact that untimely parenting has on their education and the related limitation of career opportunities. Teenage parents are more likely than those who delay childbearing to experience chronic unemployment and inadequate income. Because these young people often fare poorly in the workplace, they and their children are highly likely to become dependent on public assistance and to remain dependent longer than those who delay childbearing until their twenties. Society's economic burden in sustaining these families is substantial.

In addition, adolescents are less likely to begin prenatal care early compared to older gravidas. As shown in Fig. 4-4, only about half of all adolescents having their first birth began prenatal care by the third month, compared to nearly 80 percent of women aged 20 to 24 and 90 percent of women aged 25 and older. Whereas among all women, only 1.5 percent received no prenatal care during their first pregnancy in 1986, this figure doubled (2.9%) for adolescents aged 15 to 19 [15].

The Older Gravida

Two major factors have influenced the changing pattern of childbearing in the United States. First, due to the rapid rise in the birth rate in the 1950s and 1960s followed by a sharp decline in the 1970s, **the largest proportion of women of childbearing age are 35 years of age or older** (Table 4-4). In 1986, for example, more than 29 percent of all childbearing women were 35 years of age or older, compared to 18 to 19 percent aged 20 to 34 and 16 percent aged 19 or younger [15]. Second, more women are choosing to delay childbearing in favor of professional and educational accomplishments. Whereas only 20 percent of all births in the United States in 1980 were to women aged 30 and older, this number rose to 25 percent in 1985 and 28 percent in 1988 [16, 51].

Figure 4-1 shows that the rate of first births for women aged 30 and older has risen dramatically between 1970 and 1986 [15]. For women aged 30 to 34, the rate has increased nearly 140 percent; for women aged 35 to 39, it has increased 124 percent; and for women aged 40 to 44, it has increased 50 percent. During the same years, the changes in the first birth rate for younger women have been much less, including a 24 percent increase for women aged 25 to 29, and decreases of 33 percent for women aged 20 to 24 and 27 percent for women aged 15 to 19.

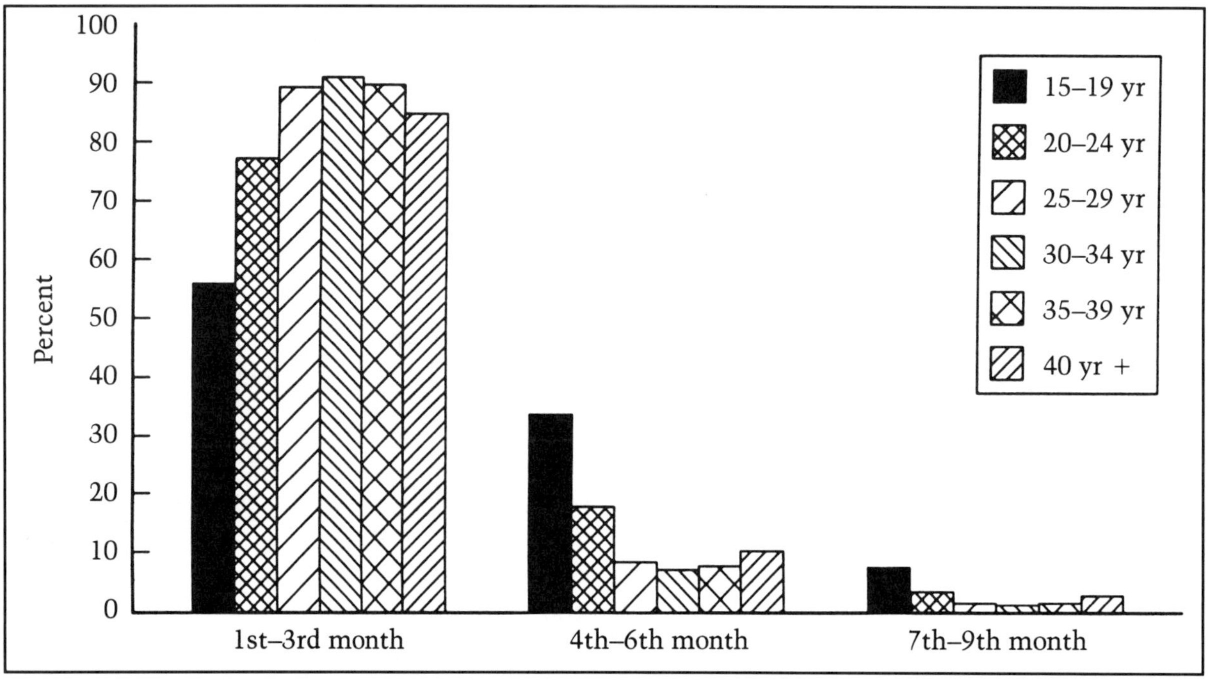

Fig. 4-4
Percent distribution of first births by month of pregnancy prenatal care began, by age of mother, United States, 1986. (Adapted from SJ Ventura, Trends and variations in first births to older women, 1970–86. *Vital and Health Statistics*, Series 21, No. 47. National Center for Health Statistics, 1989.)

Table 4-4
The proportion of women of childbearing age, by maternal age, United States, 1970–1986

	Year				
Age (yr)	*1970*	*1975*	*1980*	*1985*	*1986*
All ages	100.0	100.0	100.0	100.0	100.0
15–19	22.2	22.0	19.5	16.0	15.9
20–24	20.0	20.3	20.1	18.5	17.7
25–29	16.2	18.2	18.6	19.1	19.1
30–34	13.7	15.1	16.9	17.9	18.1
35–39	13.4	12.5	13.5	15.8	16.5
40–44	14.5	12.0	11.3	12.6	12.7
≥35	27.9	24.4	24.8	28.4	29.2

Source: Adapted from SJ Ventura, Trends and variations in first births to older women, 1970–86. *Vital and Health Statistics*, Series 21, No. 47. DHHS Pub. No. (PHS) 89-1925, 1989.

The number of multiple births (twins, triplets, and higher-order multiples) is also increased among older mothers, partially due to delaying childbirth and partially due to the use of fertility-enhancing agents (see Chap. 12). With increasing maternal age the rate of twin births (Fig. 4-5), and triplets and higher-order births (Fig. 4-6), rises dramatically, with a generally higher twin rate for blacks at all maternal ages and a higher triplet rate for whites at all maternal ages.

Two additional effects of delaying childbirth are that older mothers tend to have more education and fewer children. Whereas in 1970 only about one fourth of women having their first child at age 30 or older were college graduates (16 years of education), by 1985 that proportion had increased to nearly one half (Fig. 4-7). Among women aged 25 to 39, there is a trend toward smaller family size, although this is most evident among women aged 30 and older (Fig. 4-8). Among women aged 30 to 34, the proportion with two children or less doubled between 1970 and 1985 (28.4 to 60.7%); in contrast, the proportion with three or more children has declined by nearly one half (71.7 to 39.3%). A similar trend is seen among women aged 35 to 39, with the number of families having two or less children nearly doubling (17.4% in 1970 vs. 47% in 1985) and the number of families having three or more children declining by about one third (82.5% in 1970 vs. 53% in 1985) [15].

As with adolescent pregnancies, one of the major risks of pregnancy at the other extreme of the childbearing years is purely biologic. The risk of congenital anomalies in the newborn is greatly increased with advancing maternal age. The incidence of congenital malformations rises steeply for mothers aged 35 and older, and is particularly high for women aged 40 and older [52]. Children born to women in this latter age group are twice as likely to have a birth defect as children born to women aged 25 to 29, the age group with the lowest incidence of malformations (1710.5/100,000 live births vs. 779.5/100,000 live births). This pattern of increasing risk with increasing maternal age is similar for births to both white and black women, although the incidence is higher for whites at each category of maternal age. Of all birth defects studied, Down's syndrome is the most striking example of the increased risk to older women [53]. The incidence of this birth defect is 33 times greater for infants born to women aged 40 to 49 than infants born to women aged 20 to 24 (670.5/100,000 live births vs. 20.2/100,000 live births).

The presence of congenital anomalies can be assessed in the majority of cases using a variety of prenatal testing techniques, including

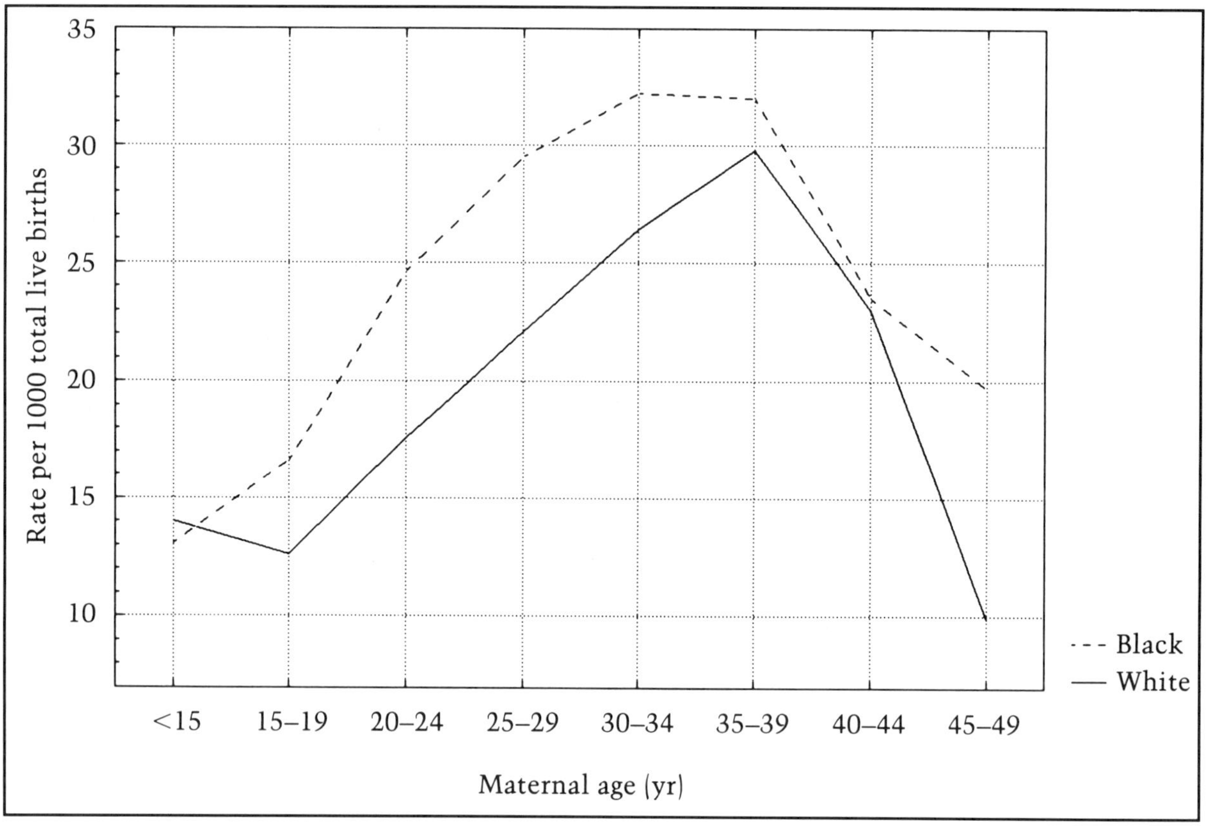

Fig. 4-5
Rate of twin births by maternal age and race, United States, 1988. (Adapted from National Center for Health Statistics: Vital Statistics of the United States, 1988. Vol. 1, *Natality. Public Health Service*. Washington, DC: Government Printing Office, 1990. P. 241.)

amniocentesis, chorionic villus sampling, ultrasound, and alpha-fetoprotein determinations. The combination of prenatal diagnosis and appropriate antepartum and intrapartum management greatly reduces the problems associated with older maternal age [54].

In summary, compared to adolescents, women who begin having their children at older ages tend to be relatively privileged, with greater social than biologic advantages. Adolescents, on the other hand, may have more biologic advantages than their older counterparts, but are at greater social disadvantage. It is this combination of social and biologic advantage and disadvantage, mediated through the associated factors of diet and nutrition, income and family support, and access to care, that influence pregnancy outcome at the extremes of the childbearing years.

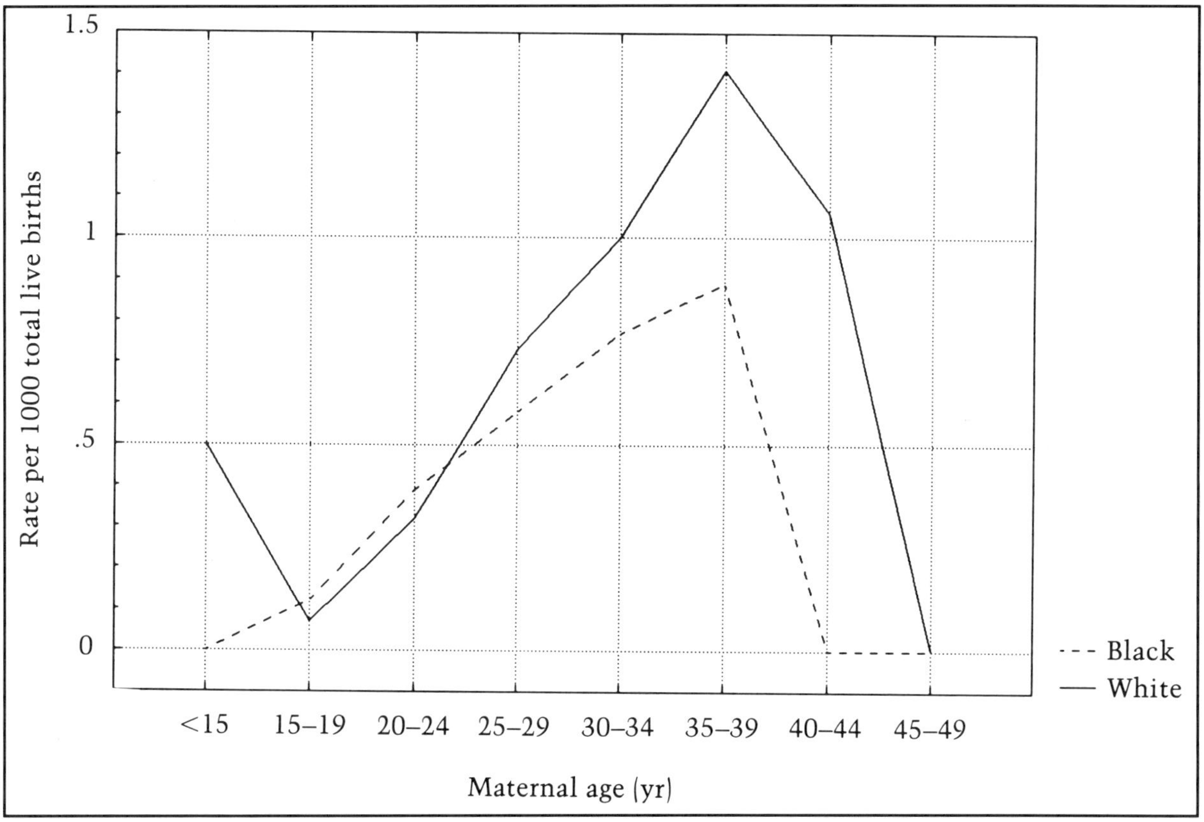

Fig. 4-6
Rate of triplet and higher-order births by maternal age and race, United States, 1988. (Adapted from National Center for Health Statistics: Vital Statistics of the United States, 1988. Vol. 1, *Natality. Public Health Service*. Washington, DC: Government Printing Office, 1990. P. 241.)

Race and Ethnicity

Racial, ethnic, and cultural influences also affect patterns of childbearing in the United States, including rates of first births by maternal age (adolescent pregnancies), childbirth to unmarried women, and biologic differences in length of gestation and birthweight distributions. The influence of genetic versus environmental factors on pregnancy outcome, particularly among new immigrants to the United States, has also received attention in recent years.

The definition of race and ethnicity is basic to identifying their effects on pregnancy rates and outcomes. Federal health statistics on births and infant deaths, as well as health status, are based on information on race and ethnicity. Birth and infant death informa-

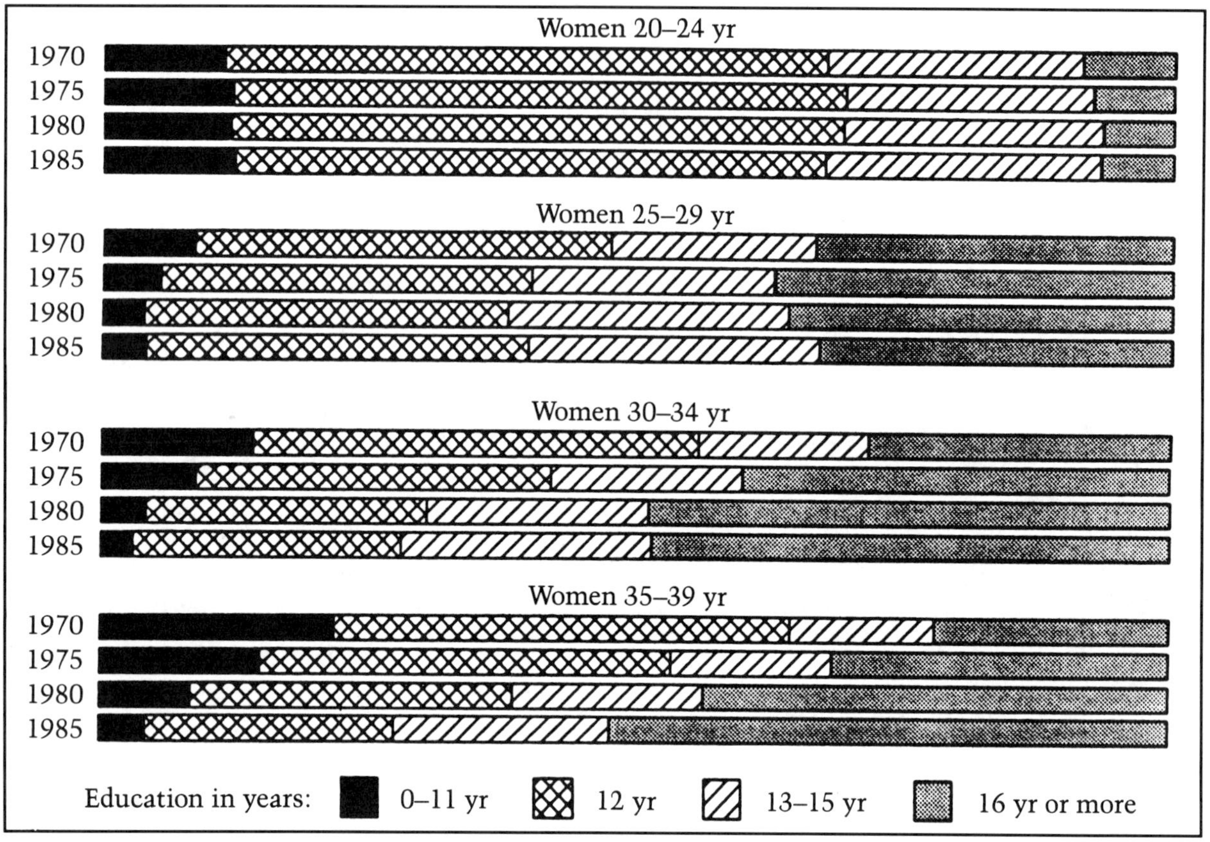

Fig. 4-7
Percent distribution of first births by mother's age and education, United States, 1970 to 1985. (Adapted from SJ Ventura, Trends and variations in first births to older women, 1970–86. *Vital and Health Statistics*, Series 21, No. 47. National Center for Health Statistics, 1989.)

tion is derived from linked birth and death certificates [55]; health status data rely on national health and examination surveys. In a recent review of state and Federal statistics based on racial and ethnic considerations, Hahn [56] stated:

> Long-standing conceptual difficulties in the definition of "race" and "ethnicity" pose a challenge to the surveillance of health in US "racial" and "ethnic" groups. The validity of the concept of "race," for example, has been questioned, and biological notions of "race" may be confused with cultural and behavioral notions of "ethnicity." Lack of scientific consensus has hindered the establishment of firm principles for surveillance of the health of racial and ethnic groups. Surveillance is also made difficult by multiple and changing perceptions of social identity in different segments of the population and by interests not consistent with scientific goals.

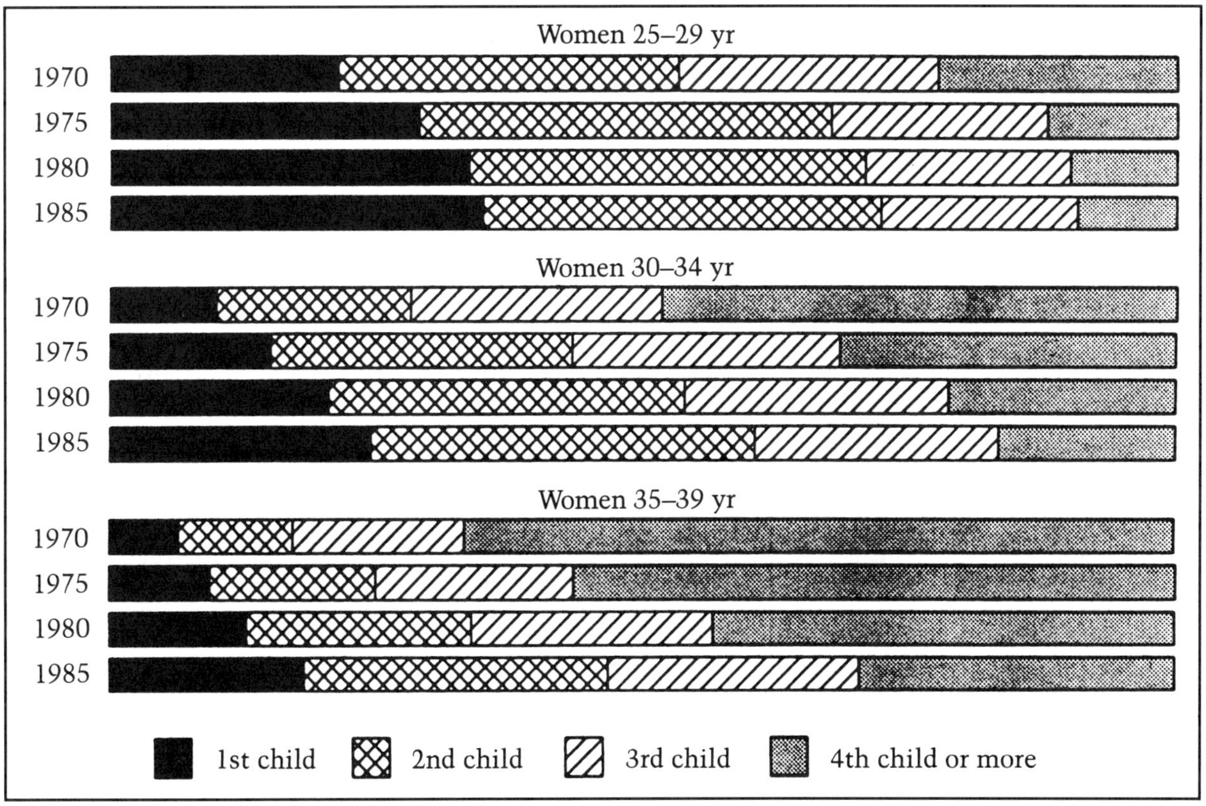

Fig. 4-8
Percent distribution of births by birth order according to age of mother, United States, 1970 to 1985. (Adapted from SJ Ventura, Trends and variations in first births to older women, 1970–86. *Vital and Health Statistics*, Series 21, No. 47. National Center for Health Statistics, 1989.)

Differences between white and black pregnancy rates and outcomes have been studied extensively for nearly 50 years, and whites and blacks continue to be the most frequently studied racial groups in the United States [57–62]. Recently, however, studies of specific ethnic influences on pregnancy outcome within the black race (foreign-born vs. US-born) have indicated that differences exist even within this single racial group [63, 64]. Interest in evaluating the health status of other racial and ethnic groups increased in the 1970s and 1980s as the proportion of different minorities in the United States changed. For example, a Hispanic Health and Nutrition Examination Survey (HHANES), conducted in 1982 to 1984, sampled three separate Latino populations (Cuban, Mexican, and Puerto Rican) in the United States [65]. In addition, Hispanic origin was added to the 1989 revision of the US standard certificate of live birth [66]. The health status of Southeast Asian immigrants and their children has also been the focus of recent research [67, 68]. Other indigenous groups, such as American Indians and native Alaskans, have also been the topic of special interest in recent years [69].

According to the National Center for Health Statistics, births to the major racial and ethnic groups in the United States in 1988 included whites (77.9%), blacks (17.2%), Asian or Pacific Islander (3.6%), and American Indian (1.2%). Most Hispanics consider themselves white, and they represent 11.5 percent of births in the United States [16]. A distribution of live births by racial and ethnic group in the United States in 1988 is shown in Table 4-5.

As shown in Fig. 4-9, there are wide variations in the age at childbearing by racial and ethnic group. The distribution of live births by maternal age is shifted farthest to the left (youngest age categories)

Table 4-5
Percent distribution of live births by race and ethnicity, United States, 1988

	All live births	
Race/ethnic group	*Number*	*Percent*
All groups	3,909,510	100.0
White	3,046,162	77.9
Black	671,976	17.2
Hispanic*	449,604	11.5
Mexican	271,170	6.9
Puerto Rican	46,232	1.2
Cuban	10,189	0.3
Central/South American	57,610	1.5
Other Hispanic	64,403	1.6
American Indian	45,871	1.2
Asian or Pacific Islander	142,258	3.6
Chinese	22,904	0.6
Japanese	10,483	0.3
Hawaiian	7,661	0.2
Filipino	24,612	0.6
Other Asian	76,598	2.0

*Most Hispanics consider themselves white.

Source: Adapted from Advance report on final natality statistics, 1988. *Monthly Vital Statistics Report*, Vol. 39, No. 4, Supplement, August 15, 1990.

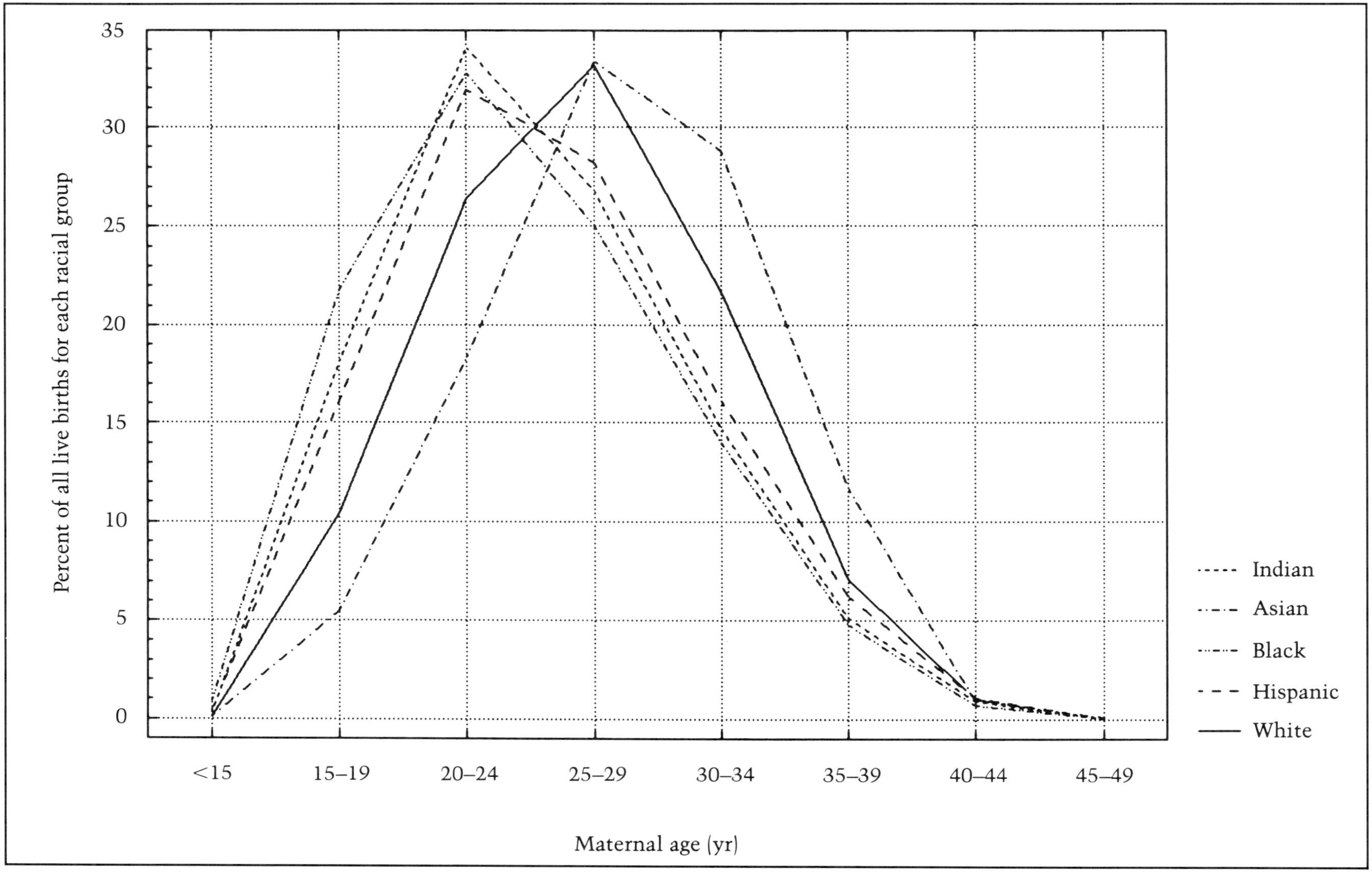

Fig. 4-9
Percent distribution of all live births by maternal age and race, United States, 1988. (Adapted from National Center for Health Statistics: Vital Statistics of the United States, 1988. Vol. 1, *Natality. Public Health Service*. Washington, DC: Government Printing Office, 1990. P. 93.

for blacks and farthest to the right (oldest age categories) for Asians. Births to women less than 20 years of age accounted for 5.7 percent of Asian births, 10.5 percent of white births, 16.4 percent of Hispanic births, 18.4 percent of American Indian births, and 22.7 percent of black births. Births to women aged 30 and older included 41.6 percent of Asian births, 30 percent of white births, 23.5 percent of Hispanic births, 20.7 percent of American Indian births, and 19.6 percent of black births.

Pregnancy outcomes also vary widely by racial and ethnic groups. The low birthweight (<2500 gm) rate is lowest among infants of whites (5.6%), American Indians (6.1%), and Asian and Hispanic (6.2% each); it is highest among blacks (13%). The duration of gestation also varies among ethnic and racial groups, with black women having a shorter natural length of gestation than whites [70], but twice the rate of preterm births [71]. Biologic differences that may account for some of this variation include variations in maternal glucose levels and body habitus [72], hemoglobin and hematocrit levels, and dietary intake. The majority of difference, though, is due to associated factors of socioeconomic status and related health knowledge and behavior [73, 74]. Even after adjusting for factors related to maternal age, education, and socioeconomic status, the odds ratio of very preterm birth was 1.9 for blacks, 1.53 for Asians, and 1.3 for Mexican-Americans, compared to 1.0 for whites [71]. For preterm births, the odds ratio was 1.79 for blacks, 1.61 for Asians, and 1.42 for Mexican-Americans, compared to 1.0 for whites [71].

Largely as a reflection of lower birthweight and shorter gestation, infant mortality varies widely between racial and ethnic groups in the United States. Based on data from the 1983 to 1984 U.S. birth cohorts, infant mortality ranged from 6 per 1000 live births among Japanese to 18.7 per 1000 live births among blacks [75] (Table 4-6). When infant mortality is examined using race-specific rates, the effect of inadequate birthweight is magnified. Compared to white infants, three times as many black infants had birthweights less than 1500 gm in 1980 [60]. Deaths to black infants in this birthweight group amounted to 50 percent during infancy. In comparison, deaths to white infants with birthweights less than 1500 gm totaled 37 percent during infancy. Birthweights less than 2500 gm accounted for 11 percent of all black infants in 1980, compared to 5 percent of all white infants. Within this birthweight group, 71 percent of black infants died during infancy, compared to 54 percent of white infants [60].

Table 4-6
Live births and infant mortality by racial and ethnic groups, United States, 1983 to 1984

		Mortality[a]		
Race/ethnic group	*Live births*	*Infant*	*Neonatal*	*Postneonatal*
All races	7,308,382	10.7	7.0	3.7
Black	1,126,605	18.7	12.2	6.5
American Indian	65,722	14.3	6.9	7.4
Puerto Rican[b]	68,196	12.9	8.7	4.2
White	5,884,364	9.1	6.0	3.2
Mexican[b]	447,743	9.0	5.8	3.2
Other Asian	115,480	9.0	5.8	3.2
Filipino	34,612	8.5	5.4	3.0
South American[b]	67,622	8.4	5.8	2.5
Chinese	27,563	8.3	4.9	3.4
Cuban[b]	19,210	7.8	5.7	2.1
Japanese	14,663	6.0	3.6	2.4

[a]Per 1000 live births.
[b]Based on data from the 23 states in which data on Hispanic origin are collected.

Source: Adapted from JC Kleinman, Infant mortality among racial/ethnic minority groups, 1983–1984. *Morbid. Mortal. Weekly Rep.*, Vol. 39, No. SS-3, 1990. Pp. 31–39.

In a recent analysis of black and white differences in the incidence of low birthweight, Kleinman and Kessel [58] suggest that:

> The large racial differences observed, even among married college graduates, emphasize the need for more in-depth research that goes beyond the traditional risk factors. There are many possible economic, social, environmental, and medical differences between blacks and whites, even in groups that appear homogeneous. Data from the 1983 National Health Interview Survey show that among married women 20 to 44 years of age who had graduated from college, 23% of whites, as compared with 35% of blacks, had an annual family income below $25,000. There are also likely to be substantial differences between low-risk black and low-risk white mothers with respect to current health status, childhood and adolescent health history, stress, nutrition, parents' and grandparents' socioeconomic status, and quality of medical care during pregnancy. Future investigations of racial differences need to consider these variables.

Socioeconomic Status

As discussed earlier, the term *socioeconomic status* reflects a myriad of economic, behavioral, environmental, and medical factors, each of which influences pregnancy outcome. In a 1962 British study of the effect of social class on prematurity (<2500 gm), Sir Dugald Baird [76] demonstrated that a combination of physical and social factors influenced pregnancy outcome, with taller women in the upper classes having the lowest rates of prematurity and the shortest women in the lowest classes having the highest rates.

More recent research has confirmed that social class, or socioeconomic status in the United States, has a powerful effect on pregnancy outcome. In an analysis of the 1976 birth cohort, Taffel [77] reported that although the incidence of low birthweight varied widely by race, maternal age, marital status, place of residence, birthplace, and pregnancy history, the socioeconomic status of the family, as measured by the mother's educational attainment, was one of the most critical factors determining birthweight. The proportion of low-birthweight infants born to women who were college graduates was half that of infants born to women with less than 9 years of education (4.9 vs. 9.9%).

Three important factors — smoking, weight gain, and prenatal care — are strongly linked to pregnancy outcome [78], and are indirectly related to education. Higher maternal educational level is associated with better health knowledge and behavior. Data from the 1985 National Health Interview Survey showed that the percentage of adult women who had an annual Papanicolaou smear and breast examination by a health professional increased with increasing level of education [48]. Among women with less than 12 years of education compared to those with 16 years or more, the percentage who had a Pap smear increased from 35 to 56 percent, and the percentage who had a breast examination increased from 42 to 60 percent. Knowledge regarding how to perform a breast self-examination also paralleled increasing education level, from 77 percent for women with less than 12 years of education to 94 percent for those with 16 years or more.

Better health knowledge and behaviors during pregnancy are also associated with better education, as shown by data from several national studies. Data from the 1985 National Health Interview Survey also showed that **knowledge about the fetal alcohol syndrome** increased with education [48] (Table 4-7). Within each age category, the proportion of women who had heard about the fetal alcohol syndrome increased twofold with increasing years of education. Data from this survey also indicated that the proportion of women who **quit smoking once they became pregnant** also paralleled education, ranging from three- to sixfold increases with greater educa-

Table 4-7
Percentage of women aged 18 to 44 years who have heard of the fetal alcohol syndrome by age, race, education, income, and marital and employment status (1985 National Health Interview Survey)

	Age (yr)				
Characteristic	*18–24*	*25–29*	*30–34*	*35–44*	*Total*
All women	56.1	64.5	68.6	61.7	62.1
Race					
White	59.7	67.7	72.6	64.0	65.3
Black	39.8	52.5	50.6	50.4	47.6
Hispanic	36.6	41.9	40.3	31.7	37.1
Education (yr)					
<12	35.4	41.0	43.4	40.3	39.3
12	54.8	61.7	65.5	55.7	58.5
13–15	65.9	69.9	73.4	70.1	69.4
≥16	78.6	79.8	83.9	81.9	81.5
Income					
<$10,000	57.5	49.1	51.3	45.5	52.6
10,000–19,999	54.9	62.2	63.6	54.6	58.2
20,000–34,999	59.9	69.4	70.8	62.4	65.4
35,000–49,999	52.8	76.1	77.2	70.3	69.8
≥50,000	63.6	70.7	76.6	70.9	70.6
Marital status					
Married	59.5	67.9	69.8	62.6	65.0
Single	54.3	57.1	61.8	55.0	55.5
Employment status					
Employed	58.2	65.5	70.4	63.1	63.8
Unemployed	55.5	61.1	63.0	60.3	59.3

Source: Adapted from CA Schoenborn, Health promotion and disease prevention: United States, 1985. *Vital and Health Statistics*, Series 10, No. 163, DHHS Pub. No. (PHS) 88-1591. Public Health Service. Washington, DC: US Govt. Printing Office, 1988. P. 47.

tional levels (see Table 4-3). Other studies have also shown the prevalence of smoking during pregnancy to drop by one half to three fourths among women with less than 12 years of education compared to those with more than 12 years of education [79, 80]. Data from the 1980 National Natality Survey showed that the proportion of women who had **low weight gains** (≤20 lb) was twice as great among women with less than 9 years of education as women with 16 or more years of education (37.4 vs. 16.1%) [81].

Early initiation of prenatal care is associated with better pregnancy outcomes as well as higher maternal education. Even after adjustment for maternal education, the incidence of low birthweight is lowest among women initiating prenatal care during the first and second months of pregnancy [77]. Recent studies with diverse populations have demonstrated the positive effect of early prenatal care on pregnancy outcome [82, 83]. Data from 1985 U.S. births indicated that prenatal care was begun during the first or second month of pregnancy by twice as many women with 16 years or more of education as women with less than 9 years of education [84] (Fig. 4-10).

Socioeconomic status is also linked with employment status and income level. Women's participation in the work force nearly doubled between 1960 and 1988, increasing from 30.5 to 56.5 percent among married women and 44.1 to 65.2 percent among single women

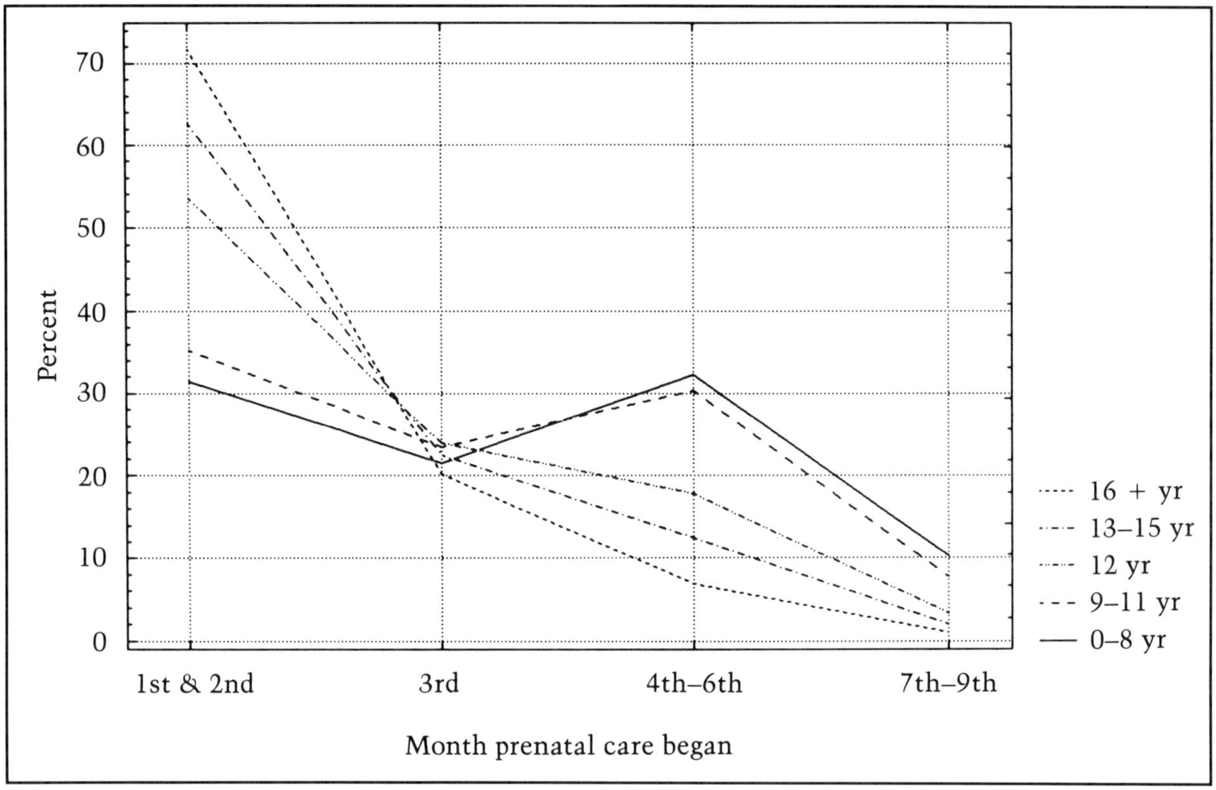

Fig. 4-10
Percent distribution of live births by month prenatal care began and education (yr) of mother, United States, 1985. (Adapted from National Center for Health Statistics: Vital Statistics of the United States, 1985, Vol. 1. *Natality. Public Health Service*, Washington, DC: Government Printing Office, 1988. P. 272.)

[85]. Work force participation also parallels increasing age. For example, among married women in 1988, 46.8 percent of those aged 16 to 19 were working, increasing to 72.7 percent of those aged 35 to 44. Although physical exertion does not appear to be detrimental during pregnancy, strenous physical activity and prolonged standing have been associated with preterm birth and lower birthweights [86–88]. Most studies that have evaluated the association between work and pregnancy, however, have not controlled for potentially confounding factors [89]. An analysis of the 1980 National Natality Survey reported that 90 percent of women aged 30 to 34 who had their first birth in 1980 were employed before delivery, and half of these women were in professional occupations [90]. These investigators concluded that professionally employed women generally have the best pregnancy outcomes, particularly if they are nonsmokers.

In conclusion, there is strong evidence that the maternal factors of age, race, and socioeconomic status influence pregnancy outcome. Modification of the potential adverse effects of each of these factors and their associated factors can be achieved through better maternal education, including improved weight gain, cessation of smoking, and early initiation of prenatal care. Biologic disadvantages of the extremes of maternal age can largely be overcome through early and comprehensive prenatal care. Some of the adverse effects of race can be overcome through better health care and nutritional status, although many questions remain regarding the relative influence of environment versus genetics.

References

1. Fedrick, J, and Anderson, ABM: Factors associated with spontaneous pre-term birth. *Br. J. Obstet. Gynaecol.* 83:342–350, 1976.
2. Fedrick, J, and Adelstein, P: Factors associated with low birth weight of infants delivered at term. *Br. J. Obstet. Gynaecol.* 85:1–7, 1978.
3. Eisner, V, Brazie, JV, Pratt, MW, and Hexter, AC: The risk of low birthweight. *Am. J. Public Health* 69:887–893, 1979.
4. Abrams, B, and Newman, V: Small-for-gestational-age birth: Maternal predictors and comparison with risk factors of spontaneous preterm delivery in the same cohort. *Am. J. Obstet. Gynecol.* 164:785–790, 1991.
5. Kramer, MS: Intrauterine growth and gestational duration determinants. *Pediatrics* 80:502–511, 1987.
6. Bakketeig, LS, Hoffman, HJ, and Harley, EE: The tendency to repeat gestational age and birth weight in successive births. *Am. J. Obstet. Gynecol.* 135:1086–1103, 1979.
7. Goldenberg, RL, Hoffman, HJ, Cliver, SP, et al. The influence of previous low birth weight on birth weight, gestational age, and anthro-

pometric measurements in the current pregnancy. *Obstet. Gynecol.* 79:276–280, 1992.
8. Hobel, CJ, Hyvarinen, MA, Okada, DM, and Oh, W: Prenatal and intrapartum high-risk screening. I. Prediction of the high-risk neonate. *Am. J. Obstet. Gynecol.* 117:1–9, 1973.
9. Hobel, CJ, Youkeles, L, and Forsythe, A: Prenatal and intrapartum high-risk screening. II. Risk factors reassessed. *Am. J. Obstet. Gynecol.* 135:1051–1056, 1979.
10. Baruffi, G, Strobino, DM, and Dellinger, WS: Definitions of high risk in pregnancy and evaluation of their predictive validity. *Am. J. Obstet. Gynecol.* 148:781–786, 1984.
11. Papiernik, E, and Kaminski, M: Multifactorial study of the risk of prematurity at 32 weeks of gestation. *J. Perinatal Med.* 2:30–36, 1974.
12. Creasy, RK, Gummer, BA, and Liggins, GC: System for predicting spontaneous preterm birth. *Obstet. Gynecol.* 55:692–695, 1980.
13. Main, DM, Richardson, D, Gabbe, SG, et al. Prospective evaluation of a risk scoring system for predicting preterm delivery in black inner city women. *Obstet. Gynecol.* 69:61–66, 1987.
14. Kaminski, M, Goujard, J, and Rumeau-Rouquette, C: Prediction of low birthweight and prematurity by a multiple regression analysis with maternal characteristics known since the beginning of the pregnancy. *Int. J. Epidemiol.* 2:195–204, 1973.
15. Ventura, SJ: Trends and variations in first births to older women, 1970–86. *Vital and Health Statistics*, Series 21, No. 47. National Center for Health Statistics, 1989.
16. Advance report of final natality statistics, 1988. *Monthly Vital Statistics Report*, Vol. 39, No. 4, Supplement, 1990.
17. Sukanich, AC, Rogers, KD, and McDonald, HM: Physical maturity and outcome of pregnancy in primiparas younger than 16 years of age. *Pediatrics* 78:31–36, 1986.
18. Harrison, KA, Fleming, AF, Briggs, ND, and Rossiter, CE: Growth during pregnancy in Nigerian teenage primigravidae. *Br. J. Obstet. Gynaecol.* 5 (Suppl.):32–39, 1985.
19. Harrison, KA, Rossiter, CE, and Chong, H: Relations between maternal height, fetal birthweight and cephalopelvic disproportion suggest that young Nigerian primigravidae grow during pregnancy. *Br. J. Obstet. Gynaecol.* 5 (Suppl.):40–48, 1985.
20. Scholl, TO, Hediger, ML, and Ances, IG: Maternal growth during pregnancy and decreased infant birth weight. *Am. J. Clin. Nutr.* 51:790–793, 1990.
21. Bayley, N: Size and body build of adolescents in relation to rate of skeletal maturing. *Child Dev.* 14:47–90, 1943.
22. Stevens-Simon, C, Forbes, GB, Kreipe, RE, and McAnarney, ER: A comparison of chronologic age and gynecologic age as indices of biologic maturity. *Am. J. Dis. Child.* 140:702–705, 1986.
23. Moerman, ML: Growth of the birth canal in adolescent girls. *Am. J. Obstet. Gynecol.* 143:528–532, 1982.

24. Garn, SM, LaVelle, M, Pesick, SD, and Ridella, SA: Are pregnant teenagers still in rapid growth? *Am. J. Dis. Child.* 138:32–34, 1984.
25. Duenhoelter, JH, Jimenez, JM, and Baumann, G: Pregnancy performance of patients under fifteen years of age. *Obstet. Gynecol.* 46:49–52, 1975.
26. Zlatnik, FJ, and Burmeister, LF: Low "gynecologic age": An obstetric risk factor. *Am. J. Obstet. Gynecol.* 128:183–186, 1977.
27. Graham, D: The Obstetric and Neonatal Consequences of Adolescent Pregnancy. In ER McAnarney and G Stickle (eds.), *Pregnancy and Childbearing During Adolescence: Research Priorities for the 1980s.* March of Dimes Birth Defects Foundation: Birth Defects: Original Article Series, Vol. XVII, No. 3, 1981. Pp. 49–67.
28. Naeye, RL: Teenaged and pre-teenaged pregnancies: Consequences of the fetal-maternal competition for nutrients. *Pediatrics* 67:146–150, 1981.
29. Frisancho, AR, Matos, J, and Bollettino, LA: Influence of growth status and placental function on birth weight of infants born to young still-growing teenagers. *Am. J. Clin. Nutr.* 40:801–807, 1984.
30. Frisancho, AR, Matos, J, and Flegel, P: Maternal nutritional status and adolescent pregnancy outcome. *Am. J. Clin. Nutr.* 38:739–746, 1983.
31. Pipe, NGJ, Smith, T, Halliday, D, et al: Changes in fat, fat-free mass and body water in human normal pregnancy. *Br. J. Obstet. Gynaecol.* 86:929–940, 1979.
32. Taggart, NR, Holliday, RM, Billewicz, WZ, et al: Changes in skinfolds during pregnancy. *Br. J. Nutr.* 21:439–451, 1967.
33. Bissenden, JG, Scott, PH, Hallum, J, et al: Anthropometric and biochemical changes during pregnancy in Asian and European mothers having well grown babies. *Br. J. Obstet. Gynaecol.* 88:992–998, 1981.
34. Bissenden, JG, Scott, PH, King, J, et al: Anthropometric and biochemical changes during pregnancy in Asian and European mothers having light for gestational age babies. *Br. J. Obstet. Gynaecol.* 88:999–1008, 1981.
35. Viegas, OAC, Cole, TJ, and Wharton, BA: Impaired fat deposition in pregnancy: An indicator for nutritional intervention. *Am. J. Clin. Nutr.* 45:23–28, 1987.
36. Maso, MJ, Gong, EJ, Jacobson, MS, et al: Anthropometric predictors of low birth weight outcome in teenage pregnancy. *J. Adolesc. Health Care* 9:188–193, 1988.
37. Horon, IL, Strobino, DM, and MacDonald, HM: Birth weights among infants born to adolescent and young adult women. *Am. J. Obstet. Gynecol.* 146:444–449, 1983.
38. Meserole, LP, Worthington-Roberts, BS, Rees, JM, and Wright, LS: Prenatal weight gain and postpartum weight loss patterns in adolescents. *J. Adolesc. Health Care* 5:21–27, 1984.
39. Scholl, TO, Decker, E, Karp, RJ, et al: Early adolescent pregnancy: A comparative study of pregnancy outcome in young adolescents and mature women. *J. Adolesc. Health Care* 5:167–171, 1984.

40. Metcoff, J, Costiloe, P, Crosby, WM, et al: Effect of food supplementation (WIC) during pregnancy on birth weight. *Am. J. Clin. Nutr.* 41:933–947, 1985.
41. Edozien, JC, Switzer, BR, and Bryan, RB: Medical evaluation of the special supplemental food program for women, infants, and children. *Am. J. Clin. Nutr.* 32:677–692, 1979.
42. Scholl, TO, Salmon, RW, Miller, LK, et al: Weight gain during adolescent pregnancy: Associated maternal characteristics and effects on birth weight. *J. Adolesc. Health Care* 9:286–290, 1988.
43. Hediger, ML, Scholl, TO, Belsky, DH, et al: Patterns of weight gain in adolescent pregnancy: Effects on birth weight and preterm delivery. *Obstet. Gynecol.* 74:6–12, 1989.
44. Position of the American Dietetic Association: Nutrition management of adolescent pregnancy. *J. Am. Diet. Assoc.* 89:104–109, 1989.
45. Loris, P, Dewey, KG, and Poirier-Brode, K: Weight gain and dietary intake of pregnant teenagers. *J. Am. Diet. Assoc.* 85:1296–1305, 1985.
46. Paige, DM, Cordano, A, Mellits, ED, et al: Nutritional supplementation of pregnant adolescents. *J. Adolesc. Health Care* 1:261–267, 1981.
47. Tobacco use among high school students—United States, 1990. *Morbid. Mortal. Weekly Rep.* 40:617–619, 1991.
48. Schoenborn, CA: Health promotion and disease prevention: United States, 1985. *Vital and Health Statistics*, Series 10, No. 163. DHHS Pub. No. (PHS) 88-1591. Public Health Service. Washington, DC: US Govt. Printing Office, 1988.
49. Wen, SW, Goldenberg, RL, Cutter, GR, et al: Smoking, maternal age, fetal growth, and gestational age at delivery. *Am. J. Obstet. Gynecol.* 162:53–58, 1990.
50. National Academy of Sciences: *Risking the Future: Adolescent Sexuality, Pregnancy, and Childbearing.* Washington, DC: National Academy Press, 1987.
51. National Center for Health Statistics: Advance report of final natality statistics, 1985. *Monthly Vital Statistics Report* Vol. 36, Suppl., July 17, 1987.
52. Taffel, S: Congenital anomalies and birth injuries among live births: United States, 1973–74. *Vital and Health Statistics*, Series 21, No. 31. DHEW Pub. No. (PHS) 79-1909, 1978.
53. Shuttleworth, GE: Mongolian imbecility. *Br. Med. J.* 2:661–665, 1909.
54. Fonteyn, VJ, and Isada, NB: Nongenetic implications of childbearing after age thirty-five. *Obstet. Gynecol. Surv.* 43:709–720, 1988.
55. Hahn, RA, Mulinare, J, and Teutsch, SM: Inconsistencies in coding of race and ethnicity between birth and death in US infants. *J.A.M.A.* 267:259–263, 1992.
56. Hahn, RA: The state and federal health statistics on racial and ethnic groups. *J.A.M.A.* 267:268–271, 1992.

57. Erhardt, CL, Joshi, GB, Nelson, FG, et al: Influence of weight and gestation on perinatal and neonatal mortality by ethnic group. *Am. J. Public Health* 54:1841–1855, 1964.
58. Kleinman, JC, and Kessel, SS: Racial differences in low birth weight: Trends and risk factors. *N. Engl. J. Med.* 317:749–753, 1987.
59. Mayberry, RM, and Lewis, RF: Ten-year changes in birthweight distributions of black and white infants, South Carolina. *Am. J. Public Health* 80:724–726, 1990.
60. National birthweight-specific infant mortality surveillance: Preliminary analysis—United States, 1980. *Morbid. Mortal. Weekly Rep.* 35:269–273, 1986.
61. Collins, JW, and David, RJ: The differential effect of traditional risk factors on infant birthweight among blacks and whites in Chicago. *Am. J. Public Health* 80:679–681, 1990.
62. Kleinman, JC, Fingerhut, LA, and Prager, K: Differences in infant mortality by race, nativity status, and other maternal characteristics. *Am. J. Dis. Child.* 145:194–199, 1991.
63. Cabral, H, Fried, LE, Levenson, S, et al: Foreign-born and US-born black women: Differences in health behaviors and birth outcomes. *Am. J. Public Health* 80:70–72, 1990.
64. Ethnic variation and maternal risk characteristics among blacks—Massachusetts, 1987 and 1988. *Morbid. Mortal. Weekly Rep.* 40:403–411, 1991.
65. National Center for Health Statistics: Plan and operation of the Hispanic Health and Nutrition Examination Survey, 1982–84. *Vital and Health Statistics*, Series 1, No. 19. DHHS Pub. No. (PHS) 85-1321, 1985.
66. Luke, B, and Keith, LG: The United States standard certificate of live birth: A critical commentary. *J. Reprod. Med.* 36:587–591, 1991.
67. Li, D-K, Ni, H, Schwartz, SM, and Daling, JR: Secular change in birthweight among Southeast Asian immigrants to the United States. *Am. J. Public Health* 80:685–688, 1990.
68. Yip, R, Scanlon, K, and Trowbridge, F: Improving growth status of Asian refugee children in the United States. *J.A.M.A.* 267:937–940, 1992.
69. Taffel, SM: Characteristics of American Indian and Alaska Native births: United States, 1984. *Monthly Vital Statistics Report*, Vol. 36, No. 3, Suppl., June 19, 1987.
70. Alexander, GR, Tompkins, ME, Altekruse, JM, and Horung, CA: Racial differences in the relation of birth weight and gestational age to neonatal mortality. *Public Health Rep.* 100:539–547, 1985.
71. Shino, PH, and Klebanoff, MA: Ethnic differences in preterm and very preterm delivery. *Am. J. Public Health* 76:1317–1321, 1986.
72. Green, JR, Schumacher, LB, Pawson, IG, et al. Influence of maternal body habitus and glucose tolerance on birth weight. *Obstet. Gynecol.* 78:235–240, 1991.
73. Rogers, RG, and Crank, J: Ethnic differences in smoking patterns:

Findings from NHIS. *Public Health Rep.* 103:387–393, 1988.
74. Novotny, TE, Warner, KE, Kendrick, JS, and Remington, PL: Smoking by blacks and whites: Socioeconomic and demographic differences. *Am. J. Public Health* 78:1187–1189, 1988.
75. Infant mortality—United States, 1988. *Morbid. Mortal. Weekly Rep.* 40:644–646, 1991.
76. Baird, D: Environmental and obstetrical factors in prematurity, with special reference to experience in Aberdeen. *Bull. W.H.O.* 26:291–295, 1962.
77. Taffel, SM: Factors associated with low birth weight, United States, 1976. *Vital and Health Statistics*, Series 21, No. 37. DHEW Pub. No. (PHS) 80-1915, 1980.
78. Guyer, B, Wallach, LA, and Rosen, SL: Birth-weight-standardized neonatal mortality rates and the prevention of low birth weight: How does Massachusetts compare with Sweden? *N. Engl. J. Med.* 306:1230–1233, 1982.
79. Kleinman, JC, and Kopstein, A: Smoking during pregnancy, 1967–80. *Am. J. Public Health* 77:823–825, 1987.
80. Cigarette smoking among reproductive-aged women—Idaho and New York. *Morbid. Mortal. Weekly Rep.* 39:659–662, 1990.
81. Taffel, SM: Maternal weight gain and the outcome of pregnancy, United States, 1980. *Vital and Health Statistics*, Series 21, No. 44. DHHS Pub. No. (PHS) 86-1922, 1986.
82. Foster, DC, Guzick, DS, and Pulliam, RP: The impact of prenatal care on fetal and neonatal death rates for uninsured patients: A "natural experiment" in West Virginia. *Obstet. Gynecol.* 79:40–45, 1992.
83. Murray, JL, and Bernfield, M: The differential effect of prenatal care on the incidence of low birth weight among blacks and whites in a prepaid health care plan. *N. Engl. J. Med.* 319:1385–1391, 1988.
84. *Vital Statistics of the United States, 1985. Vol. I, Natality.* US DHHS, Public Health Service. Hyattsville, MD: US Govt. Printing Office, 1988.
85. US Bureau of the Census: *Statistical Abstract of the United States: 1990* (110th ed.). Washington, DC: US Govt. Printing Office, 1990. P. 384.
86. Mamelle, N, Laumon, B, and Lazar, P: Prematurity and occupational activity during pregnancy. *Am. J. Epidemiol.* 119:309–322, 1984.
87. McDonald, AD, McDonald, JC, Armstrong, B, et al: Prematurity and work in pregnancy. *Br. J. Intern. Med.* 45:56–62, 1988.
88. Teitelman, AM, Welch, LS, Hellenbrand, KG, and Bracken, MB: Effect of maternal work activity on preterm birth and low birthweight. *Am. J. Epidemiol.* 131:104–113, 1990.
89. Keith, L, and Luke, B: The association between women's work, working conditions and adverse pregnancy outcomes: A review of the literature and directions for future research. *Women's Health Issues* 1:113–119, 1991.

90. Ventura, SJ, and Hendershot, GE: Infant health consequences of childbearing by teenagers and older mothers. *Public Health Rep.* 99:138–146, 1984.

Woman in labor on a birth chair with attendants and astrologers watching the heavens. (From Jacobus Rueff. *De Conceptu*. Frankfurt: S. Feyerabendt, 1580.)

A COLLECTION OF EARLY OBSTETRICAL BOOKS

L I B E R

LIBER QVARTVS.

DE VARIETATIBVS NON NA-turalis partus, & earundem curis.

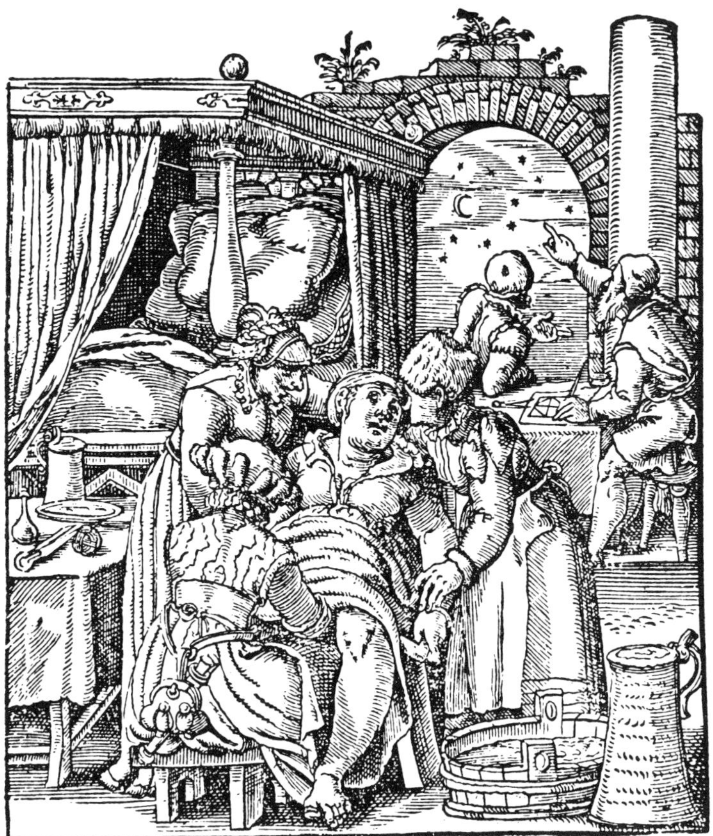

Quan-

Fig. 33. Fol. 28*v* of the 1580 edition of Jacob Rueff's "De Conceptu" (item 30), showing a room with a woman in labor on a birth chair, and astrologers watching the heavens.

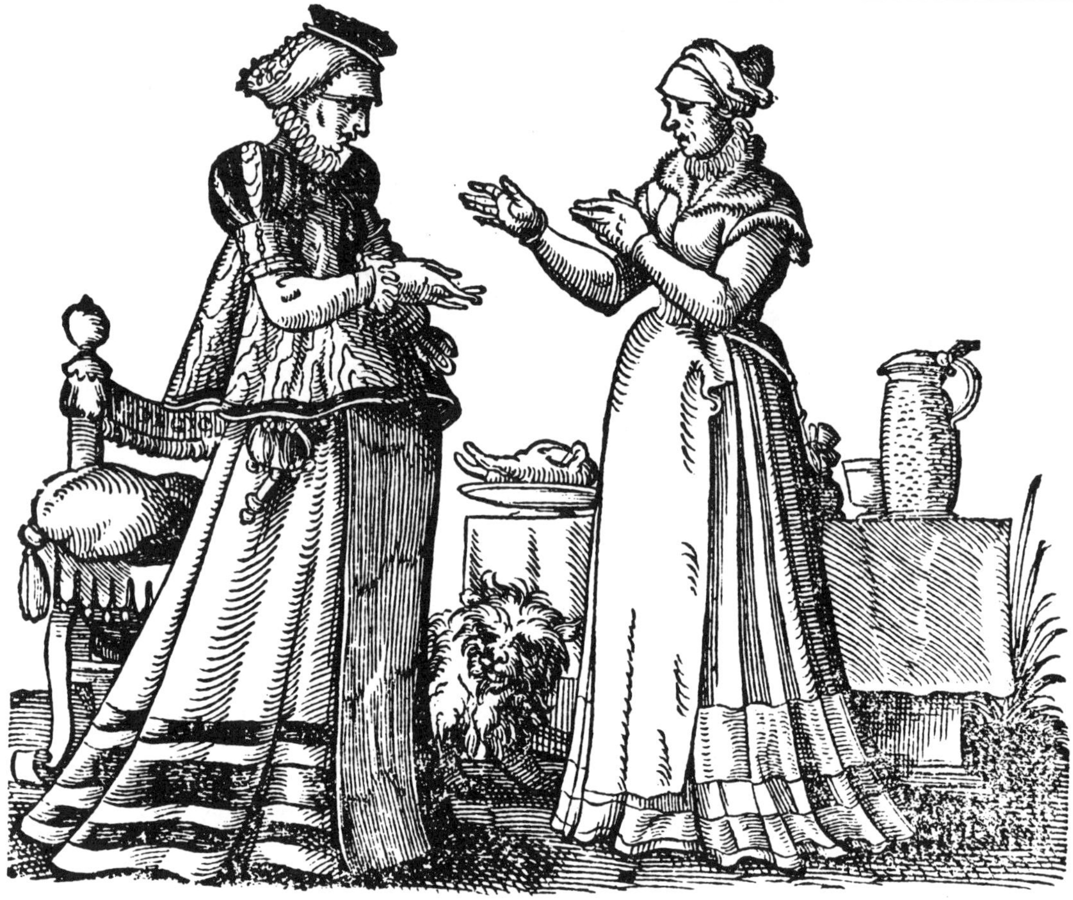

Sixteenth-century prenatal dietary advice. (From Jacobus Rueff. *De Conceptu*. Frankfurt: S. Feyerabendt, 1580.)

5

The Prenatal Diet

The underlying basis of the prenatal diet in the United States is the Recommended Dietary Allowance (RDA) of the Food and Nutrition Board of the National Academy of Sciences. The first edition of the RDAs was published in 1943, reflecting the emergence of nutrition as a separate science and in recognition of its central role in the maintenance of health [1]. The RDAs were intended to be an interpretation of the current scientific knowledge regarding nutrient requirements for healthy individuals and to serve as a guide to good nutrition. They have been revised periodically (the 10th edition was issued in 1989) and formulated as tables with specified levels of selected nutrients by gender and age, and for pregnancy and lactation.

The Most Recent RDAs

The first edition of the RDAs included only 10 nutrients; the most recent includes 19, as well as estimated minimum requirements (EMRs) of sodium, chloride, and potassium, and the estimated safe and adequate daily dietary intakes (ESADDIs) of biotin, pantothenic acid, copper, manganese, fluoride, chromium, and molybdenum. Changes from previous editions are made only if substantive new information becomes available or to correct inconsistencies in the prior evaluation of data [2].

Important changes in the 1989 RDA include a recategorization of individuals aged 19 to 22 years to include those aged 19 to 24 years, and the division of lactation into the first 6-month and second 6-month periods. The first change was made because peak bone mass, which is related to dietary calcium intake during the process of mineralization, is generally not attained before age 25. This change in age categories has resulted in higher RDAs for calcium, phosphorus, and vitamin D for individuals aged 23 and 24. The division of lactation into two periods provides higher RDAs for the initial 6 months of lactation.

Although the reference woman for the RDAs has consistently remained at 64 in. (163 cm) in height, weight varied from 55 kg (4th and 9th editions) to 56 kg (1st, 2nd, and 3rd editions) to 58 kg (5th, 6th, 7th, 8th, and 10th editions). The 1989 RDA is the first edition to be based on actual median heights and weights of American women rather than an arbitrary ideal. The heights and weights used in the 10th edition of the RDA were obtained from the second National Health and Nutrition Examination Survey (NHANES II); the differences from earlier versions include higher weights (2 kg to 10 kg) and variable heights (−1 cm to +5 cm, respectively). The higher weights resulted in higher RDAs for energy, protein, thiamin, riboflavin, and niacin.

Recommended dietary allowances were established for vitamin K and selenium in the 1989 edition. These nutrients had been introduced in the 1980 edition in the ESADDI category. The new RDA for vitamin K is 1 μg/kg body weight and, for selenium, 55 to 70 μg per day for adult women and men, respectively, representing the lower range of the 1980 ESADDI.

Other major changes in the 1989 RDA include lowered RDAs during pregnancy for folate, vitamins B_6 and B_{12}, magnesium, iron, zinc, and protein. Folate was lowered by about half based on evidence that folate status and liver stores are maintained adequately on diets containing the lower RDA for folate. For adult women the 1989 RDA for folate is 180 μg per day, 400 μg per day during pregnancy, and 280 μg per day and 260 μg per day during the first and second 6 months of lactation, respectively. Because adequate metabolic maintenance is achieved with lower levels of vitamins B_6 and B_{12}, the 1989 RDAs were reduced by one fifth and one third, respectively. The 1989 RDA for vitamin B_6 for adult women is 1.6 mg per day. During pregnancy and lactation, the 1989 RDA is 2.2 mg per day and 2.1 mg per day, respectively. The 1989 RDAs include lower levels of magnesium (280 mg/day for women, 320 mg/day during pregnancy, and 355 mg/day and 340 mg/day during the first and second 6 months of lactation, respectively) based on evidence that such levels are adequate for maintenance, growth, and support of maternal and fetal tissues.

Recommendations for zinc were lowered with the 1989 RDAs to 12 mg per day for adult women, and 19 mg per day and 16 mg per day during pregnancy and lactation, respectively. The 1989 RDA for iron was lowered to a more realistic level of 15 mg per day for adult women and during lactation, and 30 mg per day during pregnancy. The protein requirements during pregnancy were estimated using the factorial method, based on the protein content of the fetus, placenta, and maternal tissues. The resulting 1989 RDA for protein during pregnancy is 60 gm per day.

The ESADDIs for biotin, copper, manganese, and molybdenum were lower in the 1989 RDA, based on improved analytical techniques to assess intake and adequate maintenance. No changes were made in the ESADDIs for pantothenic acid, fluoride, or chromium. Electrolytes were recategorized from ESADDIs to EMRs. The 1989 EMRs for sodium, potassium, and chloride are each half of the lower range of the 1980 ESADDI. The 1989 EMRs for adults are 500 mg per day for sodium, 750 mg per day for chloride, and 2000 mg per day for potassium.

A summary of the 1989 RDAs, ESADDIs, and EMRs for adult women before and during pregnancy is given in Table 5-1. Contrary to popular belief, nutrient requirements generally do not double during gestation. Only the requirement for iron, folic acid, and vitamin D increases 100 percent over nonpregnant levels, while other nutrients, such as calcium, phosphorus, thiamin, and vitamin B_6 increase between 33 and 50 percent, respectively. Protein, zinc, and riboflavin increase about 20 to 25 percent, whereas energy, selenium, magnesium, iodine, niacin, and vitamins A, B_{12}, and C increase by 18 percent or less. **The RDAs for pregnancy have been translated into 2 weeks of menus in Table 5-2 (spring/summer) and Table 5-3 (fall/winter). The caloric content of these diets can be varied by altering the quantity of foods, but the balance of food choices provides all the RDAs during pregnancy.**

Data from national surveys of food consumption indicate that adult women in the childbearing years consume diets that meet or exceed the RDA for most nutrients (Table 5-4) [3]. The nutrients present at 80 percent or less of the RDA include vitamin B_6, calcium, magnesium, iron, zinc, and copper. Fortunately, these nutrients are present in abundant, bioavailable amounts in meat, poultry, fish, and dairy products, foods that are recommended in additional amounts during pregnancy.

Specific Dietary Requirements

Caloric Intake

Additional energy is required during pregnancy as a result of increases in the quantity of maternal tissues (principally uterus and breasts) and the growth and development of the fetus and placenta. Estimates of the quantity of these new tissues and the accompanying changes in the maternal metabolic rate differ widely in the medical literature, and calculations of the additional caloric requirement have ranged from as low as 60,000 kcal [4] and 68,000 kcal [5] to 80,000 [6] and as high as 110,000 kcal [7]. Despite these variations, it is generally agreed that adequate maternal weight gain must include some component of fat storage to ensure optimal newborn birthweight and survival, and that this energy storage is an integral part of the total energy requirement of pregnancy.

Table 5-1
Summary of the 1989 RDAs, ESADDIs, and EMRs for adult women aged 25 to 50, nonpregnant and pregnant

Nutrient	Nonpregnant levels	Pregnant levels	Percent increase
RDAs			
Folic acid	180 mcg	400 mcg	+122
Vitamin D	5 μg	10 μg	+100
Iron	15 mg	30 mg	+100
Calcium	800 mg	1200 mg	+50
Phosphorus	800 mg	1200 mg	+50
Vitamin B_6	1.6 mg	2.2 mg	+38
Thiamin	1.1 mg	1.5 mg	+36
Zinc	12 mg	15 mg	+25
Vitamin E	8 mg	10 mg	+25
Riboflavin	1.3 mg	1.6 mg	+23
Protein	50 mg	60 mg	+20
Selenium	55 μg	65 μg	+18
Iodine	150 mcg	175 mcg	+17
Vitamin C	60 mg	70 mg	+17
Energy	2200 kcal	2500 kcal	+14
Magnesium	280 mg	320 mg	+14
Niacin	15 mg	17 mg	+13
Vitamin B_{12}	2.0 mcg	2.2 mcg	+10
Vitamin A	800 μg RE	800 μg RE	No change
Vitamin K	65 μg	65 μg	No change
ESADDIs			
Biotin	30–100 μg	*	*
Pantothenic acid	4–7 mg	*	*
Copper	1.5–3.0 mg	*	*
Manganese	2.0–5.0 mg	*	*
Fluoride	1.5–4.0 mg	*	*
Chromium	50–200 μg	*	*
Molybdenum	75–250 μg	*	*
EMRs			
Sodium	500 mg	*	*
Chloride	750 mg	*	*
Potassium	2000 mg	*	*

RDAs, recommended dietary allowances; ESADDIs, estimated safe and adequate daily dietary intakes; EMRs, estimated minimum requirements; RE, retinol equivalents.
*No additional recommendations during pregnancy.

Table 5-2
Sample menus during pregnancy (spring/summer)

Breakfast	*Lunch*	*Snack*	*Dinner*	*Bedtime*
Milk[a] Grain cereal Fresh banana	Chopped liver sandwich with cheese[a] on whole wheat Lemonade	Fruit yogurt[a] Oatmeal cookies	Grilled chicken Baked potato Mixed salad Citrus juice	Fruit yogurt[a]
Fruit yogurt[a] Wheat germ Strawberries	Chef salad with ham/cheese/ turkey Salad greens Iced tea[b]	Cheddar cheese[a] Graham crackers	Grilled steak Tomatoes and corn Pasta salad/cheese[a] Iced coffee[b]	Milk[a]
Cottage cheese[a] Cracked wheat Toast Orange juice	Grilled cheese[a] sandwich with tomato on rye Lemonade	Milk[a] Graham crackers	Barbecued pork Summer squash Green beans Iced tea[b]	Milk[a]
English muffin Farmer's cheese[a] Blueberries Hot tea[b]	Chicken salad with grapes and walnuts Iced Tea[b]	Hard-boiled egg Wheat crackers Cheese[a] spread	Tuna salad with cheese[a] and pecans Dinner rolls Iced coffee[b]	Fruit yogurt[a]
Cheese[a] omelet Rye toast Fresh grapefruit Hot tea[b]	Ham and cheese[a] sandwich with tomato on wheat Lemonade	Fruit yogurt[a] Date-nut cookies	Chicken stir-fry with broccoli White rice Hot tea[b]	Milk[a]
Milk[a] Grain cereal Orange slices Hot tea[b]	Egg salad sandwich with lettuce on pumpernickel Iced tea[b]	Milk[a] Oatmeal cookies	Cold roast beef Potato/cheese[a] salad Cole slaw Iced coffee[b]	Fruit yogurt[a]
Cottage cheese[a] Cantaloupe Hot tea[b]	Sliced turkey sandwich with cranberry sauce on rye Lemonade	Fruit yogurt[a] Raisin cookies	Shish kebobs with steak, green peppers, tomatoes Baked potato with cheese[a] Citrus juice	Milk[a]

[a]Fortified with vitamin D and additional calcium.
[b]Decaffeinated.

Table 5-3
Sample menus during pregnancy (fall/winter)

Breakfast	*Lunch*	*Snack*	*Dinner*	*Bedtime*
Oatmeal Poached egg Orange juice Hot coffee[b]	Clam chowder[a] Cheese[a] sandwich Sliced apple	Rice pudding[a]	Roast turkey Cranberry sauce Wild rice Green beans Hot cider	Hot chocolate[a]
Farina Grated cheese[a] Fresh grapefruit Hot tea[b]	Vegetable soup Ham sandwich on whole wheat Fresh pear	Bread pudding[a] with raisins	Baked chicken Macaroni/cheese[a] Steamed spinach Hot tea[b]	Warm milk[a]
Wheatena cereal Hard-boiled egg Sliced banana Hot coffee[b]	Cream of tomato soup[a] Tuna salad on rye Fresh plums	Baked custard[a]	Broiled pork with apricots Baked potato Steamed broccoli with cheese[a] sauce Hot cider	Warm milk[a]
Cream of rice Scrambled egg Corn muffin Hot tea[b]	Chicken noodle soup Baked fish sticks Baked apple with cheddar[a]	Tapioca pudding[a]	Meat loaf Mashed potatoes Peas and carrots Hot tea[b]	Hot chocolate[a]
Cheese[a] omelet Citrus fruit English muffin Hot coffee[b]	Beef barley soup Peanut butter sandwich on wheat Fresh peach	Pudding with dates[a]	Spaghetti with meatballs/cheese[a] Green beans Hot tea[b]	Warm milk[a]
Waffle Fried egg/cheese[a] Orange juice Hot tea[b]	Lentil soup Grilled ham and cheese sandwich Fresh apple	Cheddar cheese[a] Graham crackers	Stuffed peppers Baked squash Mixed salad Hot tea[b]	Warm milk[a]
French toast Grapefruit Hot coffee[b]	Potato-leek soup Grilled turkey/cheese[a] sandwich on wheat Fresh orange	Baked custard[a]	Beef stew with potatoes/carrots Steamed broccoli with cheese[a] sauce Hot tea[b]	Hot chocolate[a]

[a]Fortified with vitamin D and additional calcium.
[b]Decaffeinated.

Table 5-4
Mean nutrient intakes and percent RDA of diets of women aged 19 to 50 in the CSFII[a]

Nutrient	*Daily intake*	*Percent RDA (nonpregnant levels)*
Energy	**1,528 kcal**	**69**
Protein	60.7 gm	121
Vitamin A	828 μg RE	104
Vitamin E	7.1 mg	89
Vitamin C	77 mg	128
Thiamine	1.05 mg	95
Riboflavin	1.34 mg	103
Niacin	16.1 mg	107
Vitamin B_6	**1.16 mg**	**73**
Folic Acid	189 mcg	105
Vitamin B_{12}	4.85 mcg	243
Calcium	**614 mg**	**77**
Phosphorus	966 mg	121
Magnesium	**207 mg**	**74**
Iron	**10.1 mg**	**67**
Zinc	**8.6 mg**	**72**
Copper[b]	**1.0 mg**	**67**
Sodium[c]	2368 mg	474
Potassium[c]	2066 mg	103

[a]Bolded items were ≤80% of the RDA or ESADDI.
[b]Based on ESADDI, estimated safe and adequate daily dietary intake.
[c]Based on EMR, estimated minimum requirement.

Source: Adapted from USDA, Human Nutrition Information Service, Nutrition Monitoring Division: *Nationwide Food Consumption Survey, Continuing Survey of Food Intakes by Individuals*. NFCS, CSFII Report No. 85-4. Washington, DC: US Govt. Printing Office, 1987. Pp. 46–49.

The World Health Organization estimates the energy requirement for pregnancy by dividing the gross energy cost (80,000 kcal) by the approximate duration of pregnancy (250 days following the first month) to yield an average daily increase of 300 kcal [6]. Because physical activity declines with advancing pregnancy, the National Academy of Sciences' 1989 RDAs suggest an additional 300 kcal per day during the second and third trimesters only [8]. **As recommended in the National Academy of Sciences' 1990 report on nutrition during pregnancy [9], the caloric intake during pregnancy should be based on the pregnant woman's pregravid weight and best rate of weight gain to achieve the optimal total gestational weight gain.** For women who begin pregnancy within the optimal weight-for-height (90–120%

ideal, or body mass index [BMI, weight-for-height squared, 19.8–26.0]), the recommended range of gestational weight gain is 25 to 35 lb. This weight should be gained at the rate of 3.5 lb during the first trimester and about 1 lb per week for the second and third trimesters. For women who are overweight when they begin pregnancy (20% or more above ideal, or BMI >26.0), the recommended total gestational weight gain is 15 to 25 lb, at the rate of 2 lb during the first trimester and about two thirds of a pound per week during the second and third trimesters. For women who begin pregnancy underweight (10% or more under ideal, or BMI <19.8), the recommended total gain is 28 to 40 lb, depending on the severity of the pregravid weight deficit. The recommended pattern of gestational gain for the underweight woman is 5 lb during the first trimester and slightly more than 1 lb per week during the second and third trimesters.

Protein

Protein requirements increase by 20 percent over nonpregnant levels for adult women, increasing from 50 gm to 60 gm, or about 1 gm/kg/day. This allowance must provide for both maternal physiologic adjustments and growth and development of the fetus and placenta. The RDA for protein during pregnancy is generous because of uncertainties about efficiency of protein storage and utilization during gestation, as well as the possibility of adverse effects on both mother and fetus from an inadequate intake. The richest sources of protein are meats, fish, poultry, and dairy and egg products. Legumes and grains also contribute protein to the diet, but contain binding agents that limit the bioavailability of all contained nutrients. Data from the US Department of Agriculture's 1985 Continuing Survey of Food Intake by Individuals (CSFII) indicate that the diets of adult women in the childbearing years provide adequate protein, averaging 59 to 62 gm per day [3].

Fat-Soluble Vitamins

Except for vitamin K, which is synthesized by bacteria normally present in the gastrointestinal tract, all fat-soluble vitamins are stored in the body. The fat-soluble vitamins, particularly vitamins A and D, are the most potentially toxic during pregnancy.

Vitamin A. **Vitamin A** requirements during pregnancy do not increase over nonpregnant levels, and the recommendation is 800 μg retinol equivalents per day (about 2700 IU). Vitamin A acts to maintain skin, membranes, and skeletal tissues; in the formation of sperm and maintenance of the placenta; and as a key component necessary for peripheral and color vision. Vitamin A is obtained directly from animal sources, mainly as retinol, and from vegetable sources as beta-carotene, both of which are converted to retinal in the gastrointestinal tract. The vitamin A activity in foods is expressed as retinol equivalents (RE): 1 RE is defined as 1 μg all-trans retinol, 6 μg all-trans beta-carotene, or 12 μg other provitamin A carotenoids. The richest sources of vitamin A include liver and fish liver oils, whole and fortified milk, and carrots and dark-green leafy vegetables. Data from the 1985 CSFII indicate that the dietary intake of vitamin A for adult women in their childbearing years is adequate, averaging about 800 to 850 μg RE per day (2700–2800 IU) [3]. Toxic effects occur with intakes exceeding 15,000 μg RE (50,000 IU) in adults and 6000 μg RE (20,000 IU) in infants and young children [10]. Spontaneous abortion and birth defects have been documented in the fetuses of women taking 0.5 to 1.5 mg/kg 13-cis-retinoic acid (isotretinoin) during the first trimester of pregnancy as well as those taking daily doses of 6000 μg RE or 20,000 IU retinol [11–14].

Vitamin D (Calciferol). **Vitamin D** (calciferol) is essential for the proper formation of the skeleton and for mineral homeostasis. During pregnancy the RDA for vitamin D doubles, increasing from 5 μg (200 IU) to 10 μg (400 IU). Exposure of the skin to ultraviolet light catalyzes the synthesis of vitamin D_3 (cholecalciferol) from 7-dehydrocholesterol. The other major form of the vitamin, D_2 (ergocalciferol), is the result of ultraviolet light–induced conversion of ergosterol in plants. The major dietary source of vitamin D is food fortified with this vitamin, including processed cow's milk. Excessive intakes of vitamin D are potentially toxic, and are associated with hypercalcemia and hypercalciuria, deposition of calcium in soft tissues, and irreversible renal and cardiovascular damage. Toxic effects have been documented with daily intakes as low as 45 μg (1800 IU) per day [15]. Congenital anomalies of the heart, particularly aortic stenosis, have been reported in the newborns of both humans and experimental animals with doses as low as 100 μg (4000 IU) during pregnancy [16–18]. Infants who were oversupplemented with vitamin D in England during World War II developed a syndrome known as infantile hypercalcemia, characterized by cerebral, cardiovascular, and renal changes [19].

Vitamin E. **Vitamin E** requirements during pregnancy increase by 25 percent to 10 mg per day. The most active form of vitamin E, alpha-tocopherol, is also the most abundant. The main function of vitamin E is as an antioxidant, preventing cellular membrane damage with subsequent neurologic manifestations. This cellular-level defense system is aided by two other essential nutrients: selenium and ascorbic acid. The main dietary sources of vitamin E include vegetable oils (soybean, corn, cottonseed, and safflower), wheat germ, nuts, and dark-green leafy vegetables. Dietary survey data indicate that adult women of childbearing age average dietary intakes of vitamin E of about 7 mg per day [3]. High doses of vitamin E have been used therapeutically in premature infants to prevent both retinal damage caused by oxygen therapy and lysis of red blood cells [20]. In adults, however, high doses of this vitamin can cause serious side effects, including thrombophlebitis, high blood pressure, and skin and behavioral changes [21, 22]. Although no reports have linked high doses of vitamin E during pregnancy to congenital anomalies, this complication has been demonstrated in animal studies [23].

Water-Soluble Vitamins

These vitamins, as the name implies, are soluble in water and are not stored in large amounts in the body as are the fat-soluble vitamins. This group of compounds includes ascorbic acid (vitamin C), thiamin (vitamin B_1), riboflavin (vitamin B_2), niacin, pyridoxine (vitamin B_6), folate, and cyanocobalamin (vitamin B_{12}).

Vitamin C. The RDA for **vitamin C** increases from 60 mg per day for nonpregnant adult women to 70 mg per day during pregnancy. This vitamin is essential as a cosubstrate in hydroxylations requiring molecular oxygen. The richest dietary sources of vitamin C include fruits and vegetables, particularly red and green peppers, collard greens, broccoli, spinach, tomatoes, potatoes, strawberries, oranges, grapefruit, and other citrus fruits. Data from the CSFII indicate that adult women have average dietary intakes of about 77 mg per day [3]. Large doses of vitamin C can cause the urine to become acidic, leading to the possible formation of kidney stones in susceptible individuals and interfering with urine tests for the presence of sugar [24, 25]. Other adverse effects of large doses of vitamin C include damage to the insulin-producing cells of the pancreas and altered absorption and metabolism of vitamin B_{12} [25, 26]. Cases of newborn scurvy (vitamin C deficiency) have been reported after prenatal ingestion of as little as 400 mg (less than six times the RDA for pregnancy) of vitamin C per day [27].

Thiamin. The RDA for **thiamin** during pregnancy is 36 percent above nonpregnant levels, increasing from 1.1 mg to 1.5 mg per day. The average dietary intake of thiamin among adult women is about 1.1 mg per day [3]. Thiamin, in the form of thiamin pyrophosphate, is a coenzyme required for the oxidative decarboxylation of alpha-keto acids and for the activity of transketolase in the pentose phosphate pathway. Dietary sources of thiamin include cereal grains, organ meats, pork, legumes, and seeds and nuts. Excessive amounts of thiamin have been reported to cause tachycardia and arrhythmias, but no congenital anomalies [28].

Riboflavin. Riboflavin is a water-soluble vitamin that functions primarily as a component of two coenzymes, flavin mononucleotide and flavin dinucleotide, which catalyze many oxidation-reduction reactions. The RDA for riboflavin increases by 23 percent during pregnancy, from 1.3 mg to 1.6 mg per day. Average dietary intake of riboflavin for adult women in the CSFII was 1.3 mg per day [3]. Dietary sources of riboflavin include meats, fish, poultry, dairy, and fortified grain products. Although no cases of toxicity have been reported, the safe use of high doses during pregnancy has not been established.

Niacin. Niacin is a water-soluble vitamin whose requirement is met in part by the conversion of dietary tryptophan to niacin. As a component of two enzymes, nicotinamide adenine dinucleotide (NAD) and nicotinamide adenine dinucleotide phosphate (NADP), niacin functions in many metabolic processes, including glycolysis, fatty acid metabolism, and tissue respiration. During pregnancy the RDA for niacin increases by 13 percent, from 15 mg to 17 mg. The average dietary intake of niacin of adult women in the CSFII was 16 mg per day [3]. Dietary sources of niacin include meats, nuts, and legumes. Intakes of 3 to 9 gm nicotinic acid per day result in a variety of adverse metabolic effects, including increased utilization of muscle glycogen, decreased serum lipids, and decreased mobilization of fatty acids from adipose tissue during exercise [29]. The effects of large doses of niacin during pregnancy are not known.

Vitamin B_6. Vitamin B_6, as pyridoxine, pyridoxal, and pyridoxamine, is converted in the liver, erythrocytes, and other tissues to pyridoxal phosphate (PL) and pyridoxamine phosphate (PMP). These latter compounds function as coenzymes in a variety of metabolic reactions, including transamination, decarboxylation, and other reactions with amino acids, nucleic acids, and lipids. The RDA for vitamin B_6 increases by 38 percent during pregnancy, from 1.6 mg to 2.2 mg. Average dietary intake among adult women in the CSFII was 16.1 mg [3]. Dietary sources of vitamin B_6 include poultry, fish, kidney, liver, pork, eggs, grains, and nuts. Toxic effects in adults have been reported with intakes of 7 to 10 times the RDA [30].

Folic Acid. Folic acid requirements increase more than those of any other nutrient during pregnancy, from 180 mcg to 400 mcg, or about 122 percent. Folic acid functions as a coenzyme in amino acid metabolism and nucleic acid synthesis, and this vitamin is vital to cell division and protein synthesis. Folic acid metabolism has been implicated in the occurrence of neural tube defects (see subsequent section). The average dietary intake of folic acid among adult women in the CSFII was 189 mcg [3]. Dietary sources of folic acid include liver, leafy vegetables, legumes, and fruits, although as much as half of the folic acid content of a food can be destroyed during preparation, processing, and storage. Large doses of folic acid have experimentally resulted in kidney damage and hypertrophy [31]. The effects of large doses of folic acid during pregnancy have not been established.

Vitamin B_{12}. **Vitamin B_{12}** includes the cobalt-containing substances cyanocobalamin, which is the commercially available form of vitamin B_{12}, and methylcobalamin, adenosylcobalamin, and hydroxocobalamin, which are present in plasma and tissues. During pregnancy the RDA for vitamin B_{12} increases by 10 percent, from 2.0 mcg to 2.2 mcg. Animal products are the primary dietary source of this vitamin. Supplemental vitamin B_{12} may be necessary for individuals (such as strict vegetarians) who consume diets that exclude all animal products, and for persons who lack intrinsic factor, such as after gastric surgery. No toxicity has been reported at high doses of this vitamin, but its safe and beneficial use in large amounts during pregnancy has yet to be determined.

Minerals

Calcium. **Calcium** requirements during pregnancy increase by 50 percent over nonpregnant levels, from 800 mg to 1200 mg per day. Adult women in the CSFII had an average dietary intake of only about 614 mg per day [3]. Calcium is essential for the process of skeletal formation and maintenance, as well as a factor in nerve conduction, muscle contraction, blood clotting, and membrane permeability. Calcium accretion during pregnancy totals approximately 30 gm, mostly in the fetal skeleton and deposited during the last trimester. Although calcium absorption increases and excretion decreases, additional dietary requirements are still needed to meet the demands of pregnancy. Calcium-deficient diets during gestation have been associated with decreased bone density in the newborn infant [32]. Dairy products contribute more than half of the calcium intake for the US population [33]. Other sources include green leafy vegetables (broccoli, kale, collards), calcium-precipitated tofu, calcium-fortified foods, and the soft bones of fish (cooked salmon and sardines). High calcium intakes may inhibit the absorption of iron, zinc, and other essential minerals, as well as result in hypercalciuria, hypercalcemia, and deterioration of renal function [34, 35].

The majority of the world's adult population is unable to digest unfermented dairy products due to low levels of the enzyme lactase [36–38]. Lactase is located in the brush border of the small intestine and is responsible for the hydrolysis of the disaccharide lactose, which is found exclusively in milk and milk products, into its component monosaccharides, glucose and galactose. Lactose, the main synergistic agent in milk, enhances the body's use of minerals and protein [39]. Lactose enhances animal protein absorption and utilization, and also improves the digestibility and utilization of vegetable proteins [39]. Inadequate dietary calcium and vitamin D result in biochemical changes tending toward osteomalacia in the mother and relative hypothyroidism in the infant [40, 41]. For these reasons, pregnant women with lactose intolerance should include ample amounts of low-lactose, high-calcium foods in their diets, such as aged cheeses or specially treated milks.

Phosphorus. **Phosphorus** is an essential component of bone mineral, as well as a factor in many metabolic reactions. Energy for metabolic processes is derived from the phosphate bonds of adenosine triphosphate (ATP). During pregnancy, the RDA for phosphorus increases by 50 percent to 1200 mg per day. The average phosphorus content of the diet of adult women in the CSFII was 966 mg [3]. Phosphorus is present in nearly all foods, with protein-rich foods (meats, milk, fish, poultry) and grains being the major sources. The toxic effects of excessive intakes of phosphorus during pregnancy are not known.

Magnesium. **Magnesium** is essential for all biosynthetic processes, glycolysis, formation of cyclic adenosine monophosphate (AMP), and energy-dependent membrane transport. During pregnancy the RDA for magnesium increases from 280 mg to 320 mg, about 14 percent. The diets of adult women contain, on the average, about 207 mg magnesium, or about 74 percent of the nonpregnant RDA. All unprocessed foods contain magnesium, with the highest concentration in whole seeds such as nuts, legumes, and unmilled grains [42]. More than 80 percent of magnesium is lost in processing through the removal of the germ and outer layers of cereal grains [43]. The effects of high doses of magnesium during pregnancy have not been documented, although large oral intakes may result in hypermagnesemia, with hypotension, electrocardiographic changes, and central nervous system depression [44]. Most cases of hypermagnesemia occur following the therapeutic use of magnesium-containing drugs.

Iron. The RDA for **iron** doubles during pregnancy, increasing from 15 mg to 30 mg per day. The average dietary iron content of adult women in the United States is about 10 mg, or about two thirds of the RDA [3]. As a constituent of hemoglobin, myoglobin, and a number of enzymes, iron is an essential nutrient for humans. The requirement for iron is greatest when there is rapid expansion of tissue and red cell mass, such as during infancy, childhood, and pregnancy. During pregnancy, iron needs average about 3.5 mg per day, and may reach 4 mg per day during the latter half of pregnancy. Total demands during a singleton pregnancy average 1000 to 1100 mg [45]. Iron absorption from food ranges from 1 percent with some vegetable sources to 10 to 25 percent with meats [46]. Nonanimal dietary sources of iron are also adversely affected by other dietary components, such as tea, calcium, phytates in wheat bran, and yolk phosphoprotein [47–51]. The RDA during pregnancy of 30 mg per day assumes a mixed diet (animal and vegetable sources of iron).

Zinc. **Zinc** is a vital component of enzymes involved in most major metabolic pathways. The RDA for zinc during pregnancy is 15 mg, an increase of 25 percent over the nonpregnant value of 12 mg. Data from the CSFII indicate that adult women have diets that average about 72 percent of the RDA for zinc, or about 8.6 mg [3]. About 70 percent of the zinc consumed in the US diet is provided by animal products, especially meats, whereas most of the zinc from plant sources is derived from cereals [52]. The highest bioavailability of zinc is in meats, liver, eggs, and seafood, particularly oysters, whereas grain products contain a less available form [8]. Symptoms of acute zinc toxicity have been reported with the ingestion of 2 gm or more of zinc sulfate [53]. Impaired copper status has been reported with moderately elevated intakes (18.5–25 mg/day) [54, 55]. Zinc supplementation at the level of 10 to 30 times the RDA has resulted in hypocupremia, microcytosis, neutropenia, impaired immune response, and altered lipoproteins [56–58].

Iodine. **Iodine**, as a component of the thyroid hormones thyroxine and triiodothyronine, is an essential nutrient. The RDA increases by 17 percent during pregnancy, from 150 mcg to 175 mcg. Low intakes of iodine in the United States are rare since the fortification of salt with this essential nutrient in 1924 [59]. The average dietary intake of iodine for adult women in the United States is about 170 μg per day [60]. Dietary sources of iodine include seafood, water, and iodized salt, which provides about 76 μg iodine per gram of salt [8]. Although intakes of up to 2 mg per day have not caused adverse reactions in healthy adults, the present dietary level of iodine in the US diet is considered adequate without the need for additional supplementation [8].

Selenium. **Selenium** is an important component of the enzyme glutathione peroxidase, which catalyzes the breakdown of hydroperoxides. Selenium functions in close metabolic relationship with vitamin E as an antioxidant. The RDA for selenium increases 18 percent from 55 μg to 65 μg during pregnancy. The average dietary intake for adults in the United States is 108 μg per day [61]. Good dietary sources of selenium include seafood, kidney, liver, and meats; grains and other seeds contain more variable amounts of selenium, depending on the content of the soil [62]. Selenium toxicity has been reported with daily intakes as small as 1 mg per day [8].

Use of Vitamin-Mineral Supplements

Data from national surveys indicate that the vast majority of Americans, including one half to two thirds of women of childbearing age, consume some form of vitamin-mineral supplements [3, 63–65] (Fig. 5-1). Data from the National Health Interview Survey show that vitamin-mineral use varies by gender, race, education, and income, with more females than males and more whites than blacks using supplements; use also increases with education and income [65]. These practices are in contrast with the advice currently provided from organizations of health professionals, which generally have urged consumers to obtain nutrients from a balanced and varied diet rather than through supplementation. For instance, in 1987, a task force, which included representatives from the American Dietetic Association, the Society for Nutrition Education, the American Society for Clinical Nutrition, the American Institute of Nutrition, and the American Medical Association, issued the following statement regarding use of vitamin and mineral supplements [66]:

> Healthy children and adults should obtain adequate nutrient intakes from dietary sources. Meeting nutrient needs by choosing a variety of foods in moderation, rather than by supplementation, reduces the potential risk for both nutrient deficiencies and nutrient excesses. Individual recommendations regarding supplements and diets should come from physicians and registered dietitians . . . Nutrients are potentially toxic when ingested in sufficiently large amounts. Safe intake levels vary widely from nutrient to nutrient and may vary with the age and health of the individual. In addition, high dosage vitamin and mineral supplements can interfere with the normal metabolism of other nutrients and with the therapeutic effects of certain drugs. The Recommended Dietary Allowances represent the best currently available assessment of safe and adequate intakes . . . and there are no demonstrated benefits of self supplementation beyond these allowances.

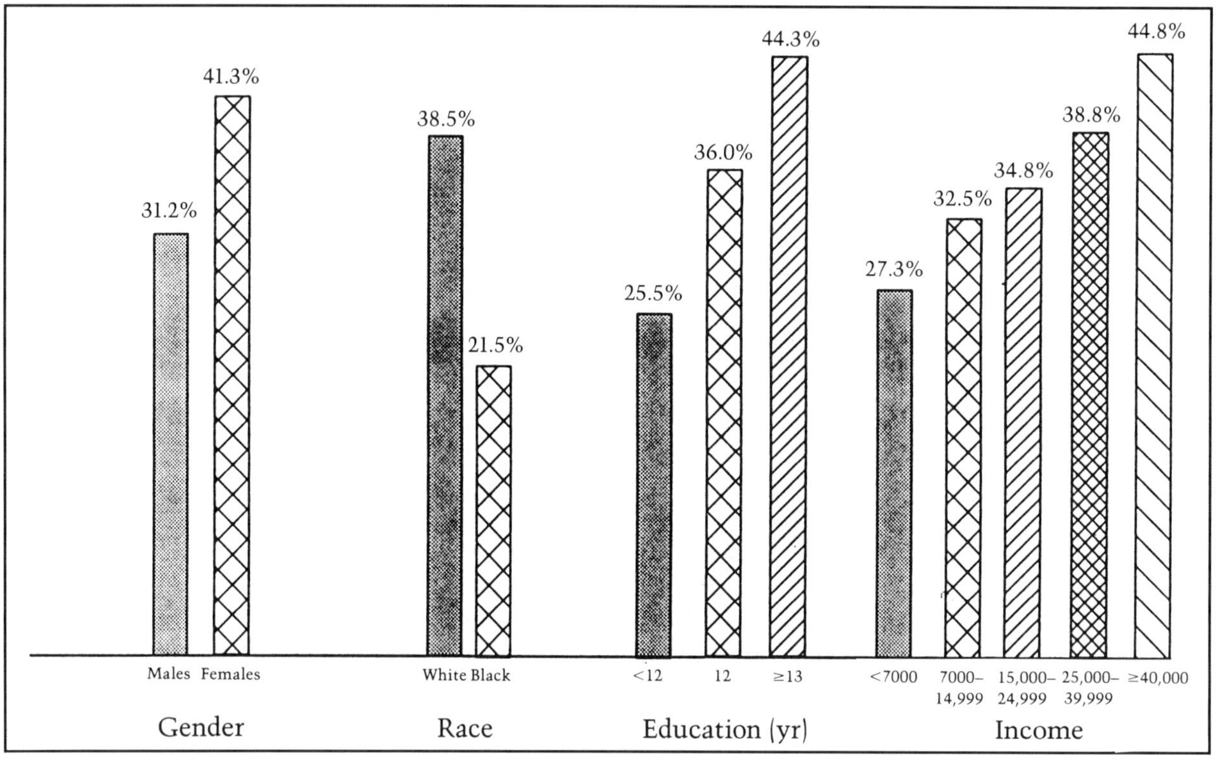

Fig. 5-1
Use of vitamin-mineral supplements by gender, race, education, and income, United States, 1986. Based on data from the National Health Interview Survey.

During recent years the use of vitamins and minerals during the periconceptional period (1–3 months before conception to 6 weeks of gestation) has attracted widespread public health interest because of its possible association with neural tube defects in the fetus.

Vitamin and Mineral Supplements and Neural Tube Defects

Neural tube defects (NTDs) include the congenital anomalies of spina bifida, anencephaly, and encephalocele. Spina bifida is a collective term for various conditions associated with incomplete closure of the spine, which in turn causes permanent damage to the spinal cord and spinal nerves [67]. Anencephaly is a lethal malformation characterized by absence of the cranial vault and cerebral hemispheres [67]. Encephalocele is a defect in the skull that results in herniation of the meninges and brain tissue [67]. Each year approximately 400,000 children with NTDs are born worldwide, including 4000 in the United States [68]. The risk of occurrence of NTD is 2 to 3 percent; the chance of a woman having a second affected child is much higher.

Neural tube defects are thought to occur as a result of an interaction between genetics and the prenatal environment. The genetic component, which may involve several genes, is not well understood. Epidemiologic, clinical, and experimental evidence has strongly implicated an environmental component. Within the environmental aspect, micronutrient metabolism during the periconception period has emerged as central to this issue, and some investigators have recommended universal periconceptional vitamin supplementation for all women of childbearing age to reduce the risk of NTDs [69, 70]. Most researchers, however, have been more cautious about interpreting present studies.

Folate is the single nutrient most strongly implicated in studies of NTDs. According to dietary data from the Second National Health and Nutrition Examination Survey conducted from 1976 to 1980 on a nationally representative sample of the US population, folate intake in the United States is low, particularly among women and blacks [71]. This study reported that approximately 50 percent of both men and women consumed less than their requirements on any given day and suggested that improvement in folate intake was needed across all age, sex, and racial groups. Studies such as the Hispanic Health and Nutrition Examination Survey have found that the prevalence of low serum folate concentrations was significantly reduced among users of vitamin supplements [72].

Animal data indicate that NTDs can result from altered folate metabolism. For example, the use of the anticonvulsant drug valproic acid during pregnancy results in a 20-fold excess risk of NTDs [73, 74]. Valproic acid impairs the activity of the enzyme that catalyzes the transformation of folic acid to its active form [75]. Data from clinical studies suggest that maternal folate metabolism may be abnormal in women who give birth to infants with NTDs, although reports are conflicting. Lower red cell folate levels [76, 77], but not serum folate levels [77, 78], were reported in women with affected infants compared to control subjects. These findings suggest that NTDs may be associated with altered folate metabolism, but not necessarily a lower dietary intake of folate.

During the past decade several large studies have attempted to clarify the role of the periconceptional use of folate in reducing the risk of NTDs. Laurence and associates [79] reported the results of a double-blind, randomized controlled trial of folate supplementation before conception and during pregnancy in southern Wales. This study was conducted with 111 women, all of whom had previously given birth to a child with an NTD. The authors reported that none of the 44 women who received folate supplementation had a recurrence, whereas 6 women among the 67 untreated cases had recurrences. The result of studies on two cohorts of women with a previous infant with an NTD was reported by Smithells and colleagues as part of the United Kingdom Multicenter Trial [80]. The recurrence rate was sevenfold higher among the nonsupplemented group (4.8%) compared to the supplemented group (0.7%). Although the results of this study are striking, its findings have been questioned because of the lack of appropriate controls [81].

In 1988, Mulinare and associates [82] reported the results of the Centers for Disease Control population-based case-control study, which retrospectively evaluated multivitamin intake. Periconceptional multivitamin use exerted a protective effect on the occurrence of NTDs, with a crude estimated relative risk of 0.40. An Australian population-based case-control study that evaluated dietary folate intake retrospectively also reported a protective effect of an increasing intake of dietary folate in the first 6 weeks of pregnancy on the prevalence of NTDs [83]. In contrast, the population-based case-control study by Mills and colleagues [84] found no evidence of a protective effect from the use of multivitamin supplementation during the periconceptional period.

The prospective cohort study by Milunsky and associates [85] reported that the prevalence of NTDs was 3.5 per 1000 live births among women who never used multivitamins before or after conception, or among those who used multivitamins before conception only, compared to 0.9 per 1000 live births for women who used folic acid–containing multivitamins during the first 6 weeks of pregnancy. For women who used multivitamins containing folic acid beginning at 7 weeks of gestation or later, the prevalences were similar to those of the nonusers.

The most recent study, which began in July 1983 and was halted in April 1991, was conducted by the British Medical Research Council (MRC) Vitamin Study Group [86]. This project, which involved 33 centers, including 17 in the United Kingdom and 16 in six other nations, studied women who had had a previous pregnancy that resulted in an infant or fetus with an NTD and who were planning a subsequent pregnancy. Each participant was randomly assigned to one of four supplementation groups: (A) 4 mg folic acid, (B) multivitamin plus 4 mg folic acid, (C) neither a multivitamin nor folic acid, and (D) multivitamin without folic acid. All capsules (including those used for placebo group C) contained ferrous sulfate and dicalcium phosphate. To test the effect of folic acid supplementation, the MRC study group compared the outcomes of groups A and B with groups C and D. To test the effect of the multivitamin preparation, the MRC study group compared the outcomes in groups B and D with those in groups A and C. NTDs recurred in 6 (1.0%) of 593 infants or fetuses of women who received folic acid (2 of 298 in group A and 4 of 295 in group B) compared with 21 (3.5%) of 602 women who did not receive folic acid (13 of 300 in group C and 8 of 302 in group D). Thus, oral supplementation with folic acid was associated with a 71 percent reduction in the recurrence of NTDs. The use of multivitamins without folic acid was not associated with a similar protective effect. NTDs recurred in 12 (2.0%) of 597 infants or fetuses of women who received multivitamins (groups B and D) compared with 15 (2.5%) of 598 women who did not receive multivitamins (groups A and C). Because of the substantial protective effect of folic acid supplementation, the MRC study group halted the study early so that all women at risk could receive the potential benefits of supplementation.

Based on these and other findings, the Centers for Disease Control recommended in August 1991 that women who have had a previous pregnancy that resulted in an infant or fetus with an NTD be given 4 mg folic acid (as a separate supplement, not as part of a multivitamin) beginning at least 4 weeks before conception and through the first 3 months of pregnancy [68]. However, the Centers for Disease Control cautioned that this dose of folic acid is 10 times the pregnancy RDA and 20 times the nonpregnant RDA for folic acid. The use of folic acid at this dosage may complicate the diagnosis of vitamin B_{12} deficiency because it may mask megaloblastic anemia while neurologic manifestations progress. In September 1992 the Centers for Disease Control recommended that women of childbearing age in the United States, who are capable of becoming pregnant, consume 0.4 mg of folic acid per day to reduce the risk of NTD [87].

Conclusions and Recommendations

An adequate and balanced prenatal diet is central to fetal growth and development, as well as the health and vitality of the mother. This diet is best obtained through the judicious choice of nourishing foods in quantities appropriate for the individual woman's caloric needs. Nutrients from dietary sources have the greatest bioavailability, and, therefore, vitamin and mineral supplements are not recommended. An exception to this rule is in women who have had a previous pregnancy in which the infant or fetus had an NTD. These women should take 4 mg folic acid, as a single supplement and not as part of a multivitamin, from 4 weeks before conception through the first 3 months of pregnancy.

References

1. Food and Nutrition Board, National Academy of Sciences: *Recommended Dietary Allowances*. Washington, DC: National Academy Press, 1943.
2. Monsen, ER: The 10th edition of the Recommended Dietary Allowances: What's new in the 1989 RDAs? *J. Am. Diet. Assoc.* 89:1748–1752, 1989.
3. US Dept. of Agriculture, Human Nutrition Information Service, Nutrition Monitoring Division: *Nationwide Food Consumption Survey, Continuing Survey of Food Intakes by Individuals*. Report No. 85-4. Hyattsville, MD: U.S. Govt. Printing Office, 1987. Pp. 46–49.
4. Durnin, JVGA: Energy requirements of pregnancy: An integration of the longitudinal data from the five-country study. *Lancet* 2:1131–1133, 1987.
5. Van Raaji, JMA, Schonk, CM, Vermaat-Miedema, SH, et al: Body fat mass and basal metabolic rate in Dutch women before, during, and after pregnancy: A reappraisal of energy cost of pregnancy. *Am. J. Clin. Nutr.* 49:765–772, 1989.
6. World Health Organization: Energy and Protein Requirements. Report of a Joint FAO/WHO/UNU Expert Consultation. Technical Report Series No. 724. Geneva, Switzerland: World Health Organization, 1985. 206 pp.
7. Forsum, E, Sadurkis, A, and Wagner, J: Resting metabolic rate and body composition of healthy Swedish women during pregnancy. *Am. J. Clin. Nutr.* 47:942–947, 1988.
8. Food and Nutrition Board, National Academy of Sciences: *Recommended Dietary Allowances* (10th ed.). Washington, DC: National Academy Press, 1989.
9. Food and Nutrition Board, National Academy of Sciences: *Nutrition During Pregnancy*. Washington, DC: National Academy Press, 1990.
10. Bauernfeind, JC: Carotenoid vitamin A precursors and analogs in foods and feeds. *J. Agric. Food. Chem.* 20:456–473, 1972.
11. Lammer, EJ, Chen, DT, Hoar, RM, et al: Retinoic acid embryopathy. *N. Engl. J. Med.* 313:837–841, 1985.
12. Costas, K, Davis, R, Kim, N, et al: Use of supplements containing high-dose vitamin A—New York State 1983–1984. *J.A.M.A.* 257:1292–1297, 1987.
13. Miller, RK, Brown, K, Cordero, J, et al: Position paper by the Teratology Society: Vitamin A during pregnancy. *Teratology* 35:267–275, 1987.
14. Stange, L, Carlstrom, K, and Erickson, M: Hypervitaminosis A in early human pregnancy and malformations of the central nervous system. *Acta Obstet. Gynecol. Scand.* 57:289–291, 1978.

15. American Academy of Pediatrics: The prophylactic requirement and toxicity of vitamin D. *Pediatrics* 31:512–525, 1963.
16. Dalerup, IM, Stockman, VA, Rechsteiner de Vos, H, et al: Survey on coronary heart disease in relation to diet in physically active farmers. *Voeding* 26:245, 1965.
17. Dalderup, IM: Vitamin D, cholesterol, and calcium. *Lancet* 1:645, 1968.
18. Seelig, MS: Vitamin D and cardiovascular, renal, and brain damage in infancy and childhood. *Ann. N. Y. Acad. Sci.* 147:537, 1969.
19. Taussig, HB: Possible injury to the cardiovascular system from vitamin D. *Ann. Intern. Med.* 65:1195, 1966.
20. Finer, N, Grant, G, Schindler, R, et al: Effect of intramuscular vitamin E on frequency and severity of retrolental fibroplasia. *Lancet* 1:1087, 1982.
21. Roberts, H: Perspective on vitamin A as therapy. *J.A.M.A.* 246:129, 1981.
22. Hook, E, Healy, K, Niles, A, et al: Vitamin E: Teratogen or anti-teratogen? *Lancet* 1:809, 1974.
23. Bencze, B, Ugrai, E, Gerloczy, F, et al: The effect of tocopherol on the embryonal development. *Int. J. Vit. Res.* 44:180, 1974.
24. Ringsdorf, W, and Cheraskin, E: Nutritional aspects of urolithiasis. *South. Med. J.* 74:41, 1981.
25. Toxicity of vitamin C megadose. *Nutrition and the MD,* Vol. 6, no. 10, 1980.
26. Herbert, V, and Jacobs, F: Destruction of B-12 by ascorbic acid. *J.A.M.A.* 230:241, 1974.
27. Cochrane, WA: Overnutrition in prenatal and neonatal life: A problem? *Can. Med. Assoc. J.* 93:893, 1965.
28. Effects of excesses of thiamine and pyridoxine. *Nutr. Rev.* 18:95, 1960.
29. Darby, WJ, McNutt, KW, and Todhunter, EN: Niacin. *Nutr. Rev.* 33:289–297, 1975.
30. Dalton, K, and Dalton, MJT: Characteristics of pyridoxine overdose neuropathy syndrome. *Acta Neurol. Scand.* 76:8–11, 1987.
31. Colman, N, and Herbert, V: Dietary Assessments with Special Emphasis on Prevention of Folate Deficiency. In MI Botez and EH Reynolds (eds.) *Folic Acid in Neurology, Psychiatry, and Internal Medicine.* New York: Raven, 1979. Pp. 23–33.
32. Krishnamachari, KAVR, and Iyengar, L: Effect of maternal malnutrition on the bone density of the neonates. *Am. J. Clin. Nutr.* 28:482, 1975.
33. Block, G, Dresser, CM, Hartman, AM, and Carroll, MD: Nutrient sources in the American diet: Quantitative data from the NHANES II survey. Vitamins and minerals. *Am. J. Epidemiol.* 122:13–26, 1985.
34. Gregor, JL: Effect of Variations in Dietary Protein, Phosphorus, Electrolytes, and Vitamin D on Calcium and Zinc Metabolism. In CE Bodwell and JW Erdman, Jr. (eds.) *Nutrient Interactions.* New York: Marcel Dekker, 1988. Pp. 205–227.

35. Avioli, LV: Calcium and Phosphorus. In ME Shils and VR Young (eds.), *Modern Nutrition in Health and Disease* (7th ed.). Philadelphia: Lea & Febiger, 1988. Pp. 142–158.
36. Bayless, TM, et al: Lactose intolerance and milk drinking habits. *Gastroenterology* 60:605, 1971.
37. McCracken, RD: Lactase deficiency: An example of dietary evolution. *Curr. Anthropol.* 12:479, 1971.
38. Simoons, FJ: New light on ethnic differences in adult lactose intolerance. *Am. J. Digest. Dis.* 18:595, 1972.
39. Sewell, RF, and West, JP: Some effects of lactose on protein utilization in the baby pig. *J. Animal Sci.* 24:239, 1965.
40. Watney, RJ, and Rudd, BT: Calcium metabolism in pregnancy and in the newborn. *J. Obstet. Gynecol. Br. Commonwlth.* 81:210, 1974.
41. Liu, SH, et al: Calcium and phosphorus metabolism in osteomalacia: XI. The pathogenetic role of pregnancy and relative importance of calcium and vitamin D supply. *J. Clin. Invest.* 20:255, 1941.
42. Seelig, MS: The requirement of magnesium by the normal adult. *Am. J. Clin. Nutr.* 14:342–390, 1964.
43. Marier, JR: Magnesium content of the food supply in the modern-day world. *Magnesium* 5:1–8, 1986.
44. Mordes, JP, and Wacker, WE: Excess magnesium. *Pharmacol. Rev.* 29:273–300, 1978.
45. Jacobs, A: Transferrin and Transferrin Iron. In A Jacobs and M Worwood (eds.), *Iron in Biochemistry and Medicine*. London: Academic, 1974.
46. World Health Organization: *Nutritional Anaemias: Report of a WHO Scientific Group*. WHO Technical Report Series No. 405, Geneva, Switzerland, 1968.
47. Bjorn-Rausmussen, E: Iron absorption from wheat bread: Influence of various amounts of bran. *Nutr. Metab.* 16:107, 1974.
48. Callender, ST, et al: Eggs and iron absorption. *Br. J. Haematol.* 19:657, 1970.
49. Conrad, ME: Factors Affecting Iron Absorption. In L Hallberg, HG Harwerth, and A Vannotti (eds.), *Iron Deficiency*. London: Academic, 1970. Pp. 87–120.
50. Turnbull, A: Iron Absorption. In A Jacobs and M Worwood (eds.), *Iron in Biochemistry and Medicine*. London: Academic, 1974. Pp. 369–403.
51. Disler, PB, et al: The effect of tea on iron absorption. *Gut* 16:193, 1975.
52. Welsh, SO, and Marston, RM: Zinc levels of the U.S. food supply: 1909–1980. *Food Technology* 36:70–76, 1982.
53. Prasad, AS: Deficiency of zinc in man and its toxicity. In AS Prasad (ed.): *Trace Elements in Health and Disease*, Vol. 1, *Zinc and Copper*. New York: Academic, 1976. Pp. 1–20.
54. Festa, MD, Anderson, HL, Dowdy, RP, and Ellersieck, MR: Effect of zinc intake on copper excretion and retention in men. *Am. J. Clin. Nutr.* 41:285–292, 1985.

55. Fischer, PWF, Giroux, A, and Abbe, MR: Effect of zinc supplementation on copper status in adult man. *Am. J. Clin. Nutr.* 40:743–746, 1984.
56. Prasad, AS, Brewer, GJ, Schoomaker, EB, and Rabbani, P: Hypocupremia induced by zinc therapy in adults. *J.A.M.A.* 240:2166–2168, 1978.
57. Chandra, RK: Excessive intake of zinc impairs immune responses. *J.A.M.A.* 252:1443–1446, 1984.
58. Hooper, PL, Visconti, L, Garry, PJ, and Johnson, GE: Zinc lowers high-density lipoprotein cholesterol levels. *J.A.M.A.* 244:1960–1961, 1980.
59. Brush, BE, and Atland, JK: Goiter prevention with iodized salt: Results of a thirty-year study. *J. Clin. Endocrinol. Metab.* 12:1380–1388, 1952.
60. Pennington, JAT, Young, BE, and Wilson, DB: Nutritional elements in U.S. diets: Results from the Total Diet Study, 1982 to 1986. *J. Am. Diet. Assoc.* 89:659–664, 1989.
61. Pennington, JAT, Wilson, RF, Harland, BF, et al: Selected minerals in foods surveys, 1974 to 1981/82. *J. Am. Diet. Assoc.* 84:771–780, 1984.
62. World Health Organization: *Selenium: Environmental Health Criteria #58: Report of the International Programme on Chemical Safety*. Geneva: World Health Organization, 1987.
63. Block, G, Cox, C, Madans, J, et al: Vitamin supplement use by demographic characteristics. *Am. J. Epidemiol.* 127:297–309, 1988.
64. Koplan, JP, Annest, JL, Layde, PM, and Rubin, GL: Nutrient intake and supplementation in the United States (NHANES II). *Am. J. Public Health* 76:287–289, 1986.
65. National Center for Health Statistics: *Advance Data from Vital and Health Statistics*. No. 174., 1987.
66. American Dietetic Association: Recommendations concerning supplement usage: ADA statement. *J. Am. Diet. Assoc.* 87:1342–1343, 1987.
67. International Clearinghouse for Birth Defects Monitoring Systems: *Congenital Malformations Worldwide: A Report from the International Clearinghouse for Birth Defects Monitoring Systems*. Amsterdam: Elsevier, 1991. Pp. 41–51.
68. Use of folic acid for prevention of spina bifida and other neural tube defects—1983–1991. *Morbid. Mortal. Weekly Rep.* 40:513–516, 1991.
69. International Conference on Prepregnancy Nutrition. White Plains, NY: March of Dimes Birth Defects Foundation, 1987.
70. Holmes, LB: Does taking vitamins at the time of conception prevent neural tube defects? *J.A.M.A.* 260:3181, 1988.
71. Subar, AF, Block, G, and James, LD: Folate intake and food sources in the U.S. population. *Am. J. Clin. Nutr.* 50:508–516, 1989.
72. Fanelli-Kuczmarski, MT, Johnson, CL, et al: Folate status of Mexican American, Cuban, and Puerto Rican women. *Am. J. Clin. Nutr.* 52:368–372, 1990.

73. Lammer, EJ, Sever, LE, and Oakley, GP: Teratogen update: Valproic acid. *Teratology* 35:465–473, 1987.
74. Trotz, M, Wegner, C, and Nau, H: Valproic acid–induced neural tube defects: Reduction by folinic acid in the mouse. *Life Sci.* 41:103–110, 1987.
75. Wegner, CHR, and Nau, H: Valproic acid–induced neural tube defects: Disturbance of the folate metabolism in day 9 mouse embryo. *Teratology* 39:488, 1989.
76. Smithells, RW, Sheppard, S, and Schorah, CJ: Vitamin deficiencies and neural tube defects. *Arch. Dis. Child.* 51:944–950, 1976.
77. Yates, JRW, Ferguson-Smith, MA, Shenkin, A, et al: Is disordered folate metabolism the basis for the genetic predisposition to neural tube defects? *Clin. Genet.* 31:279–287, 1987.
78. Molloy, AM, Kirke, P, Hillary, I, et al: Maternal serum folate and vitamin B-12 concentrations in pregnancies associated with neural tube defects. *Arch. Dis. Child.* 60:660–665, 1985.
79. Laurence, KM, James, N, Miller, MH, et al: Double-blind randomized controlled trial of folate treatment before conception to prevent recurrence of neural-tube defects. *Br. Med. J.* 282:1509–1511, 1981.
80. Smithells, RW, Nevin, NC, Seller, MJ, et al: Further experience of vitamin supplementation for prevention of neural tube defect recurrences. *Lancet* 1:1027–1031, 1983.
81. Wald, NJ, and Polani, PE: Neural-tube defects and vitamins: The need for a randomized clinical trial. *Br. J. Obstet. Gynaecol.* 91:516–523, 1984.
82. Mulinare, J, Cordero, JF, Erickson, JD, and Berry, RJ: Periconceptional use of multivitamins and the occurrence of neural tube defects. *J.A.M.A.* 260:3141–3145, 1988.
83. Bower, C, and Stanley, FJ: Dietary folate as a risk factor for neural-tube defects: Evidence from a case-control study in Western Australia. *Med. J. Aust.* 150:613–619, 1989.
84. Mills, JL, Rhoads, GG, Simpson, JL, et al: The absence of a relationship between the periconceptional use of vitamins and neural-tube defects. *N. Engl. J. Med.* 321:430–435, 1989.
85. Milunsky, A, Jick, H, Jick, SS, et al: Multivitamin/folic acid supplementation in early pregnancy reduces the prevalence of neural tube defects. *J.A.M.A.* 262:2847–2852, 1989.
86. Medical Research Council Vitamin Study Research Group: Prevention of neural tube defects: Results of the Medical Research Council Vitamin Study. *Lancet* 338:131–137, 1991.
87. Centers for Disease Control: Recommendations for the use of folic acid to reduce the number of cases of spina bifida and other neural tube defects. *MMWR 1992.* 41:RR-14. Pp. 1–7.

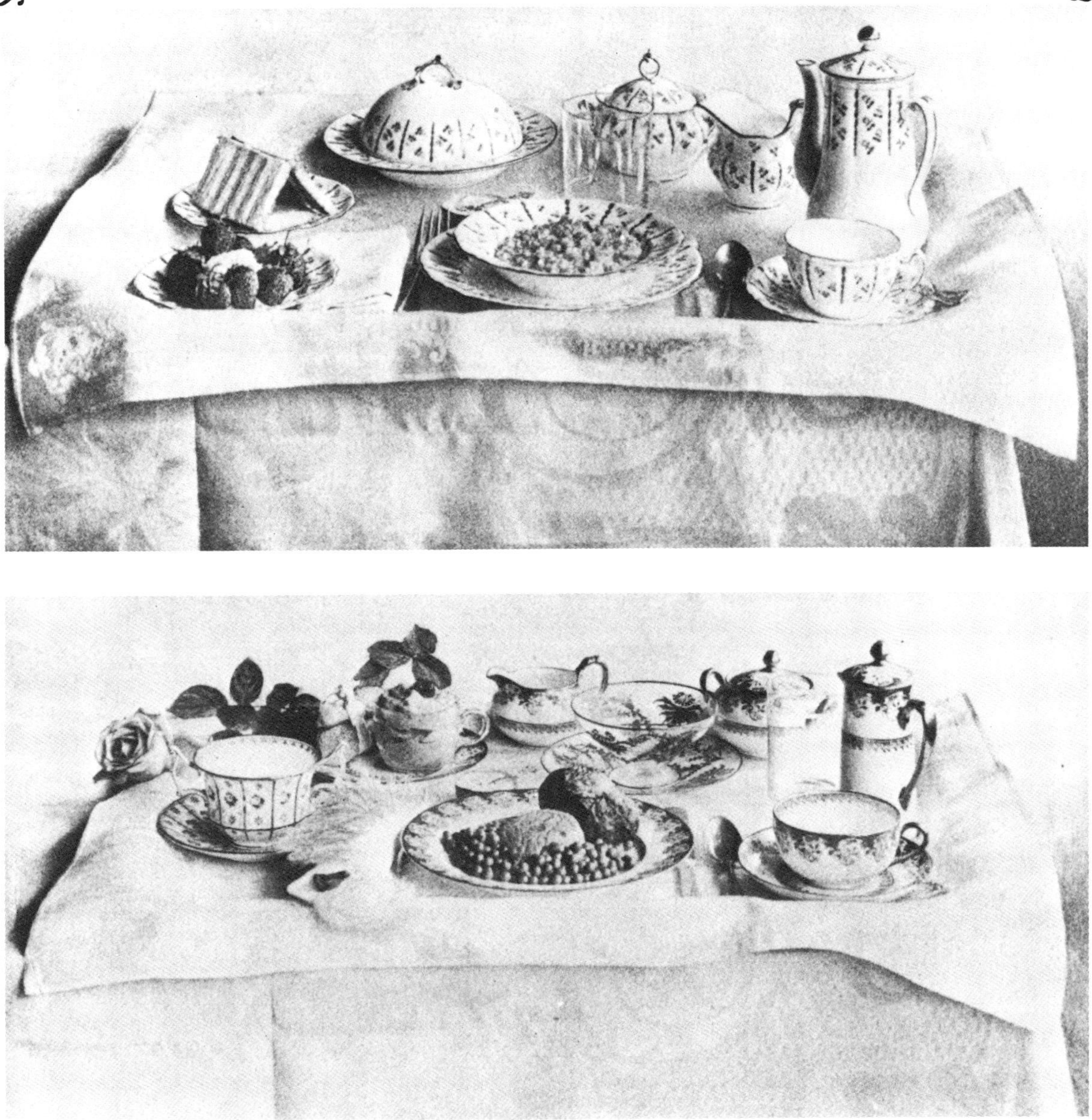

Breakfast and dinner for the convalescent. (From Fannie Farmer. *Food and Cookery for the Sick and Convalescent*. Boston: Little, Brown and Company, 1905.)

Illustration from 19th-century health and physiology guide. (From C. Audureau. *Étude sur l'Obstétrique en occident*. Dijon: Imprimerie Darantiere, 1892.)

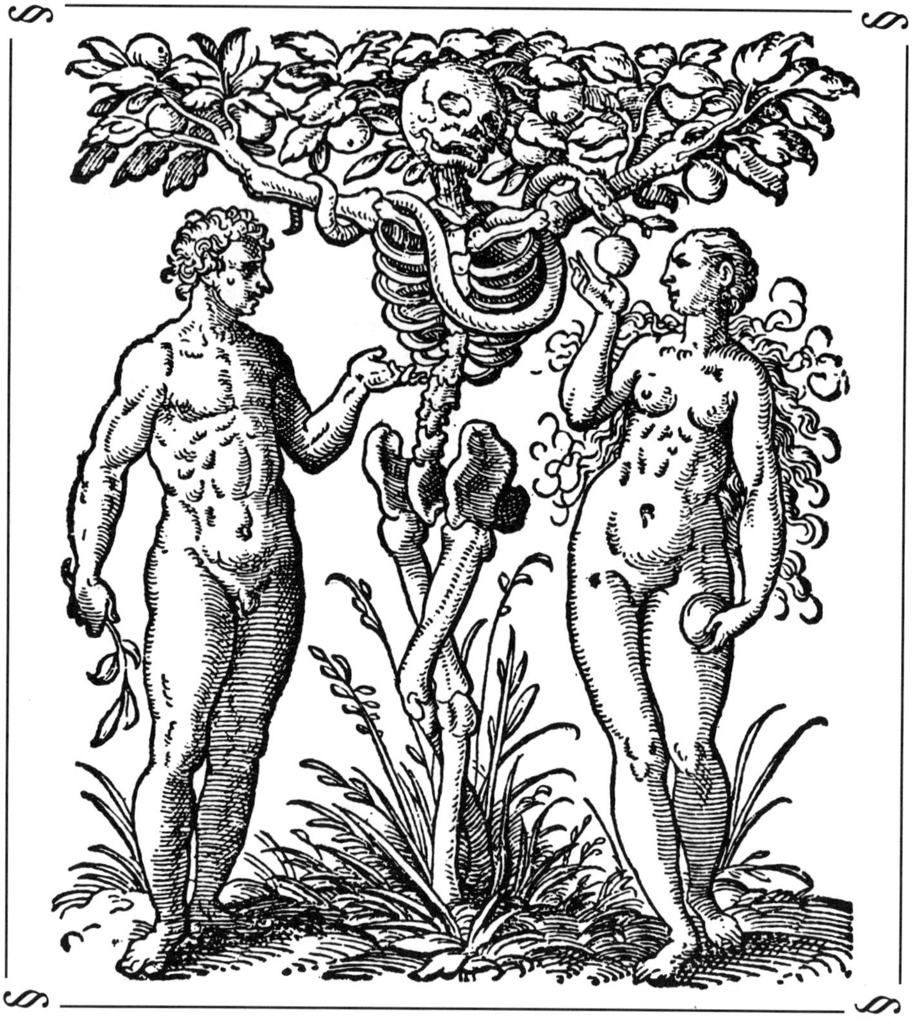

6

Bone Health and Calcium Metabolism

Calcium is one of the most plentiful and important minerals in the body. Nearly all of calcium is stored in the skeletal system, where it acts as both a structural component and a ready reserve to maintain the plasma calcium levels. During pregnancy calcium metabolism changes, facilitating dietary absorption and, across a concentration gradient, transfer from mother to fetus for ossification of fetal bones. This chapter presents a review of the literature pertaining to bone health in women, calcium absorption and metabolism, and metabolic demands during pregnancy. New research on the effect of calcium supplementation in preventing preterm birth and preeclampsia is also presented, and sources of dietary calcium and calcium supplements are discussed.

Bone Health

Bone is composed of a collagen-rich organic matrix impregnated with minerals, predominately calcium and phosphorus. The two major types of bone are cortical bone, which forms the external envelopes of the skeleton, and trabecular or medullary bone, which forms plates that traverse the internal cavities of the skeleton. The relative composition of bone depends on its site. For example, the bones in the vertebral column are composed mostly of trabecular bone, whereas the proximal femur contains mostly cortical bone. The two types of bone respond differently to metabolic influences and have different susceptibility to fracture. Trabecular bone has a much higher metabolic rate. Bone undergoes continuous remodeling or turnover throughout life. Osteoclasts resorb bone in microscopic cavities; osteoblasts then reform the bone surface, filling in the cavities. Although the processes of resorption and formation occur simultaneously, they are influenced by genetics, diet, hormones, physical activity, medications, and stage in the life cycle (Table 6-1).

During childhood and adolescence, more calcium is absorbed than is resorbed, resulting in a net growth of bone in both length and width. The degree of bone maturity at menarche (the onset of menses) may have important implications for the pregnant adolescent. Peak height velocity, which usually precedes menarche [1], is observed in girls at about age 12 compared to age 13.5 in boys. A moderately high correlation exists between age at menarche and skeletal maturity, with reduced variance in skeletal ages at the time of menarche [2, 3]. As discussed in Chaps. 2 and 5, the time interval from the first signs of puberty to complete maturity varies as much as 1.5 to 6.0 years [1], with the onset of menarche occurring toward the beginning of

Table 6-1
Factors influencing bone health

Positively associated with bone loss	*Negatively associated with bone loss*
Low dietary calcium intake	High dietary calcium intake
Alcohol use	
Cigarette smoking	
Immobility	Moderate physical activity
Hypoestrogenism	Normal estrogen levels (including postmenopausal supplementation)
Asian or white race	Black race
	Thiazide diuretic use

puberty in early-maturing girls and toward the end in late-maturing girls. As early-maturing girls approach maturity, their growth slows down and stops at an age when late-maturing girls are still growing fairly rapidly [4]. At the same skeletal age, early-maturing girls tend to be smaller than their late-maturing counterparts, and as adults these individuals remain shorter in stature. The skeletal age of early-maturing girls is significantly lower than that of late-maturing girls [4, 5].

By menarche, late-maturing girls have attained more linear and pelvic growth, and have about half as much growth remaining to complete before reaching maturity as early-maturing girls. Pregnancy in early-maturing girls of young chronologic age is associated with increased incidence of pelvic inlet contraction, cephalopelvic disproportion, forceps delivery, and cesarean section [6, 7]. Adolescence is therefore a critical period, during which inadequate calcium intake is detrimental to skeletal maturation [8, 9].

The concept of **peak bone mass**, the amount of bone present before age-related loss begins, is of vital importance in women's health. Bone mass increases during childhood, adolescence, and young adulthood. Even after closure of the epiphyseal plates, bone mass continues to increase by radial growth until about age 30, although some studies have shown continued increase midway through the fourth decade [10, 11]. The onset of age-related bone loss during the decade preceding menopause is a universal phenomenon in nearly all populations, although this loss is modified by numerous factors [12, 13]. Bone loss indicative of osteoporosis generally begins during the fourth decade, and the rate of loss is greater in females than in males [14]. Peak bone mass is important, therefore, because insufficient accumulation of skeletal mass by young adulthood predisposes a woman to fractures later in life as age-related bone loss occurs [15]. Over their lifetimes, women lose about 35 percent of their cortical bone and about 50 percent of their trabecular bone, whereas men lose only about two thirds of these amounts. A biphasic pattern of bone loss occurs for both types of bone: A protracted slow initial phase for both sexes is followed by a transient accelerated phase for women after menopause.

Many factors influence an individual's peak bone mass, including gender, race, diet, smoking and drinking habits, and exercise. During their adult life, women lose twice as much bone mass as men [12]. This is due to a combination of a lower peak bone mass and a more rapid rate of age-related loss. Over a 30-year period, women lose about 750 gm of their 3000-gm skeleton, whereas men lose 450 gm of their 4000-gm skeleton [12].

Race and Gender

Race and gender differences in bone density are present even at birth. Although blacks are generally smaller than whites as newborns, by age two they average greater height and weight [16, 17]. Through childhood and as young adults, blacks of each sex exceed whites in cortical bone mass by about 10 percent [18, 19]. Moreover, blacks also have significantly higher calcium, potassium, inorganic phosphate, sodium, and chloride than age- and gender-matched whites [20]. Total body calcium, as measured by neutron-activation analysis [20], is 22 percent higher for adult black men than adult white men and 17 percent higher for adult black women compared to adult white women. Potassium, a measure of total cellular mass, particularly muscle, is higher in blacks. This larger muscle mass in black women may in part be a determinant of greater skeletal mass, and may therefore be partially responsible for the greater resistance of black women to osteoporosis and fracture [20]. Blacks also have a lower mean rate of bone turnover, about one third that of whites [21]. Furthermore, blacks have a greater resistance to the bone-resorptive effects of parathyroid hormone and 1,25-dihydroxyvitamin D_3, allowing greater accumulation of bone during growth and lower loss during aging [22].

The bone densities of other racial and ethnic groups have also been evaluated, although not as extensively as for the black population. Chinese, Japanese, and Mexican-Americans all have been reported to have a lower cortical bone mass than whites, and far lower than blacks [23, 24].

Genetics

Studies of mother-daughter pairs provide insight regarding the relative influence of genetics versus environment on bone health [25,

26]. Women with osteoporosis have a lower bone mass, which is not only due to excessive bone loss, but results from a combination of the attainment of a lower peak bone mass in their 30s, followed by age-related bone loss [25]. Their premenopausal daughters are more likely to develop osteoporosis themselves, because they, too, have a relatively low bone mass [25]. The inheritance of bone mass in women may have at least two components, one influencing the level of peak bone mass and the other related to the rate of bone loss after menopause [26].

Diet

Dietary calcium intake is significantly associated with peak bone mass, and is most effective in the years of growth and development. In a study of two Yugoslavian districts with a twofold difference in calcium intake, Matkovic and associates [8] reported a lower metacarpal density and higher incidence of hip fractures among residents in the district with lower calcium intakes. These differences were apparent during young adulthood, but the groups did not diverge with aging, suggesting that the major effect of dietary calcium was on peak bone mass. Among adult women, recent research [27] has indicated no relationship between dietary calcium intake and bone mineral density of the lumbar vertebrae. Moreover, in the later years, calcium supplementation is not as effective as is estrogen in slowing bone loss; it has a minor effect on cortical bone and no effect on trabecular bone in postmenopausal women [28, 29].

A recent intervention study of adolescent girls reported that the main determinant of calcium balance was calcium intake, with net calcium absorption increasing with intake and no change in urinary calcium [30]. Retention of supplemental calcium averaged 200 to 500 mg per day, resulting in twice the increase in bone mass over time compared to the nonsupplemented control group (1640 mg/day vs. 750 mg/day). By age 16, adolescent girls had accumulated 90 to 97 percent of the bone mass of their premenopausal mothers. The authors of this study suggest that "because calcium intake during adolescence appears to directly influence skeletal calcium retention, calcium intake up to perhaps 1800 mg/day may be needed. Such an increase in calcium intake during adolescence could play an important role in the attainment of an optimal peak bone mass. This would translate into optimum bone status at the menopause and potentially act as prophylaxis against subsequent osteoporosis."

Dietary studies of premenopausal women aged 19 to 34 indicate that calcium intake is closely related to calcium balance [31]. Supplementation of postmenopausal women with calcium carbonate for a total intake of 1500 mg per day significantly retarded, but did not prevent, cortical bone loss [32, 33]. Studies of postmenopausal women, however, have reported a weak association between calcium intake and bone mass [34–37]. Balance studies conducted with women aged 35 to 70 have shown only a weak correlation with dietary calcium intake [31, 38]; they suggest that a calcium intake of 1000 to 1500 mg per day prevents the net loss of skeletal calcium [39]. Calcium supplementation has been shown to slow the loss of bone mass in postmenopausal women [28, 33, 40, 41].

Other studies of the effect of diet on bone mass have produced inconclusive results. No relationship exists between bone density and intakes of protein [42], phosphorus [43], or caffeine [35, 43]. Other dietary factors, such as fiber, alcohol [44], and aluminum [45], are each associated with lower bone mass and higher incidence of osteoporosis, although the exact mechanisms of their effects are not clear.

Physical Activity

Low physical activity is a significant risk factor for postmenopausal osteoporosis. Studies of athletes demonstrate a greater cortical thickness in the dominant arm of tennis players [46], as well as greater bone density in swimmers and runners [46, 47]. Among individuals with low body fat, particularly if associated with primary or secondary amenorrhea (see Chap. 2), exercise is not protective of bone mass. Studies of ballet dancers show that the incidence of scoliosis and stress fractures is inversely proportional to the incidence and duration of amenorrhea, reflecting prolonged hypoestrogenism [48]. Studies of runners also conclude that reduced levels of circulating estrogens in amenorrheic women are related to reduced bone mineral content [49, 50]. Women with anorexia nervosa have reduced bone mass secondary to amenorrhea, although a high level of physical activity is protective [51, 52].

Absorption and Metabolism

The adult human body contains about 1200 to 1250 gm calcium, 99 percent of which is bound in the hard matrix of the bones and teeth as hydroxyapatite, with small additional amounts of noncrystalline calcium phosphates, carbonates, and other calcium salts. These structures provide both a rigid framework and a ready reserve of calcium to maintain a constant blood level. These minerals in the bones and teeth comprise about 50 percent of the total skeletal mass; the remainder consists of an organic matrix of proteins, glycoproteins, and proteoglycans on which the calcium salts are deposited. Bone is constantly being remodeled, with about 700 mg calcium entering and leaving daily.

The 10 to 12 gm calcium found outside the skeletal structure is critically important to the regulation of a large number of vital cellular activities, such as nerve and muscle function, hormonal actions, blood clotting, and cellular motility. Calcium is often referred to as a "second messenger" because it is involved in the control of so many processes. The importance of calcium in so many body functions is reflected in the precision with which plasma calcium levels are regulated. Plasma calcium levels of 9 to 11 mg/100 ml are maintained by the complex regulatory actions of vitamin D, parathyroid hormone, calcitonin, and other hormones.

Calcium is absorbed by an active transport process in the duodenum and proximal jejunum by means of a calcium-binding protein synthesized in response to the action of 1,25-dihydroxycholecalciferol. Absorption of calcium is inhibited by compounds that form insoluble calcium salts (oxalates, phytates, and phosphates) and by undigested fat through formation of insoluble calcium soaps. The amount of calcium absorbed is therefore directly related and adjusted to body needs. About 30 percent of the calcium present in a mixed diet is normally absorbed by a healthy adult. The amount absorbed from individual foods ranges from 10 to 40 percent. Pregnant women and growing children absorb about 40 percent or more from foods. With a limited intake of calcium, absorption becomes more efficient, especially when an adequate amount of vitamin D is also present.

Because calcium salts are more readily soluble in an acid medium, most of the absorption occurs in the duodenum. Achlorhydria (lack of normal gastric acid) and increased intestinal motility both decrease absorption. Other factors hindering normal absorption include substances that form insoluble complexes with dietary calcium, such as phytic acid, oxalic acid, and free fatty acids. Phytic acid is an organic compound found in the outer layers of cereal grains. Oxalic acid is present in spinach, Swiss chard, beet tops, cocoa, and rhubarb. Foods high in saturated fatty acids are likely to produce free fatty acids, which will then combine with calcium to form insoluble complexes or soaps.

Factors that increase absorption include the presence of vitamin D, which facilitates the movement of calcium into the mucosal cells and increases absorption from the duodenum; high-protein diets, because of the action of specific amino acids, especially serine, arginine, and lysine; the presence of lactose, the disaccharide found exclusively in milk products; and an increase in acidophilic flora (i.e., the lactobacilli), which lowers the pH, favoring absorption. The amount of calcium in proportion to phosphorus in the diet, the calcium-phosphorus ratio, also affects absorption. An excess of animal protein, which is high in phosphorus, in the diet can cause an imbalanced ratio and result in higher calcium requirements. To maximize absorption and minimize loss from bone, the calcium-phosphorus ratio should be between 2 : 1 and 1 : 2; the recommended dietary allowances (RDAs) are based on a ratio of 1 : 1.

When the plasma calcium levels begin to fall, parathormone is secreted, which causes calcium to be released from bone, increases the reabsorption of calcium by the renal tubules, and increases the excretion of phosphates in the urine. Parathormone thus restores the plasma calcium level while maintaining the proper calcium-phosphorus ratio in the blood. The opposite effect is produced by the hormone calcitonin, which lowers the plasma calcium and phosphate levels by increasing absorption of calcium by bone and increasing the renal clearance of both calcium and phosphates. Together with vitamin D, parathormone and calcitonin maintain the plasma calcium level within relatively narrow limits.

The maintenance of the plasma calcium level is more dependent on bone than on the diet for a ready source of calcium. The calcium in the bones is constantly turning over, and in the healthy adult, the rates of mineralization (the addition of calcium to bone) and demineralization (resorption of calcium from bone) are equal. During periods of growth, the amount of calcium added to the bones exceeds that removed. When calcium needs exceed dietary intake, the calcium from bone is mobilized.

Most of the calcium eliminated from the body is excreted via the feces, with only a small amount being eliminated in the urine. Most of the calcium present in the feces is that unabsorbed from the diet. Calcium losses in sweat range from 15 to 20 mg per day and may be higher during periods of strenuous physical exercise, even when dietary intakes are low.

Lactose Intolerance

Although milk and milk products traditionally are considered the primary sources of dietary calcium, the majority of the world's adult population is unable to digest varying quantities of milk due to a low level of the enzyme lactase. This enzyme is located on the brush border of the small intestine and is responsible for the hydrolysis of the disaccharide lactase, which is found exclusively in milk and milk products, into its component monosaccharides, glucose and galactose. If the amount of lactose entering the jejunum exceeds the hydrolytic capacity of the available lactase, the excess sugar is transported undigested into the large intestine. Its presence increases the osmolarity of the intestinal fluid and thus draws water from the surrounding tissues into the intestinal lumen. In addition, undigested lactose is fermented by bacteria present in the colon, producing organic acids (lactic, pyruvic, and acetic), carbon dioxide, and hydrogen. These products, along with the large amount of water also present, are responsible for the well-known symptoms of lactose intolerance: abdominal cramps, bloating, diarrhea, and flatulence.

Although a temporary form of lactose intolerance can occur with inflammation or damage to the gastrointestinal epithelial mucosa, most cases represent primary adult low lactase activity, which occurs in young adults after a normal infancy and childhood. Most ethnic and racial groups, with the exception of northern Europeans and their descendants, have low lactase activity during adulthood. Lactose, the main synergistic agent in milk, enhances the body's use of minerals and protein. Because it is slowly hydrolyzed and absorbed, lactose promotes the proliferation of gastrointestinal flora, which lowers the pH of the gut, aiding calcium absorption. Lactose further aids calcium absorption by forming soluble nonionized complexes with calcium, preventing its chelation with insoluble compounds, such as oxalates. Individuals should determine the amount of lactose they can tolerate because of its beneficial effects on calcium metabolism and absorption. Lactose-reduced milk products are available, as are lactose-reducing tablets that can be added to foods.

Calcium Metabolism During Pregnancy

During pregnancy the fetus accumulates approximately 30 gm calcium at the rate of 1.5 gm by 20 weeks of gestation, 10 gm by 30 weeks, and 30 gm by 40 weeks [53]. Calcium, as well as phosphate and magnesium, is actively transferred across a concentration gradient from mother to fetus [54]. Changes in calcium metabolism facilitate the transfer of calcium from mother to fetus while protecting calcium levels in maternal serum and bone. These changes are mediated through the calcium-regulating hormones, which in turn affect intestinal absorption, renal reabsorption, and maternal skeletal calcium economy.

The mother and her fetus each maintain parathyroid hormone (PTH) and calcitonin levels, because neither of these hormones crosses the placenta [55, 56]. Fetal PTH tends to be lower and calcitonin levels higher than maternal levels, which is consistent with the observed differences in fetal and maternal calcium concentrations. The placenta synthesizes and transfers 1,25-cholecalciferol (vitamin D_3) and its metabolites through specific protein-binding proteins, and is responsible for the rapid mineral transfer in late pregnancy. By term, maternal levels of vitamin D_3 and its metabolites are about 40 percent higher than levels in cord blood [57]. During pregnancy there is an increased placental production of calcitriol, as well as a two- to threefold increase in vitamin D–binding protein [55, 58, 59]. In the presence of adequate vitamin D, plasma PTH and calcitonin levels rise and calcium and phosphorus absorption increases.

Maternal calcium absorption increases during pregnancy, doubling by 24 weeks of gestation and remaining at this level until term [60]. This augmentation occurs in advance of fetal needs, and by 24 weeks of gestation the level of urinary calcium also rises. As fetal demands increase, the amount of calcium deposited in both the maternal and fetal skeletons increases, and the level of calcium in the urine returns to normal or slightly lower than normal. The turnover of calcium in the mother's exchangeable pool of body calcium increases markedly, suggesting a higher metabolic activity of the skeleton in general.

The substantial amount of calcium needed by the fetus (30 gm) is provided by increased maternal efficiency of dietary calcium absorption. This is achieved through increases in calcitonin levels early in pregnancy, and elevated levels of 1,25-dihydroxycholecalciferol. Maternal calcium absorption doubles by 5 to 6 months of gestation and continues at near this level to term [60].

Calcium Supplementation During Pregnancy

Calcium has recently been used therapeutically to prevent maternal hypertension, preterm birth, and low birthweight. Studies have demonstrated a significant negative association between calcium intake and blood pressure in nonpregnant populations [61–66]. The pressure-lowering effect of calcium is believed to be mediated through alterations in plasma renin activity and parathyroid hormone, decreasing vascular sensitivity to angiotensin II and resulting in direct smooth-muscle relaxation [67]. During pregnancy, supplemental calcium has resulted in lower incidence of preterm and low birthweight [67–69].

Recommended Dietary Allowances

Although the World Health Organization recommends 400 to 500 mg per day for adults, indicating that there is no evidence of calcium deficiency in countries where this level of intake is common and that persons can maintain calcium balance with intakes as low as 200 to 400 mg per day, the Food and Nutrition Board of the National Academy of Sciences (NAS) argues that there are no advantages to such low recommendations. The NAS recommended dietary allowances are given in Table 6-2.

During pregnancy, about 30 mg is mobilized for the calcification of the fetal skeleton, mostly during the last third of fetal life. Calcium absorption is increased and calcium excretion decreased during pregnancy. Calcium is stored in the maternal skeleton in early pregnancy to be mobilized later when needed. About 300 mg per day above nonpregnant level is actually needed by the pregnant woman, but to provide for individual variation, 400 mg per day, for a total of 1200 mg per day, is recommended. Data from calcium balance studies suggest increasing the RDA for calcium from 800 mg to 1000 mg for premenopausal women and to 1500 mg for postmenopausal women [70].

Table 6-2
Recommended dietary allowances for calcium

Age (yr)	*mg/day*	*mg/kg*	*(mg/lb)*	*mg/100 kcal*
Infants 0–0.5	400	67	(30.8)	61.5
0.5–1.0	600	67	(30)	70.6
Children 1–3	800	62	(27.6)	61.5
4–6	800	40	(18.2)	44.4
7–10	800	29	(12.9)	40
Females 11–14	1200	26	(11.9)	54.5
15–18	1200	22	(10)	54.5
19–24	1200	21	(9.4)	54.5
25–50	800	13	(5.8)	36.4
51 +	800	12	(5.6)	42.1
Pregnant	1200	18	(8.3)	48
Lactating	1200	13	(8.7)	44.4

Source: Adapted from National Academy of Sciences, *The Recommended Dietary Allowances* (10th ed.). Washington, DC: National Academy Press, 1989.

Food Sources

About 60 percent of the calcium intake in the United States is derived from milk and dairy products. Ounce per ounce, milk and cheese are the richest sources of calcium in the diet. Calcium is also found in such foods as mustard greens, turnip greens, kale, and collard greens. Spinach also contains considerable amounts of calcium, but the presence of oxalates prevents much of its calcium from being absorbed. Shrimp, clams, oysters, and salmon eaten with the bones also provide some calcium. A summary of calcium-rich foods is given in Table 6-3.

Recent changes in the consumption of dairy products are reflective of changes in American dietary practices as a whole. For example, between 1945 and 1985, per capita consumption of milk dropped by one third, from 167 qt to 114 qt. During these years, whole-milk consumption fell by 57 percent (from 150 qt to 64 qt), whereas the intake of skim and low-fat milks rose by 200 percent (from 17 qt to 50 qt) [71]. At the same time, per capita consumption of whole- and part-skim milk cheeses increased 214 percent, from 7 lb to 22 lb. Other indicators of changing food habits, motivated to a large degree by the desire to reduce calories and diminish cholesterol intake, include a 55 percent drop in per capita consumption of butter, from 11 lb to 5 lb, and a 19 percent decline in per capita consumption of eggs, from 313 in 1965 to 255 per year in 1985 [71]. The per capita consumption of sodas, which are high in phosphates, more than doubled between 1965 and 1985, from less than 20 gal to more than 45 gal (Fig. 6-1). Other calcium-rich foods that have gained renewed popularity include yogurt. Per capita consumption of yogurt increased 12-fold between 1965 and 1985 (0.3 lb to 4.0 lb) [72].

Despite these positive changes, most women in the childbearing years do not meet their dietary requirements for calcium. Data from the Continuing Survey of Food Intake by Individuals (CSFII), a component of the National Nutrition Monitoring System, which provides dietary information on women aged 19 to 50 and their children aged 1 to 5, demonstrates this trend. Milk and milk products account for 76.2 percent of the calcium, 20 percent of the magnesium and zinc, and 11 percent of the vitamin B_6 in the total US food supply [72]. However, data from the CSFII indicate that milk and milk products contributed only 42 percent of the calcium, less than 15 percent of the magnesium and zinc, and less than 10 percent of the vitamin B_6 in the diets of adult women [73].

Table 6-3
Calcium-rich foods

Food	*Calcium content (mg)* Per 100 gm	*Calcium content (mg)* Per 100 kcal
Cheddar	729	177
Cottage cheese (4% fat)	60	57
(2% fat)	69	76
Feta cheese	500	187
Mozzarella (whole milk)	525	184
(part skim)	740	259
Parmesan	1393	300
Provolone	764	214
Ricotta (whole milk)	207	118
(part skim)	272	197
Swiss	971	259
Pasteurized process	582	172
Milk (whole, 3.5% fat)	119	194
(2% fat)	122	248
(1% fat)	123	300
(skim)	123	355
Ice cream	132	65
Yogurt (low fat)	152	150
Oysters	94	141
Salmon, canned	196	139
Sardines, canned	436	212
Shrimp, canned	115	98
Figs, dried	144	57
Apricots, dried	45	19
Oranges, fresh	40	85
Peaches, dried	28	12
Raisins, seedless	49	16
Almonds	266	45
Brazil nuts	279	153

Source: Adapted from US Department of Agriculture, Human Nutrition Information Service, *Nutritive Value of Foods*, Home and Garden Bulletin No. 72. Washington, DC: US Govt. Printing Office, 1985.

Calcium Supplements

Calcium supplements may be useful adjuncts to dietary calcium in women with lactose intolerance or milk allergy, or in those who choose not to include dairy products in their diet. Calcium carbonate provides the most concentrated source of elemental calcium

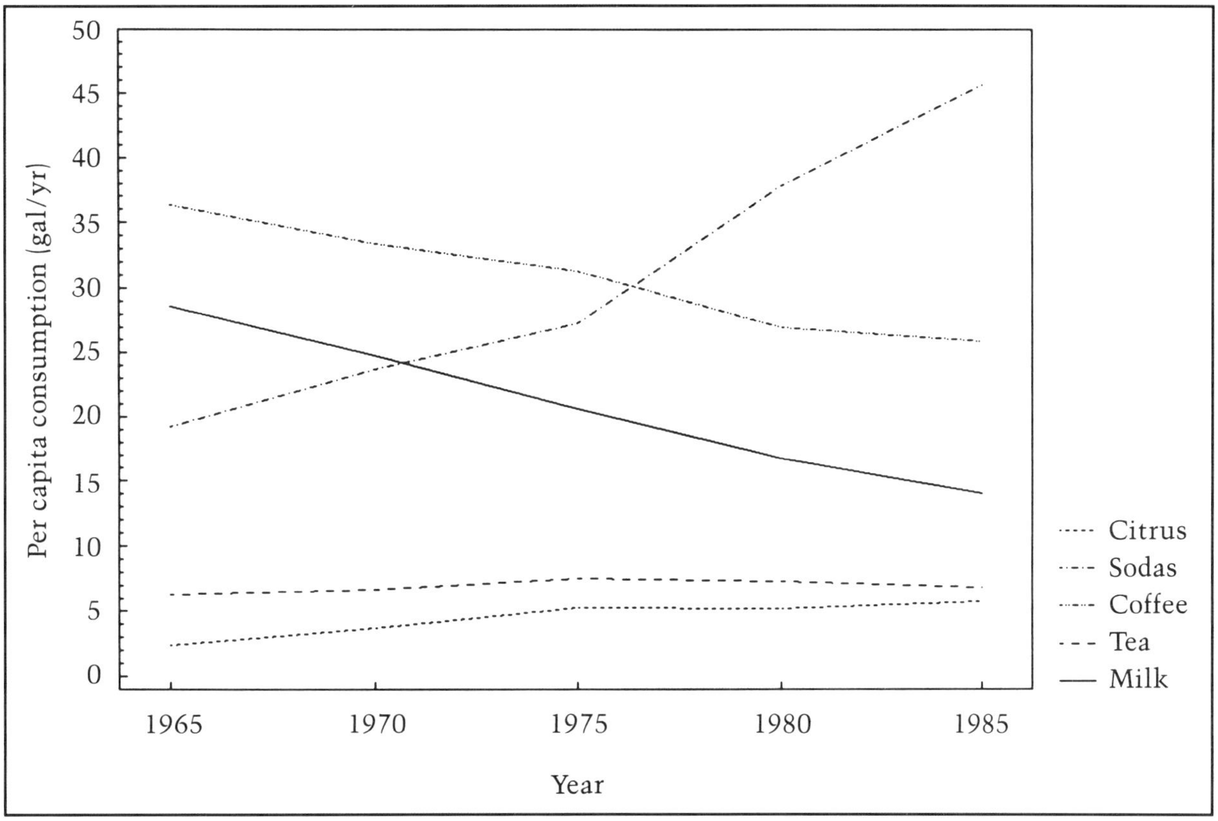

Fig. 6-1
Per capita consumption of beverages, United States, 1965 to 1985. (Adapted from K Bunch, Food Consumption, prices, and expenditures 1985. National Economics Division, Economic Research Service, US Department of Agriculture, Statistical Bulletin No. 749, 1987.)

(2.5 mg/mg elemental calcium), followed by calcium citrate (4.2 mg/mg), calcium lactate (7.7 mg/mg), and calcium gluconate (11 mg/mg). Calcium carbonate supplements, however, are associated with a higher frequency of gastrointestinal disturbances, including constipation and abdominal distention [74]. Calcium supplements inhibit the absorption of dietary nonheme iron and iron supplements [75]. Calcium citrate and calcium phosphate reduce iron absorption significantly by 49 and 62 percent, respectively. All calcium supplements inhibit iron absorption when taken with food.

Other studies have shown that calcium added to flour reduces phytate degradation by 50 percent, thus increasing phytate content of bread and interfering with iron absorption [76]. Calcium also has a direct dose-related inhibiting effect on iron absorption. Iron absorption is reduced by 50 to 60 percent at doses of 300 to 600 mg calcium, or as calcium in milk or cheese. Absorption of heme as well as nonheme iron is inhibited by calcium, suggesting that the effect is related to the mucosal transfer of iron.

Conclusions and Recommendations

In summary, optimal bone health is associated with regular menses, appropriate body weight, adequate dietary intake of calcium and protein through age 35 to 40, moderate exercise, and nonsmoking and minimal or no alcohol intake. Peak bone mass is extremely important in long-term bone health, particularly in women. Dietary intake of calcium-rich foods during childhood and adolescence is of vital importance in establishing optimal peak bone mass and in minimizing the incidence and severity of osteoporosis and age-related bone loss during adulthood. Pregnancy induces changes in calcium metabolism, favoring calcium absorption and retention. Adequate calcium intake during pregnancy is essential in the maintenance of maternal bone health and for fetal bone ossification.

Dietary sources of calcium are preferred because of the presence of other nutrients and better absorption. When dietary sources of calcium cannot be tolerated, due to milk allergy or lactose intolerance, calcium supplements can be used, but should be taken between meals to minimize their adverse effects on other components of the diet.

References

1. Marshall, WA, and Tanner, JM: Variations in pattern of pubertal changes in girls. *Arch. Dis. Child.* 44:291–303, 1969.
2. Tanner, JM: *Growth at Adolescence* (2nd ed.). London: Blackwell Scientific, 1962.
3. Malina, RM: Adolescent growth and maturation: Selected aspects of current research. *Yearbook Phys. Anthropol.* 21:63–94, 1978.
4. Bayley, N: Size and body build of adolescents in relation to rate of skeletal maturing. *Child Dev.* 14:47–90, 1943.
5. Stevens-Simon, C, Forbes, GB, Kreipe, RE, and McAnarney, ER: A comparison of chronologic age and gynecologic age as indices of biologic maturity. *Am. J. Dis. Child.* 140:702–705, 1986.
6. Duenhoelter, JH, Jimenez, JM,and Baumann, G: Pregnancy performance of patients under fifteen years of age. *Obstet. Gynecol.* 46:49–52, 1975.
7. Graham, D: The obstetric and neonatal consequences of adolescent pregnancy. *Birth Defects: Original Article Series*, Vol. XVII, No. 3, 1981. Pp. 49–67.

8. Matkovic, V, Kostial, K, Simonovic, I, et al. Bone status and fracture rates in two regions of Yugoslavia. *Am. J. Clin. Nutr.* 32:540–549, 1979.
9. Sandler, RB, Slemenda, C, LaPorte, RE, et al: Postmenopausal bone density and milk consumption in childhood and adolescence. *Am. J. Clin. Nutr.* 42:270–274, 1985.
10. Rodin, A, Murby, B, Smith, A, et al: Premenopausal bone loss in the lumbar spine and neck of femur: A study of 225 Caucasian women. *Bone* 11:1–5, 1990.
11. Mazess, RB, and Barden, HS: Bone density in premenopausal women: Effects of age, dietary intake, physical activity, smoking, and birth-control pills. *Am. J. Clin. Nutr.* 53:132–142, 1991.
12. Garn, SM, Rohmann, CG, and Wagner, B: Bone loss as a general phenomenon in man. *Fed. Proc.* 26:1729–1736, 1967.
13. Garn, SM: Bone-loss and Aging. In R Goldman and M Rockstein (eds.), *The Physiology and Pathology of Human Aging.* New York: Academic, 1975. Pp. 39–57.
14. Nordin, BEC: International patterns of osteoporosis. *Clin. Orthop.*, 45:17–30, 1966.
15. Riggs, BL, and Melton, LJ: Involutional osteoporosis. *N. Engl. J. Med.* 314:1676–1686, 1986.
16. Owen, GM, and Lubin, LH: Anthropometric differences between black and white preschool children. *Am. J. Dis. Child.* 126:168–169, 1973.
17. Garn, SM, and Clark, DC: Nutrition, growth, development and maturation: Findings from the Ten-State Survey 1968–70. *Pediatrics* 56:306–319, 1975.
18. Schulte, JE, Townsend, EJ, Hugg, J, et al: Density of lean body mass is greater in blacks than in whites. *J. Appl. Physiol.* 56:1647–1649, 1984.
19. Garn, SM, Nagy, JM, and Sandusky, ST: Differential sexual dimorphism in bone diameters of subjects of European and African ancestry. *Am. J. Phys. Anthropol.* 37:127–130, 1972.
20. Cohn, SH, Abesamis, C, Zanzi, I, et al: Body elemental composition: Comparison between black and white adults. *Am. J. Physiol.* 232:E419–422, 1977.
21. Weinstein, RS, and Bell, NH: Diminished rates of bone formation in normal black adults. *N. Engl. J. Med.* 319:1698–1701, 1988.
22. Bell, NH, Greene, A, Epstein, S, et al: Evidence for alteration of the vitamin D–endocrine system in blacks. *J. Clin. Invest.* 76:470–473, 1985.
23. Garn, SM, Pao, EM, and Rihl, ME: Compact bone in Chinese and Japanese. *Science* 143:1439–1440, 1964.
24. Garn, SM, Poznanski, AK, and Larson, K: Metacarpal Lengths, Cortical Diameters and Areas from the Ten-State Nutrition Survey. In ZFC Jaworski (ed.), *Proceedings of the First Workshop on Bone Morphometry.* Ottawa: University of Ottawa Press, 1976. Pp. 367–391.

25. Seeman, E, Hopper, JL, Bach, LA, et al: Reduced bone mass in daughters of women with osteoporosis. *N. Engl. J. Med.* 320:554–558, 1989.
26. Lutz, J, and Tesar, R: Mother-daughter pairs: Spinal and femoral bone densities and dietary intakes. *Am. J. Clin. Nutr.* 52:872–877, 1990.
27. Mazess, RB, Barden, H, and Green, G: Bone mineral density of the spine. *J. Bone Mineral Res.* 2 (Suppl.):330, 1987 (abstract).
28. Riis, B, Thomsen, K, and Christiansen, C: Does calcium supplementation prevent postmenopausal bone loss? *N. Engl. J. Med.* 316:173–177, 1987.
29. Riggs, BL, Wahner, HW, Melton, LJ, et al: Dietary calcium intake and rates of bone loss in women. *J. Clin. Invest.* 80:979–982, 1987.
30. Matkovic, V, Fontana, D, Tominac, C, et al: Factors that influence peak bone mass formation: A study of calcium balance and the inheritance of bone mass in adolescent females. *Am. J. Clin. Nutr.* 52:878–888, 1990.
31. Lakshmanan, FL, Rao, RB, and Church, JP: Calcium and phosphorus intakes, balances, and blood levels of adults consuming self-selected diets. *Am. J. Clin. Nutr.* 40:1368–1379, 1984.
32. Recker, RR, Saville, PD, and Heaney, RP: Effect of estrogens and calcium carbonate on bone loss in postmenopausal women. *Ann. Intern. Med.* 87:649–655, 1977.
33. Horsman, A, Gallagher, JC, Simpson, M, and Nordin, BEC: Prospective trial of oestrogen and calcium in postmenopausal women. *Br. J. Med.* 2:789–792, 1977.
34. Garn, SM, Solomon, MA, and Friedl, J: Calcium intake and bone health in the elderly. *Ecol. Food Nutr.* 10:131–134, 1981.
35. Yano, K, Heibrun, LK, Wasnich, RD, et al: The relationship between diet and bone mineral content of multiple skeletal sites in elderly Japanese-American men and women living in Hawaii. *Am. J. Clin. Nutr.* 42:877–888, 1985.
36. Riggs, BL, Kelley, PJ, Kinney, VR, et al: Calcium deficiency and osteoporosis. *J. Bone Joint Surg.* 49A:915–924, 1967.
37. Sowers, MR, Wallace, RB, and Lemke, JH: Correlates of mid-radius bone density among postmenopausal women: A community study. *Am. J. Clin. Nutr.* 41:1045–1053, 1985.
38. Recker, RR, and Heaney, RP: The effect of milk supplements on calcium metabolism, bone metabolism and calcium balance. *Am. J. Clin. Nutr.* 41:254–263, 1985.
39. Heaney, RP, Recker, RR, and Saville, PD: Menopausal changes in calcium balance performance. *J. Lab. Clin. Med.* 92:953–963, 1978.
40. Polley, KJ, Nordin, BEC, Baghurst, PA, et al: Effect of calcium supplementation on forearm bone mineral content in postmenopausal women: A prospective, sequential controlled trial. *J. Nutr.* 117:1929–1935, 1987.
41. Smith, EL, Gilligan, C, Smith, PE, and Sempos, CT: Calcium supplementation and bone loss in middle-aged women. *Am. J. Clin. Nutr.* 50:833–842, 1989.

42. Spencer, H, Kramer, L, and Osis, D: Factors contributing to calcium loss in aging. *Am. J. Clin. Nutr.* 36:776–787, 1982.
43. Heaney, RP, and Recker, RR: Effects of nitrogen, phosphorus, and caffeine on calcium balance in women. *J. Lab. Med.* 99:46–55, 1982.
44. Dalen, N, and Lamke, B: Bone mineral losses in alcoholics. *Acta Orthop. Scand.* 47:469–471, 1976.
45. Heaf, JG, Podenphant, J, and Anderson, JR: Bone aluminum deposition in maintenance dialysis patients treated with aluminum-free dialysate: Role of aluminum hydroxide consumption. *Nephron* 42:210–216, 1986.
46. Jacobson, PC, Beaver, C, Grubb, SA, et al: Bone density in women: College athletes and older athletic women. *Orthop. Res.* 2:328–332, 1984.
47. Smith, EL, and Raab, DM: Osteoporosis and physical activity. *Acta Med. Scand.* 711 (Suppl.):149–156, 1986.
48. Warren, MP, Brooks-Gunn, J, Hamilton, LH, et al: Scoliosis and fractures in young ballet dancers. *N. Engl. J. Med.* 314:1348–1353, 1986.
49. Fisher, EC, Nelson, ME, Frontera, WR, et al: Bone mineral content and levels of gonadotropins and estrogens in amenorrheic running women. *J. Clin. Endocrinol. Metab.* 62:1232–1236, 1986.
50. Drinkwater, BL, Nilson, K, Chestnut, CH, et al: Bone mineral content of amenorrheic and eumenorrheic athletes. *N. Engl. J. Med.* 311:277–281, 1984.
51. Crosby, LO, Kaplan, FS, Pertschuk, MJ, and Mullen, JL: The effect of anorexia nervosa on bone morphometry in young women. *Clin. Orthop.* 201:271–277, 1985.
52. Rigotti, NA, Nussbaum, SR, Herzog, DB, and Neer, RM: Osteoporosis in women with anorexia nervosa. *N. Engl. J. Med.* 311:1601–1606, 1984.
53. Hytten, FE, and Leitch, I: *The Physiology of Human Pregnancy* (2nd ed.). London: Blackwell Scientific, 1971. P. 383.
54. Reitz, RE, Daane, TA, Woods, JR, and Weinstein, RL: Calcium, magnesium, phosphorus and parathyroid hormone inter-relationships in pregnancy and newborn infants. *Obstet. Gynecol.* 50:701–705, 1977.
55. Northrop, G, Misenhimer, HR, and Becker, FO: Failure of parathyroid hormone to cross the nonhuman primate placenta. *Am. J. Obstet. Gynecol.* 129:449–453, 1977.
56. Milhaud, G, Moukhtar, MS, Perault-Staub, AM, et al: Studies in Thyrocalcitonin. In S Taylor and GV Foster (eds.), *Calcitonin.* Proceedings of the Second International Conference. London: Heinemann, 1969. P. 182.
57. Weisman, Y, Occhipinti, M, Knox, G, et al: Concentrations of 24,25-dihydroxyvitamin D and 25-hydroxyvitamin D in paired maternal-cord sera. *Am. J. Obstet. Gynecol.* 130:704–707, 1978.
58. Hillman, LS, and Haddad, JG: Perinatal vitamin D metabolism: Factors influencing late gestational human serum 25-hydroxyvitamin D. *Am. J. Obstet. Gynecol.* 125:196–200, 1976.
59. Barragry, JM, Corless, D, Auton, J, et al: Plasma vitamin D–binding

globulin in vitamin D deficiency, pregnancy and chronic liver disease. *Clin. Chim. Acta* 87:359–365, 1978.
60. Heaney, RP, and Skillman, TG: Calcium metabolism in normal human pregnancy. *J. Clin. Endocrinol. Metab.* 33:661–670, 1971.
61. Iso, H, Kitamura, A, Sato, S, et al: Calcium intake and blood pressure in seven Japanese populations. *Am. J. Epidemiol.* 133:776–783, 1991.
62. McCarron, DA, Morris, CD, and Cole, C: Dietary calcium in human hypertension. *Science* 217:267–269, 1982.
63. Ackley, S, Barrett-Connor, E, and Suarez, L: Dairy products, calcium and blood pressure. *Am. J. Clin. Nutr.* 38:457–461, 1983.
64. Harlan, WR, Hull, AL, Schmouder, RL, et al: Blood pressure and nutrition in adults. The National Health and Nutrition Examination Survey. *Am. J. Epidemiol.* 120:17–28, 1984.
65. Trevisan, M, Krogh, V, Farinaro, E, et al: Calcium-rich foods and blood pressure: Findings from the Italian National Research Council Study. *Am. J. Epidemiol.* 127:1155–1163, 1988.
66. Garcia-Palmieri, MR, Costas, R, Cruz-Vidal, M, et al: Milk consumption, calcium intake, and decreased hypertension in Puerto Rico. *Hypertension* 6:322–328, 1984.
67. Repke, JT, and Villar, J: Pregnancy-induced hypertension and low birth weight: The role of calcium. *Am. J. Clin. Nutr.* 54:237S–241S, 1991.
68. Repke, JT: Prevention of preeclampsia. *Clin. Perinatol.* 18:779–792, 1991.
69. Villar, J, and Repke, JT: Calcium supplementation during pregnancy may reduce preterm delivery in high-risk populations. *Am. J. Obstet. Gynecol.* 163:1124–1131, 1990.
70. Heaney, RP, Recker, RR, and Saville, PD: Calcium balance and calcium requirements in middle-aged women. *Am. J. Clin. Nutr.* 30:1603–1611, 1977.
71. Bunch, K: Food consumption, prices, and expenditures 1985. National Economics Division, Economic Research Service, US Department of Agriculture, Statistical Bulletin No. 749, 1987.
72. National Academy of Sciences: *Designing Foods: Animal Product Options in the Marketplace.* Washington, DC: National Academy Press, 1988. P. 37.
73. Nationwide Food Consumption Survey: Continuing Survey of Food Intakes by Individuals. US Department of Agriculture, Human Nutrition Information Service, Nutrition Monitoring Division, Report No. 85-4, 1987.
74. Wardlaw, G: The effects of diet and life-style on bone mass in women. *J. Am. Diet. Assoc.* 88:17–25, 1988.
75. Cook, JD, Dassenko, SA, and Whittaker, P: Calcium supplementation: Effect on iron absorption. *Am. J. Clin. Nutr.* 53:106–111, 1991.
76. Hallberg, L, Brune, M, Erlandsson, M, et al: Calcium: Effect of different amounts on nonheme- and heme-iron absorption in humans. *Am. J. Clin. Nutr.* 53:112–119, 1991.

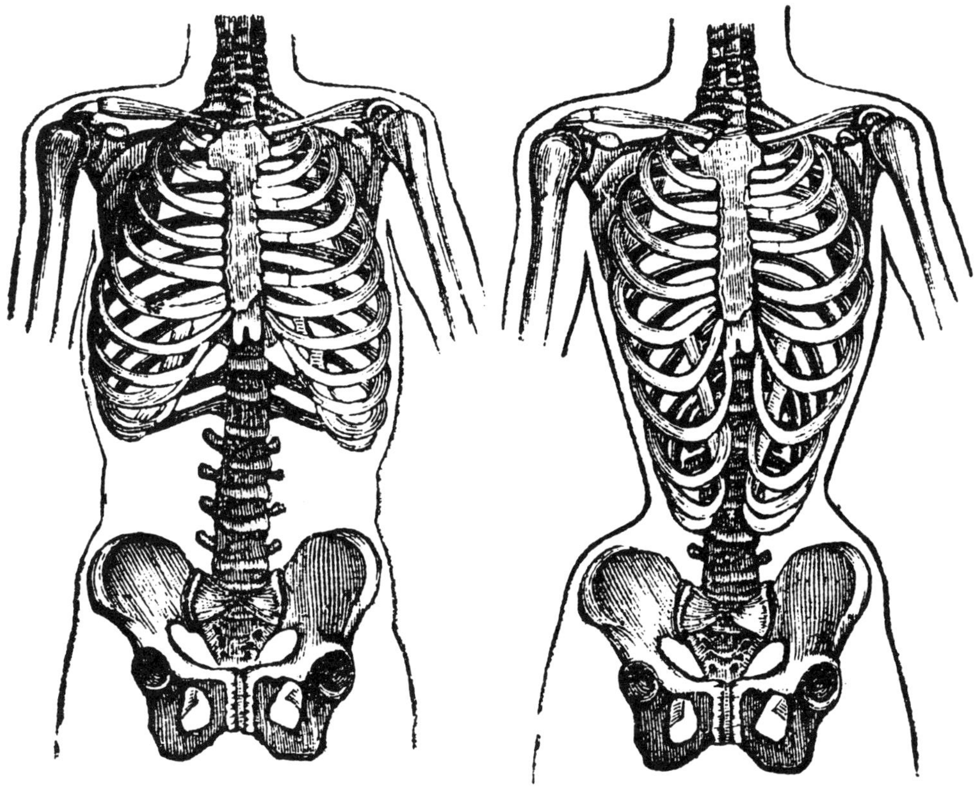

The effect of tight corseting on bones of the ribcage.

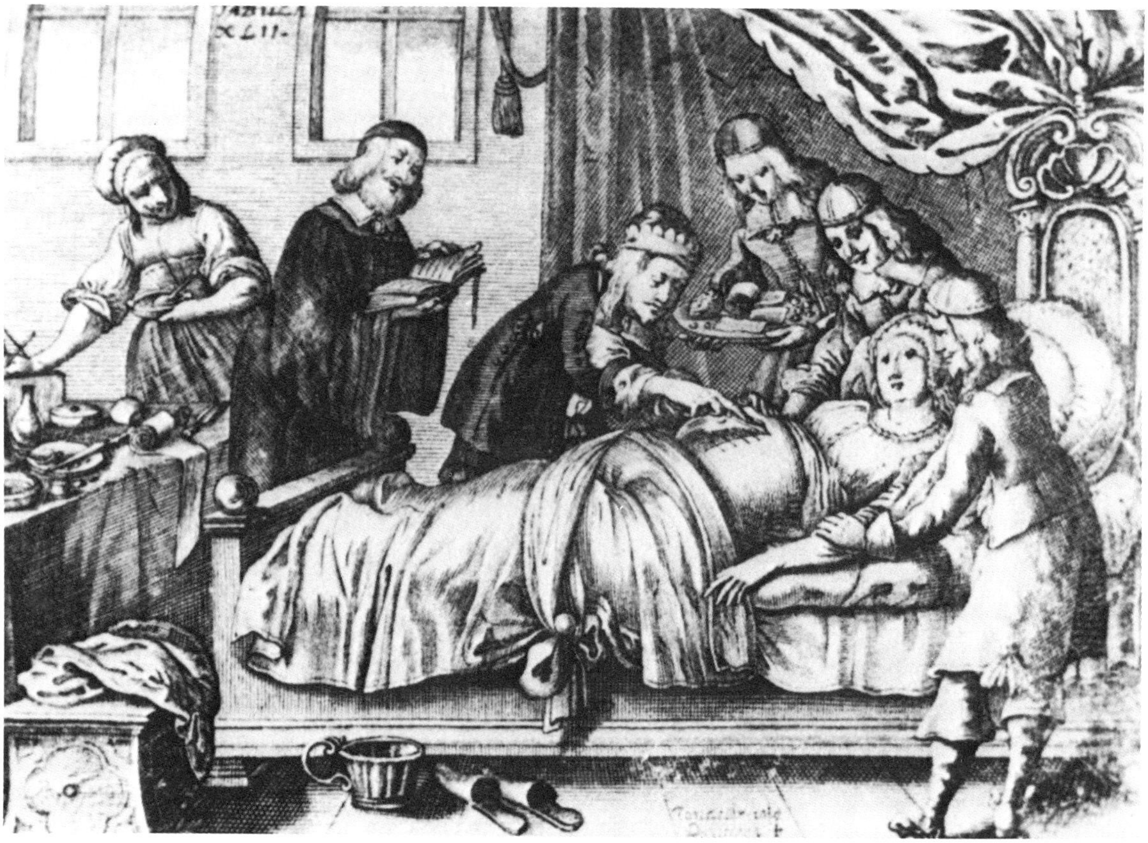

Cesarean section. (From Johannes Scultetus. *Auctarium ad armamentarium chirurgicum*. Leyden, 1653.)

7 Iron Metabolism

Iron is one of the most plentiful elements on earth, making up about 5 percent of its crust and an even greater part of its core. According to the Ebers papyrus, iron was first used as a medicine around 1500 BC to treat parasitic infections and a variety of other ailments. In the 18th century its presence was demonstrated in animal tissue, and blood was found to contain iron. Most of what is known about iron, including its important interactions with other elements, has been learned in this century. This chapter is divided into three sections: an overview, including the metabolism, requirements, and dietary sources of iron; iron balance in pregnancy, including iron hematologic changes; and iron deficiency in pregnancy, including prevalence, consequences, and therapy.

Overview

Function and Distribution

Iron is a constituent of hemoglobin, myoglobin, and a number of enzymes, and is therefore an essential nutrient for humans. This trace element accounts for about 35 mg/kg body weight in these forms, and an additional 5 to 20 mg/kg stored in ferritin and hemosiderin. Iron in the body is almost exclusively involved in the uptake and release of oxygen at the cellular level. The average adult body contains about 4 gm iron: 3 gm in active or functional form and about 1 gm in storage or transport form. Most of the active iron, as components of porphyrin, forms integral parts of hemoglobin, myoglobin, and the enzymes cytochrome, catalase, and peroxidase. The majority of this iron is found in the hemoglobin of red blood cells. Hemoglobin's ability to take up and release oxygen and carbon dioxide is dependent on the presence of iron.

Metabolism and Dietary Iron

Iron balance is dependent on several factors: iron requirements for hemoglobin production, iron losses from physiologic and pathologic processes, and the amount of iron absorbed from the intestine. The requirements for hemoglobin synthesis are greatest when there is rapid expansion of tissue and red cell mass, that is, during infancy, childhood, and pregnancy. During gestation the greatest blood volume expansion and therefore greatest iron need occurs in women of low pregravid weight with large weight gains [1].

Healthy men lose about 1 mg iron per day through physiologic means. In contrast, women experience an additional loss of about 0.5 mg per day: the amount of iron in the menstrual flow averaged over one month. During pregnancy, iron requirements average about 4 mg per day, rising from 2.8 mg per day for the nonpregnant woman to 6.6

mg per day in the last few weeks of pregnancy [2]. Pathologic losses from menorrhagia average as much as 57 mg per month [3]. Diseases of the gastrointestinal tract can also represent a major factor in negative iron balance among males and females. The most important pathologic iron loss is hookworm infestation [4]; losses can average from 2 ml blood per day from infestation with *Necator americanus* to about 4.5 ml blood per day with *Ancylostoma duodenale* [5].

Iron is unique among mineral elements in that there is no physiologic mechanism for regulating increases or decreases in its excretion. Iron balance is primarily controlled at the site of intestinal absorption. No physiologic mechanism exists for the excretion of absorbed iron, and losses occur entirely through elimination of iron-containing cells such as blood or epithelium. Absorption of iron is influenced by several factors [6]: the integrity of the intestinal mucosa, the amount and chemical nature of iron in the ingested food, and the numerous and varied dietary factors that increase or decrease the availability of iron for absorption. Iron is absorbed only when needed, a circumstance that prevents excessive storage of iron in the body. Ferrous, or oxidized, iron (Fe^{++}) is more easily absorbed than is ferric, or reduced, iron (Fe^{+++}). The absorption of heme or organic iron, found only in animal sources, is unaffected by other dietary components. In contrast, nonheme or inorganic iron, present in vegetable and medicinal sources, is profoundly affected by other components of the diet. Absorption of nonheme iron is enhanced by an acid medium, which may aid in the conversion of ferric to ferrous iron. Absorption is more efficient in the presence of ascorbic acid, sulfhydryl compounds, and other reducing substances. Heme-rich dietary sources of iron are given in Table 7-1.

The efficiency of nonheme dietary iron absorption is also influenced by the form in which the iron is present and the foods with which it is eaten. Thus, the amount of iron absorbed from a meal is the net effect of a variety of factors that either enhance or inhibit iron absorption. Iron absorption from dietary sources ranges from 1 percent for some vegetables to 10 to 25 percent from meat [7]. The small amount of iron absorbed from vegetables suggests that they contain inhibitors of iron absorption. Phosphates in carbonated beverages, oxalates in chocolate, and phytates in whole grains form insoluble complexes with iron, preventing its absorption [8]. Iron from animal sources (primarily heme iron) is absorbed better than iron from vegetable sources (nonheme iron), although when both are eaten at the same time, absorption from vegetable sources is enhanced. Dietary fiber also decreases the absorption of iron, as well as

Table 7-1
Heme-rich dietary sources of iron

Food and method of preparation	Iron content (mg) Per 100 gm	Per 100 kcal
Pork sausage (Braunschweiger)	9.3	2.6
Chicken liver (cooked)	8.5	5.7
Oysters (breaded, fried)	6.7	3.3
Oysters (raw)	6.5	9.8
Beef liver (fried)	6.2	2.9
Clams (canned)	4.1	4.1
Sirloin steak (lean, broiled)	3.3	1.6
Sardines (canned)	3.1	1.5
Duck (roasted)	2.7	1.3
Turkey (dark meat, roasted)	2.4	1.3
Lamb chops (lean, broiled)	2.0	0.9
Shrimp (canned)	1.6	1.4
Ocean perch (breaded, fried)	1.4	0.6
Turkey (light meat, roasted)	1.3	0.8
Fried chicken	1.3	0.5
Ham (lean, roasted)	1.1	0.6
Roasted chicken	1.0	0.6
Veal cutlet (broiled)	0.9	0.4
Canadian bacon (fried)	0.9	0.5
Tuna (solid white, canned)	0.7	0.4

Source: Calculated from US Dept. of Agriculture, Human Nutrition Information Service, *Nutritive Value of Foods*, Home and Garden Bulletin No. 72. Washington, DC: US Govt. Printing Office, 1985.

zinc and calcium. Tea inhibits the absorption of nonheme iron by forming insoluble iron-tannate complexes. Both tea and coffee decrease iron absorption in a dose-dependent manner [9–12]. In patients with iron overload, such as those with thalassemia syndromes, tea produces a 41 to 95 percent inhibition of iron absorption [13]. Calcium also inhibits iron absorption. When added as a fortifying agent to wheat flour, or as a component of other foods, such as milk and cheese, calcium reduces the absorption of iron by 50 percent [14]. Milk and eggs also interfere with absorption [14, 15].

Amino acids in animal proteins form soluble complexes with iron and aid its absorption [16–18]. Ascorbic and citric acids, as well as fructose, also form soluble complexes with inorganic iron that enhance its absorption. Ascorbic acid enhances the absorption of nonheme iron, as do fruits in proportion to their ascorbate content

[14, 19]. Vitamin C increases iron absorption from iron-enriched foods [20].

The amount of iron absorbed from any given meal is largely dependent on the composition of the meal and the iron status of the individual. During states of iron balance, only about 10 percent of dietary iron is absorbed. This figure can increase by a factor of two or three during periods of iron deficiency. Iron absorption increases with physiologic need, such as during periods of rapid growth in infancy, childhood, adolescence, and pregnancy; as a result of blood loss; and at high altitudes.

From the intestinal lumen, iron is absorbed in the ferrous (Fe^{++}) oxidation state into the cells of the intestinal mucosa. Within the mucosal cells it is oxidized to the ferric (Fe^{+++}) form and then combines with a specific protein (apoferritin) to form an iron–protein complex, **ferritin**. When iron is needed by the body, ferritin releases its iron component into the bloodstream: The ferric iron within the mucosal cell is reduced to the ferrous form and released. The apoferritin in the mucosal cell can then combine with dietary iron absorbed in the intestines. If all the mucosal cells are saturated (their apoferritin components have been changed to ferritin), no further iron will be absorbed. In the bloodstream, the released ferrous iron is reoxidized to ferric iron, which then combines with another specific protein compound to form **transferrin**, the transport form of iron in which it is carried to various tissues. Most of the iron in the bloodstream is utilized by the bone marrow to synthesize hemoglobin, although some is used by other tissues in the formation of enzymes. Of the 3.5 to 4.0 gm iron present in the adult human body, about one fourth, or 1 gm, is stored, mainly in the liver and spleen. Other storage iron is found within cells as part of an iron–protein complex, **hemosiderin**. These forms are readily mobilized when iron is needed.

Erythrocytes require about 7.5 days for maturation and function for about 120 days. After that time they are broken down and the iron is efficiently conserved. New hemoglobin is synthesized to replace that of matured erythrocytes. Normal losses of iron occur daily in sweat, hair, desquamated epithelial and mucosal cells, and urine. Menstrual losses, pregnancy, blood donations, and injury with bleeding add to iron losses.

Requirements and Recommended Allowances

Because iron is efficiently conserved and reutilized in the body, the daily physiologic requirements are small. According to the most recent World Health Organization estimates, only 10 to 15 percent of iron is available (absorbed) from the diets of individuals in the industrialized nations [21]. For men the recommended dietary allowance (RDA) is 10 mg per day; for nonpregnant women it is 15 mg per day [22]. During pregnancy, the RDA doubles to 30 mg per day. The recommended energy intake during pregnancy is 2200 kcal during the first trimester and 2500 kcal during the second and third trimesters. To meet the RDA for iron during pregnancy from foods alone, the iron density of the diet would have to be between 12.0 and 13.6 mg iron/1000 kcal. Data from national dietary surveys indicate that the iron density of the diets of women of childbearing age is only about 7 mg/1000 kcal [23]. Because the increased pregnancy requirement for iron cannot be easily met by diet alone, daily iron supplements are usually recommended.

Iron Balance in Pregnancy

Iron Demands

During pregnancy, demands are made on iron stores by the growing fetus and placenta, the expanding maternal blood volume and red cell mass, and blood losses at delivery. These demands are superimposed on the nonpregnant baseline needs, and although they are in part offset by pregnancy amenorrhea and increased iron absorption, it is doubtful that they can be met by dietary sources alone [6]. Total iron demands during pregnancy with a single fetus average 1000 to 1100 mg [24].

The fetus and placenta both effectively abstract folate and iron from the mother, even if her iron stores are grossly deficient [3]. Iron is transferred to the fetus against a concentration gradient; the placenta and fetus receive about one sixth of the total iron passing through the maternal plasma each day. The total iron drain becomes maximal after the 20th week of pregnancy. Maternal excretion accounts for about 240 mg; about 350 mg is transferred to the fetus, placenta, and its contained blood; and about 450 mg is utilized to increase the maternal blood volume [25]. The mode of delivery also greatly influences iron balance: Vaginal delivery is associated with a blood loss of at least 500 ml blood or over 200 mg iron; cesarean section is associated with at least 1000 mg blood loss, or more than 400 mg iron [26].

A portion of these requirements for iron can be met by mobilization of body iron stores. In males, iron stores range from 500 to 1500 mg, but in females they tend to be much lower [7]. Kitay and Harbort [3] summarize the clinical possibilities as follows:

> It is, therefore, entirely reasonable to assume that a large percentage of women enter pregnancy with compromised iron status only to be con-

fronted by the large gestational physiological iron drain. The otherwise normal pregnant woman, assuming a state of excellent nutrition, will finish pregnancy with an iron store deficit (if not supplemented), and if nutrition was suboptimal prior to pregnancy and iron stores minimal to absent, frank iron deficiency will develop.

Blood Volume Changes

Plasma Volume. The rise in the plasma volume occurs earlier than that of the erythrocyte mass, resulting in a temporary fall in hematocrit between 24 to 32 weeks' gestation [3]. Dilutional anemia of pregnancy results from the combination of the early expansion of plasma volume followed by a later and considerably smaller rise in total red cell mass [2]. Red cell mass expansion occurs late in pregnancy, mostly during the last 8 to 10 weeks. As the red cell mass increases, the hematocrit rises to normal levels toward the end of pregnancy. The hematocrit also rises 3 to 5 percent on the second or third postpartum day as a result of physiologic diuresis and contraction of blood volume [3]. The packed red cell volume, or the hematocrit, is an indirect measurement of the oxygen-carrying capacity of the blood. In the healthy, nonpregnant woman, it is 38 to 45 percent. It may fall as low as 34 percent, reflecting the physiologic hydremia of pregnancy, rather than a decrease in oxygen-carrying capacity or true anemia [3]. On the other hand, values less than 34 percent are reflective of true anemia.

The increase in plasma volume is about 50 percent, with a range of 20 to 100 percent above normal, nonpregnant blood volume [26]. These changes amount to at least 1250 ml above the average nonpregnant level, and result in a final plasma volume of about 2600 ml [27]. Little increase is noted before the first 10 weeks; after that a progressive rise is followed by a plateau at about 30 to 34 weeks. The extent of the plasma volume increase is related to the clinical condition. Larger increases are associated with multiple pregnancy and larger infants. Smaller increases are associated with preeclampsia, and women with a history of habitual abortions or stillbirths often have little or no increase [27]. In the presence of iron-deficiency anemia, a smaller increase in plasma volume and red cell volume occurs during the pregnancy.

Erythrocyte Volume. The rise in the erythrocyte volume begins sometime between 10 and 20 weeks, and continues progressively to term [2]. In the non–iron-supplemented gravida, the erythrocyte volume rises from a nonpregnant value of about 1400 ml to about 1650 ml, an increase of 250 ml, or 18 percent. In the iron-supplemented gravida, increases of 400 to 450 ml, or about 30 percent over nonpregnant values, occur. The magnitude of these changes is dependent on the clinical situation, as with the plasma volume. In warm climates, there is a larger increase in plasma volume to provide a greater peripheral circulation for heat loss. At high altitudes, there is a greater rise in the circulating erythrocyte mass to increase oxygen transport.

Plasma volume is increased because more circulation is needed in the skin to dissipate fetal heat and in the kidneys to increase filtration. Erythrocyte volume increases to meet the needs of the fetus and the additional, metabolizing maternal tissue.

Pregnancy-Induced Hematologic Changes

The plasma erythropoietin activity increases steadily during pregnancy [3]. The hormone placental lactogen augments the action of erythropoietin, similar to the action of testosterone. It also stimulates aldosterone secretion. Prolactin additionally enhances the effect of erythropoietin. Estrogen antagonizes the erythropoietin-augmenting effects of placental lactogen. It inhibits utilization of erythropoietin by the marrow stem cell, and also impairs its production. Progesterone preserves the erythropoietic effect of placental lactogen. It also blocks estrogen inhibition of stem cell erythropoietin utilization.

During normal pregnancy, hematologic values change substantially. For women with adequate iron stores, hemoglobin and hematocrit values begin to decline during the first trimester, reach a nadir by the end of the second trimester, and gradually rise again during the third trimester [28–31]. However, because of the concomitant changes in hemoglobin and hematocrit during pregnancy, iron-deficiency anemia ideally should be characterized according to the specific stage of gestation. Table 7-2 gives the mean hemoglobin values by week of gestation, as well as cutoff values of hemoglobin and hematocrit defining anemia as suggested by the Centers for Disease Control.

Effect of Altitude and Smoking

Hemoglobin and hematocrit values should also be adjusted for the factors of altitude and smoking when normal values during pregnancy are defined. Individuals residing at high altitudes (>3300 ft) have higher hemoglobin and hematocrit values than those residing at sea level, because of the lower oxygen partial pressure, a reduction in the oxygen saturation of the blood, and a compensatory increase in red cell production to ensure adequate oxygenation. The upward shift in hemoglobin and hematocrit distributions caused by higher altitudes may result in underdiagnosis of anemia if sea-level cutoffs are

Table 7-2
Pregnancy month-specific hemoglobin and hematocrit cutoffs

Gestation (wk)	Mean hemoglobin (gm/100 ml)	5th percentile hemoglobin (gm/100 ml)	5th percentile hematocrit (%)
12	12.2	11.0	33.0
16	11.8	10.6	32.0
20	11.6	10.5	32.0
24	11.6	10.5	32.0
28	11.8	10.7	32.0
32	12.1	11.0	33.0
36	12.5	11.4	34.0
40	12.9	11.9	36.0

Source: Adapted from CDC criteria for anemia in children and childbearing-aged women. *MMWR* 38:400–404, 1989.

Table 7-3
Altitude adjustments for hemoglobin (Hgb) and hematocrit (Hct) cutoffs

Altitude (ft)	Hgb (gm/100 ml)	Hct (%)
<3000	0.0	0.0
3000–3999	+0.2	+0.5
4000–4999	+0.3	+1.0
5000–5999	+0.5	+1.5
6000–6999	+0.7	+2.0
7000–7999	+1.0	+3.0
8000–8999	+1.3	+4.0
9000–9999	+1.6	+5.0
>10,000	+2.0	+6.0

Source: Adapted from CDC criteria for anemia in children and childbearing-aged women. *MMWR* 38:400–404, 1989.

applied. Accurate diagnosis of anemia for individuals living at high altitudes requires an altitude-specific adjustment of hemoglobin and hematocrit cutoffs (Table 7-3).

The changes in hemoglobin and hematocrit values induced by altitude are similar to those caused by smoking. The higher hemoglobin and hematocrit values of smokers result from an increased level of carboxyhemoglobin, secondary to the inhalation of carbon monoxide. Because carboxyhemoglobin has no oxygen-carrying capacity, its presence causes an upward shift in the distribution of hemoglobin and hematocrit values. As is the case with altitude, a smoking-specific adjustment is required for the accurate diagnosis of anemia in smokers (Table 7-4). It is important to remember that the

Table 7-4
Smoking adjustments for hemoglobin (Hgb) and hematocrit (Hct)

Characteristic	*Hgb (gm/100 ml)*	*Hct (%)*
Nonsmoker	0.0	0.0
Smokers (all)	+0.3	+1.0
½–1 pack/day	+0.3	+1.0
1–2 packs/day	+0.5	+1.5
>2 packs/day	+0.7	+2.0

Source: Adapted from CDC criteria for anemia in children and childbearing-aged women. *MMWR* 38:400–404, 1989.

altitude and smoking adjustments are additive, and both must be taken into account when diagnosing anemia.

Iron Deficiency in Pregnancy

Development of Iron-Deficiency Anemia

The first stage in the development of iron-deficiency anemia occurs when more iron is lost than enters the body and iron stores are mobilized. As iron stores decrease, iron absorption from the gastrointestinal tract increases. After iron stores are depleted, marrow staining is low to absent. With continued depletion, serum transferrin begins to rise. Elevated serum transferrin is directly reflected by an increased total iron-binding capacity (TIBC) as a compensatory response to iron depletion. As a result of depleted iron stores, fewer red cells are produced by the marrow in an attempt to conserve iron. The morphology of a peripheral smear during the first stage of iron deficiency is that of a normocytic, normochromic anemia.

The second stage of iron-deficiency anemia occurs with continued iron depletion, when the marrow is forced to produce red cells with lower levels of hemoglobin; the peripheral smear is normocytic, hypochromic. The third and final stage of iron-deficiency anemia occurs after further depletion; this is characterized by deterioration of both the quality and quantity of the erythrocytes, that is, smaller cells of lowered hemoglobin concentration; the peripheral smear reflects a microcytic, hypochromic anemia. Fewer than 20 percent of all gravidas progress to the third stage of iron-deficiency anemia; either normochromic or mildly normocytic, hypochromic red cell indices are present in more than 80 percent of cases [32].

Prevalence and Consequences of Iron Deficiency During Pregnancy

Iron deficiency is the most common nutritional disorder and the most important cause of anemia in the world [33]. Approximately 5 percent of nonpregnant women of reproductive age in the United States have anemia, but the true prevalence during pregnancy is unclear [34]. Data from the Pregnancy Nutrition Surveillance System of the Centers for Disease Control for 1987 indicated that among low-income women the rate of anemia varied by trimester and maternal race [35]. Among white gravidas, the prevalence of anemia was 3.5, 6.4, and 18.8 percent, respectively, during the first, second, and third trimesters. Among black gravidas, the prevalence was 12.7, 17.8, and 38.1 percent, respectively, during the first, second, and third trimesters. The high prevalence of anemia during the third trimester indicates that many low-income women have poor iron stores both before and during pregnancy. Data from the 1976 to 1980 National Health and Nutrition Examination Survey (NHANES) and the 1982 to 1984 Hispanic HANES previously had indicated that risk factors for iron deficiency included low socioeconomic status, low level of education, black or Hispanic background, and high parity [25, 34].

Anemia causes a reduction in the capacity to do energy-requiring tasks by imposing a limit on the oxygen transport to the tissues. Iron deficiency may cause systemic effects by impairing the immune response and the ability of an individual to resist infection [36, 37]. Imposed on the physiologic stresses of pregnancy, severe anemia increases maternal morbidity and mortality, and also increases the risk to the fetus [38, 39]. Anemic gravidas are less able to withstand serious hemorrhage; the risk of maternal death from hemorrhage in the presence of iron-deficiency anemia has been established. These women also have a greater incidence of premature deliveries associated with increased stillbirth and perinatal mortality, as well as low birth weight [38, 39].

Anemia may cause more direct pathology during pregnancy. Reduced oxygen tension in the amniotic fluid, hypertrophy of the placenta, low estriol excretion, and placental insufficiency have all been associated with iron-deficiency anemia. An increased incidence of urinary tract infections and pyelonephritis has been reported among anemic gravidas, as well as preeclampsia and pica [3, 40].

Diagnosis of Iron Deficiency in Pregnancy

If iron-deficiency anemia is suspected during pregnancy, a thorough review of the dietary history should be initiated to include past and present patterns of food preferences and specific items such as fad and reducing diets and food allergies. A thorough menstrual history should also be documented, including menstrual blood losses and type of previous contraception. The obstetric history is also important; blood losses with previous pregnancies should be noted. Intercurrent respiratory/urinary tract infections should be ruled out. Patients with acute pyelonephritis should not be considered iron deficient until the infection has been treated and resolved, and the studies repeated.

A normal increase in erythrocyte volume and a large increase in plasma volume result in a low hemoglobin concentration without anemia. A small rise in plasma volume may lead to the maintenance of a normal hemoglobin concentration in the gravida who is iron deficient. A lowered hematocrit or packed cell volume may fail to detect up to 25 percent of pregnant women with deficient iron stores [3]. The Centers for Disease Control recommended cutoff values to define anemia are: first and third trimesters, hemoglobin less than 11 gm/100 ml or hematocrit less than 33 percent; second trimester, hemoglobin less than 10.5 gm/100 ml or hematocrit less than 32 percent [41].

The **percent saturation** of the serum transferrin, expressed as the serum iron/TIBC × 100, is also useful to diagnose iron deficiency. Iron saturation of transferrin is a valid predictor of iron status in pregnancy. In the nonpregnant woman with iron deficiency, the percent saturation is below 16 percent. During pregnancy, a decrease in the percent saturation of transferrin below 16 percent indicates insufficient iron stores. Increased estrogen levels induce a rise in transferrin during pregnancy; serum iron is not so affected. The blood specimens for serum iron/TIBC should be drawn in the morning because of the diurnal fluctuation in circulating iron, with lower values in the afternoon and evening hours.

The **total iron binding capacity (TIBC)** rises in iron deficiency; it also normally rises in the iron-sufficient pregnant woman. The normal range is between 250 and 450 μg/100 ml. With chronic infection, chronic inflammatory disease, and malignancy, the percent saturation is depressed below 16 percent, with the TIBC less than 300 μg/100 ml (low-normal to depressed). A TIBC value greater than 350 μg/100 ml represents a combination of iron deficiency and pregnancy-induced iron-binding capacity elevation. The usual rise during pregnancy from 3 mg per liter to 5 to 6 mg per liter is only slightly reduced with therapeutic iron.

A **serum iron** value of less than 42 μg/100 ml is indicative of iron deficiency and correlates with a red blood cell count of less than 4,000,000/cu mm [3]. The fall in serum iron can be modified but not fully prevented by therapeutically ingested iron.

A **mean corpuscular volume (MCV)** of less than 82 cuμ is indicative of iron deficiency [3]. In pure iron deficiency, the MCV is decreased; in folate deficiency, it is increased; and in the presence of both (dimorphic), it is normal.

Storage iron has been related to **plasma ferritin** [42]. Eight micrograms of storage iron was found to be equivalent to 1 μg ferritin per liter of plasma. To meet the iron requirements of pregnancy (1100 mg), 138 μg ferritin per liter would be required. The storage ferritin in the nonpregnant population studied by Walters and associates [43] was 31.5 μg per liter. The serum ferritin seems to be the most sensitive, noninvasive method developed within recent years for identifying iron deficiency. Good correlation exists between serum ferritin concentration and the size of body iron stores (as measured by repeated phlebotomies) [43, 44], as well as bone marrow hemosiderin [42]. An inverse correlation occurs between serum ferritin and iron absorption in normal subjects [45]. The World Health Organization [46] has stated that ". . . the serum ferritin measurement may prove to be the single most effective tool for evaluating the iron status of different population groups and especially those in which anemia is not prevalent."

The concentration of **free protoporphyrin** in the erythrocytes is increased in pregnancy. The rise in iron deficiency is much greater, from 0.5 mg per liter to 3 mg per liter erythrocytes.

Therapy

The two principal goals of therapy for the treatment of iron-deficiency anemia are correction of the iron deficit and replenishment of the iron stores. The absorption of iron supplements is influenced by the solubility of the compound, dosage, timing of administration (with or between meals), concurrent medications (alone or as part of a vitamin-mineral supplement), and extent of physiologic iron stores. The therapeutic dosage of iron supplements should be evaluated in terms of the amount of iron in the compound, the equivalent in elemental iron, and the presence of additional ingredients that could potentially reduce iron absorption. Hydrated ferrous sulfate contains 20 percent iron by weight, and therefore 60 mg elemental iron in a 300-mg tablet [26]. Since ferrous gluconate contains 12 percent iron by weight and ferrous fumarate contains 32 percent iron by weight, a 300-mg tablet would contain, respectively, 36 mg and 96 mg elemental iron. The highest availability of therapeutic iron derives from ferrous sulfate and such organic complexes or chelates of iron as the ascorbate, fumarate, and citrate complexes; reduced (metallic) iron is intermediate. Iron phosphates, carbonates, or ethylenediaminetetraacetic acid (EDTA) complexes exhibit poor bioavailability. The absorption of iron is much greater when the supplement contains only an iron salt than when the iron is part of a vitamin-mineral compound [47]. Calcium carbonate, citrate, and phosphate all have been shown to inhibit iron absorption [47, 48], as do magnesium [47] and zinc [49–51]. Although ascorbic acid (vitamin C) increases the absorption of nonheme iron [7], excessive amounts can cause serious side effects. For example, large doses of vitamin C can interfere with vitamin B_{12} absorption and metabolism, an effect that cannot be overcome by higher vitamin B_{12} supplementation [52]. Healthy adults can become conditioned to high doses of vitamin C (500–1500 mg/day) over a period as short as 2 weeks, with resultant abnormally low serum and leukocyte ascorbic acid levels when they resume normal dietary intake of vitamin C [53]. Rebound scurvy during the neonatal period has been reported in infants whose mothers ingested 400 mg (less than six times the RDA) vitamin C during pregnancy [54].

The Institute of Medicine's 1990 report on nutrition during pregnancy [26] recommended the routine use of 30 mg ferrous iron per day beginning at about the 12th week of gestation. The iron supplement should include a type of iron that has a high bioavailability (ferrous sulfate or fumarate), is free from additional ingredients that could lower the absorption of iron (such as calcium, magnesium, or zinc), and, if part of a multivitamin, does not contain excessive levels of additional vitamins or minerals. A comparison of iron supplements is given in Table 7-5.

Conclusions and Recommendations

Pregnancy imposes special demand for iron that may not be adequately met in women with low or absent iron stores. A thorough hematologic evaluation is important to establish the extent of iron stores at the onset of pregnancy and to prescribe appropriate therapy. Animal sources of iron are the best-absorbed dietary sources because of their content of heme iron. Ferrous sulfate has the highest bioavailability of the medicinal forms of iron. Because iron-deficiency anemia during pregnancy is associated with an increased risk of morbidity and mortality for both the mother and her unborn child, assessment of iron status and provision of appropriate therapy are important considerations of optimal prenatal care.

Table 7-5
Comparison of iron supplements

Supplement and manufacturer	*Iron content type*	*Equivalent elemental Fe (mg)*	*Inhibiting factors*			*Additives in excess of twice the RDA**
			Ca	*Mg*	*Zn*	
Berocca Plus Roche	Ferrous fumarate	27	–	+	+	1, 2, 3, 4, 5, 6
Ferancee Johnson & Johnson	Ferrous fumarate	134	–	+	–	1
Ferancee-HP Johnson & Johnson	Ferrous fumarate	110	–	–	–	1
Fero-Folic-500 Abbott	Ferrous sulfate	105	+	+	–	1
Fero-Grad-500 Abbott	Ferrous sulfate	105	–	+	–	1
Fero-Gradumet Abbott	Ferrous sulfate	105	–	+	–	1
Ferro-Sequels Lederle	Ferrous fumarate	150	–	+	–	0
Iberet Abbott	Ferrous sulfate	105	+	+	–	3, 4, 5, 6
Iberet-500 Abbott	Ferrous sulfate	105	+	+	–	1, 3, 4, 5, 6
Iberet-Folic-500 Abbott	Ferrous sulfate	105	+	+	–	1, 3, 4, 5, 6
Irospan Fielding	Ferrous sulfate	200	–	–	–	0
Materna Lederle	Ferrous fumarate	60	+	+	+	3, 5, 6
Mevanin-C Beutlich	Ferrous sulfate	65	+	+	+	1
Natalins Mead Johnson	Ferrous fumarate	110	+	+	+	0
Natalins Rx Mead Johnson	Ferrous fumarate	60	+	+	+	0
Peritinic Lederle	Ferrous fumarate	100	–	+	–	1, 3, 4, 5, 6
Pramet FA Ross	Ferrous sulfate	60	+	+	–	0
Pramilet FA Ross	Ferrous fumarate	40	+	+	+	0

Table 7-5
Comparison of iron supplements (continued)

Supplement and manufacturer	*Iron content type*	*Equivalent elemental Fe (mg)*	*Inhibiting factors*			*Additives in excess of twice the RDA**
			Ca	*Mg*	*Zn*	
Prenate 90 Bock	Ferrous fumarate	90	+	−	+	0
Stuart Formula Stuart	Ferrous fumarate	18	+	+	−	0
Stuart Prenatal Johnson & Johnson	Ferrous fumarate	60	+	−	+	0
Stuartinic Johnson & Johnson	Ferrous fumarate	100	+	−	−	1, 3, 4, 6
Stuartnatal 1 + 1 Stuart	Ferrous fumarate	65	+	−	+	5, 6
Zenate Reid-Rowell	Ferrous fumarate	65	+	+	+	5, 6

*Code for additives in excess of twice the RDA (recommended dietary allowance): 0, none; 1, vitamin C; 2, niacin; 3, thiamin; 4, riboflavin; 5, pyridoxine; 6, cyanocobalamin.

The Institute of Medicine [25] recommends the following clinical regimen to prevent iron deficiency during pregnancy:

1. The routine use of 30 mg ferrous iron per day beginning at about the 12th week of gestation, in conjunction with a well-balanced diet that contains enhancers of iron absorption (ascorbic acid, meats).
2. The supplemental iron should be taken between meals with liquids other than milk, tea, or coffee.
3. Hemoglobin or hematocrit should be routinely determined at the first prenatal visit in order to detect preexisting anemia. A hemoglobin level below 11 gm/100 ml during the first or third trimesters or below 10.5 gm/100 ml during the second trimester is defined as anemia. Anemia accompanied by a serum ferritin concentration less than 12 μg/100 ml can be presumed to be iron-deficiency anemia and requires treatment with 60 to 120 mg ferrous iron daily. When the hemoglobin concentration becomes normal for the stage of gestation, the iron dose can be decreased to 30 mg per day.

References

1. American Medical Association Committee on Iron Deficiency: Iron deficiency in the United States. *J.A.M.A.* 203:407, 1968.
2. Letsky, E: The Haematological System. In F Hytten and G Chamberlain (eds.), *Clinical Physiology in Obstetrics* (2nd ed.). London: Blackwell Scientific, 1991. Pp. 39–82.
3. Kitay, DZ, and Harbort, RA: Iron and folate deficiency in pregnancy. *Clin. Perinatol.* 2:225, 1975.
4. Roche, M, and Layrisse, M: The nature and causes of hookworm anemia. *Am. J. Trop. Med. Hyg.* 15:1031, 1966.
5. *Nutritional Anaemias: Report of a WHO Scientific Group.* WHO Technical Report Series No. 405, Geneva, Switzerland, 1968.
6. Food and Nutrition Board, Institute of Medicine: Trace Elements, Iron. In *Recommended Dietary Allowances* (10th ed.). Washington, DC: National Academy Press, 1989. Pp. 195–205.
7. Monsen, ER: Iron nutrition and absorption: Dietary factors which impact iron availability. *J. Am. Diet. Assoc.* 88:786–790, 1988.
8. Rossander, L, and Bjorn-Rasmussen, E: Absorption of iron from breakfast meals. *Am. J. Clin. Nutr.* 32:2484–2489, 1979.
9. Disler, PB, et al: The effect of tea on iron absorption. *Gut* 16:193, 1975.
10. Morck, TA, Lynch, SR, and Cook, JD: Inhibition of food iron absorption by coffee. *Am. J. Clin. Nutr.* 37:416–420, 1983.
11. Munoz, LM, Lonnerdal, B, Keen, CL, and Dewey, KG: Coffee consumption as a factor in iron deficiency anemia among pregnant women and their infants in Costa Rica. *Am. J. Clin. Nutr.* 48:645–651, 1988.
12. Hallberg, L, and Rossander, L: Effect of different drinks on the absorption of non-heme iron from composite meals. *Hum. Nutr. Appl. Nutr.* 36A: 116–123, 1982.
13. de Alarcon, PA: Iron absorption in the thalassemia syndromes and its inhibition by tea. *N. Engl. J. Med.* 300:5, 1979.
14. Hallberg, L, Brune, M, Erlandsson, M, et al: Effect of different amounts of nonheme- and heme-iron absorption in humans. *Am. J. Clin. Nutr.* 53:112–119, 1991.
15. Callender, ST, et al: Eggs and iron absorption. *Br. J. Haematol.* 19:657, 1970.
16. Layrisse, M, et al: Measurement of the total daily dietary iron absorption by the extrinsic tag method. *Am. J. Clin. Nutr.* 27:152, 1974.
17. Martinez-Torres, C, and Layrisse, M: Effect of amino acids on iron absorption from a staple vegetable food. *Blood* 35:669, 1970.
18. Martinez-Torres, C, and Layrisse, M: Iron absorption from veal muscle. *Am. J. Clin. Nutr.* 24:531, 1971.
19. Hallberg, L, et al: Iron absorption from Southeast Asian diets. *Am. J. Clin. Nutr.* 27:826, 1974.
20. Sayers, MH, et al: Iron absorption from rice meals cooked with fortified salt containing ferrous sulfate and ascorbic acid. *Br. J. Med.* 31:367, 1974.

21. Food and Agriculture Organization: *Requirements of Vitamin A, Iron, Folate, and Vitamin B-12*. Report of a Joint FAO/WHO Expert Consultation. FAO Food and Nutrition Series No. 23. Rome: Food and Agriculture Organization, 1988.
22. National Academy of Sciences: *Recommended Dietary Allowances* (10th ed.). Washington, DC: National Academy Press, 1989.
23. United States Department of Agriculture, Human Nutrition Information Service: *Nationwide Food Consumption Survey. Continuing Survey of Food Intakes by Individuals*. NFCS, CSFII, Rep. Nos. 86-1 and 86-2, 1987.
24. Hallberg, L: Iron Balance in Pregnancy. In H Berger (ed.), *Vitamins and Minerals in Pregnancy and Lactation*. New York: Raven, 1988. Pp. 115–127.
25. Food and Nutrition Board, Institute of Medicine: Iron Nutrition During Pregnancy. In *Nutrition During Pregnancy*. Washington, DC: National Academy Press, 1990. Pp. 272–298.
26. Scott, DE, and Pritchard, JA: Anemia in pregnancy. *Clin. Perinatol.* 1:491, 1974.
27. Hytten, FE, and Lind, T: *Diagnostic Indices in Pregnancy*. Basel, Switzerland: CIBA-GEIGY, 1973. P. 36.
28. Svanberg, B, Arvidsson, B, Norrby, A, et al: Absorption of supplemental iron during pregnancy: A longitudinal study with repeated bone-marrow studies and absorption measurements. *Acta Obstet. Gynecol. Scand. Suppl.* 48:87–108, 1975.
29. Sjostedt, JE, Manner, P, Nummi, S, and Ekenved, G: Oral iron prophylaxis during pregnancy: A comparative study on different dosage regimens. *Acta Obstet. Gynecol. Scand. Suppl.* 60:3–9, 1977.
30. Puolakka, J, Janne, O, Pakarinen, A, et al: Serum ferritin as a measure of iron stores during and after normal pregnancy with and without iron supplements. *Acta Obstet. Gynecol. Scand. Suppl.* 95:43–51, 1980.
31. Taylor, DJ, Mallen, C, McDougall, N, and Lind, T: Effect of iron supplementation on serum ferritin levels during and after pregnancy. *Br. J. Obstet. Gynecol.* 89:1011–1017, 1982.
32. Carr, MC: Managing iron deficiency in pregnancy. *Contemp. Obstet. Gynecol.* 4:15, 1974.
33. DeMaeyer, D, and Adiels-Tegman, M: The prevalence of anaemia in the world. *World Health Stat. Q.* 38:302–316, 1985.
34. Dallman, PR, Yip, R, and Johnson, C: Prevalence and causes of anemia in the United States, 1976 to 1980. *Am. J. Clin. Nutr.* 39:437–445, 1984.
35. Anemia during pregnancy in low-income women—United States, 1987. *MMWR* 39:73–81, 1990.
36. Chandra, RK: Iron and immunocompetence. *Nutr. Rev.* 34:129, 1976.
37. The relationship between infection and the iron status of an individual. *Nutr. Rev.* 33:103, 1975.
38. Murphy, JF, O'Riordan, J, Newcombe, RG, et al: Relation of haemo-

globin levels in first and second trimester to outcome of pregnancy. *Lancet* 1:992–995, 1986.

39. Garn, SM, Ridella, SA, Petzold, AS, and Falkner, F: Maternal hematologic levels and pregnancy outcomes. *Semin. Perinatol.* 5:155–162, 1981.
40. Danford, DE: Pica and nutrition. *Ann. Rev. Nutr.* 2:303–322, 1982.
41. Centers for Disease Control: CDC criteria for anemia in children and childbearing aged women. *MMWR* 38:400–404, 1989.
42. Lipschitz, DA, et al: A clinical evaluation of serum ferritin as an index of iron stores. *N. Engl. J. Med.* 209:1213, 1974.
43. Walters, GO, Miller, FM, and Worwood, M: Serum ferritin concentration and iron stores in normal subjects. *J. Clin. Pathol.* 26:770, 1973.
44. Jacobs, A, et al: Ferritin in the serum of normal subjects and patients with iron deficiency and iron overload. *Br. Med. J.* 4:206, 1972.
45. Cook, JD, et al: Serum ferritin as a measure of iron stores in normal subjects. *Am. J. Clin. Nutr.* 27:681, 1974.
46. *Control of Nutritional Anaemia With Special Reference to Iron Deficiency.* WHO Technical Report Series No. 580, Geneva, Switzerland, 1975.
47. Seligman, PA, Caskey, JH, Frazier, JL, et al: Measurements of iron absorption from prenatal multivitamin-mineral supplements. *Obstet. Gynecol.* 61:356–362, 1983.
48. Babior, BM, Peters, WA, Briden, PM, and Cetrulo, CL: Pregnant women's absorption of iron from prenatal supplements. *J. Reprod. Med.* 30:355–357, 1985.
49. Crofton, RW, Gvozdanovic, D, Gvozdanovic, S, et al: Inorganic zinc and the intestinal absorption of ferrous iron. *Am. J. Clin. Nutr.* 50:141–144, 1989.
50. Sandstrom, B, Davidsson, L, Cederblad, A, and Lonnerdal, B: Oral iron, dietary ligands and zinc absorption. *J. Nutr.* 115:411–414, 1985.
51. Solomons, NW: Competitive interaction of iron and zinc in the diet: Consequences for human nutrition. *J. Nutr.* 116:927–935, 1986.
52. Herbert, V, and Jacob, E: Destruction of vitamin B-12 by ascorbic acid. *J.A.M.A.* 230:241, 1974.
53. Rhead, WJ, and Schrauzer, GN: Risks of long-term ascorbic acid overdosage. *Nutr. Rev.* 29:262, 1971.
54. Cochrane, WA: Overnutrition in prenatal and neonatal life: A problem? *Can. Med. Assoc. J.* 93:893, 1965.

Advertisement in *Practical Dietetics with Reference to Diet in Disease*. (From AF Pattee. *Practical Dietetics with Reference to Diet in Disease*. [5th ed.]. New York: Pattee, 1905.)

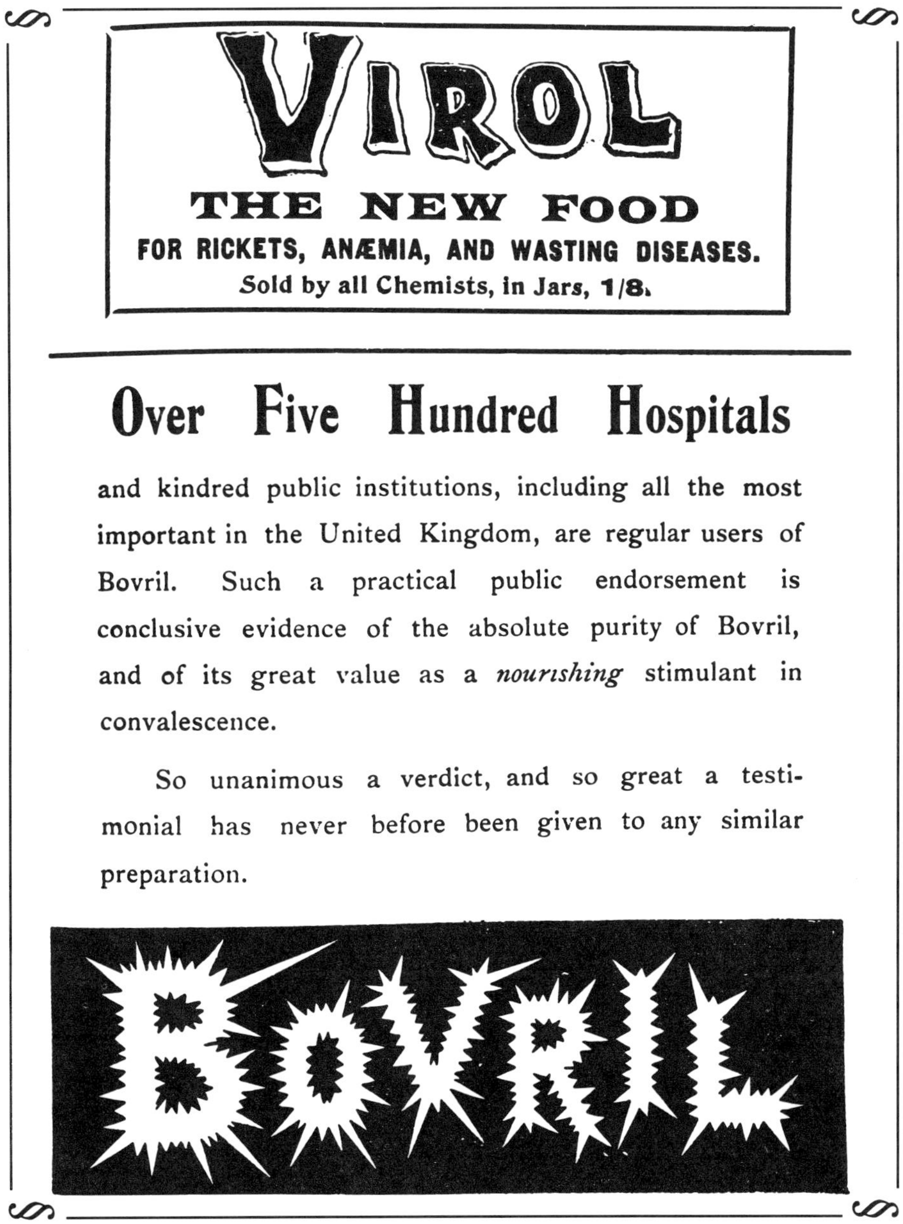

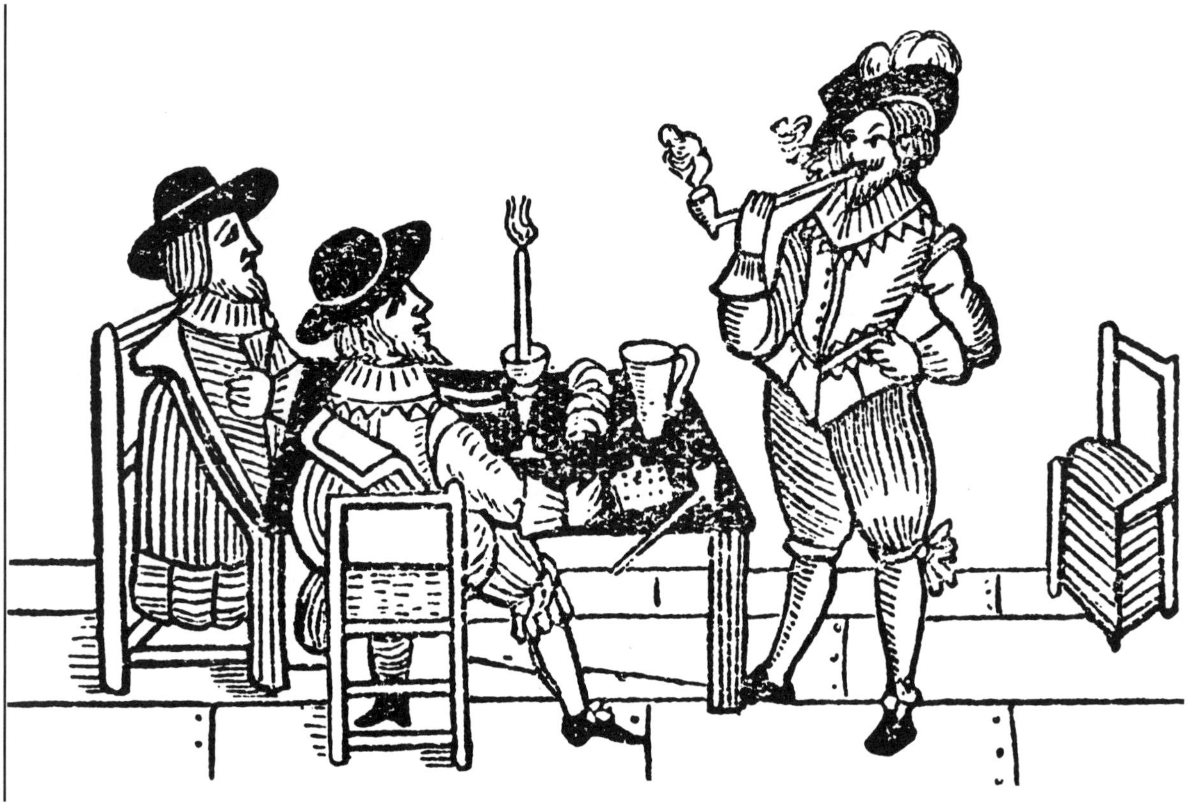

St. Nicotine of the Peace Pipe. (From E. Heward. *St. Nicotine of the Peace Pipe*. London: George Routledge, 1909.)

8 Smoking

Smoking during pregnancy induces a unique spectrum of metabolic and biochemical changes in the mother and adaptive responses in the fetus and placenta. This altered prenatal environment results in increased maternal complications, as well as a special type of fetal malnutrition, the long-term consequences of which are not completely known. Although the overall prevalence of smoking in the United States has declined in the past 20 years, it is still a fairly common practice among pregnant women. Between 1965 and 1987, the proportion of women of childbearing age who smoked decreased from 40 percent to 30 percent [1]. Data from two national samples of live births to married women (the 1967 and 1980 National Natality Surveys) indicate that the prevalence of smoking during pregnancy has decreased during this time [2]. Among women aged 20 and older, the prevalence of smoking during pregnancy decreased from 40 percent to 25 percent among whites and 33 percent to 23 percent among blacks. Women with 16 years of education (college graduates) showed the greatest reduction in smoking during pregnancy over this time period, from 38 percent to 15 percent. Data from the Behavioral Risk Factor Surveillance System in 1985 and 1986 indicate that the overall prevalence of smoking in pregnancy was 21 percent, with higher rates for unmarried women (36%) compared to married women (18%) [3].

Since the late 1950s and early 1960s, many studies have concluded that maternal smoking exerts numerous adverse effects on reproduction and fetal growth [4–8]. First, a reduction in birthweight ranging from 150 to 325 gm is the most consistently reported observation [9–12]. Second, a mother who smokes is nearly twice as likely to deliver a low-birthweight infant (<2500 gm) as is a nonsmoking mother [12]. Third, the influence of smoking is dose-related, with the number of cigarettes smoked per day inversely proportional to birthweight. Infants of "heavy" smokers are more affected than those of "light" smokers, and smoking during "whole" pregnancy is worse than smoking during "part" pregnancy. Further, "active" smoking is worse than "passive" smoking [13–16]. In addition, the effects of maternal smoking appear to be independent of other factors, such as race, parity, socioeconomic status, pregravid weight, and gestational weight gain. Evidence also suggests that the adverse effects of smoking demonstrate a cause-and-effect relationship and are not due to differences in the characteristics of smokers and nonsmokers. Other adverse effects of maternal smoking include increased rates of stillbirth, neonatal mortality, and prematurity, as well as increased bleeding during pregnancy, spontaneous abortion, ectopic and tubal pregnancies, premature rupture of the membranes, and placental complications (abruptio placentae, placenta previa) [9, 14–19]. This increased mortality and morbidity may stem from the effects of cigarette smoke and its components on the infant, the placenta, hemodynamic relationships, maternal-fetal nutrition, or any combination of these factors.

Physiologic Effects of Carbon Monoxide from Cigarette Smoke

Cigarette smoke contains approximately 5 percent carbon monoxide (CO) by volume. Hemoglobin has an affinity of 210 times greater for CO than for oxygen, combining to form the inactive, stable pigment **carboxyhemoglobin** (COHb). Hemoglobin partially linked to CO releases its oxygen at a lower partial pressure (a proportionate decrease in the oxygen-carrying capacity of the blood), resulting in a shift to the left of the adult oxygen dissociation curve (Haldave-Smith effect). The mean COHb level in nonsmokers is 1.2 percent; for smokers, it ranges from 4.1 to 8.0 percent [20, 21].

There is a positive correlation between the number of cigarettes smoked per day and the COHb level. Because carboxyhemoglobin results in elevated hemoglobin concentrations in smokers in proportion to the number of cigarettes smoked per day, the Centers for Disease Control recently recommended higher hemoglobin and hematocrit cutoff values in identifying the risk of anemia for smokers [22] (Table 8-1). Chronic hypoxia due to increased COHb levels triggers numerous homeostatic mechanisms in the maternal-fetal

Table 8-1
Cutoff values for anemia in women: nonpregnant and pregnant, smokers and nonsmokers

	Hemoglobin (gm/100 ml)			*Hematocrit (%)*		
	Nonsmokers	*Smokers*		*Nonsmokers*	*Smokers*	
		*10–20**	*21–40**		*10–20**	*21–40**
Nonpregnant	12.0	12.3	12.5	36.0	37.0	37.5
Pregnant						
1st trimester	11.0	11.3	11.5	33.0	34.0	34.5
2nd trimester	10.5	10.8	11.0	32.0	33.0	33.5
3rd trimester	11.0	11.3	11.5	33.0	34.0	34.5

*Number of cigarettes smoked per day.

Source: Adapted from Centers for Disease Control criteria for anemia in children and childbearing-aged women. *MMWR* 38:400–404, 1989.

unit to guarantee a continuous supply of oxygen in the respective compartments of the maternal-fetal-placental unit: **maternal:** increased ventilation, cardiac output, changes in the distribution of blood flow; **placental:** increased size and surface area, increased vascularity, decreased diffusion distance; **fetal:** increases in hemoglobin and hematocrit, decreased oxygen consumption, and redistribution of blood flow in favor of the most vital organs [11]. The chronic hypoxia caused by altitude is also reflected in birthweight: As the elevation increases, birthweight decreases and the ratio of placental weight to birthweight increases [23]. A low arterial oxygen tension (PO_2) in the mother, and presumably the fetus, leads to growth retardation. The placental ratio (placental weight–birthweight) increases in proportion to smoking level [24]. In animal studies a direct correlation has been shown between fetal oxygen consumption and birthweight [25]. Inhalation of CO results in a fall in arterial oxygen tension and therefore a lower oxygen saturation in the blood. The presence of CO can reduce tissue oxygenation by combining with a portion of the hemoglobin, causing a reduction in the total oxygen-carrying capacity of both the mother and the fetus. Also, the oxygen dissociation of the remaining active hemoglobin is impaired by the presence of CO. The resultant tissue hypoxia, together with a reduction in fetal and maternal oxygen-carrying capacity and in maternal arterial oxygen tension, is a contributing factor in the low birthweights and other reported consequences of smoking during pregnancy. The lower fetal weight and higher placental ratio may aid in fetal survival by increasing oxygen exchange and decreasing oxygen demand under conditions of reduced partial pressure. The infants of smokers have a significantly higher hemoglobin concentration and red cell volume than infants of nonsmokers, indicating a compensatory response to chronic prenatal oxygen deprivation [26]. The growth-retarding effects of cigarette smoking are dose-dependent, with reductions in birthweight of 5 to 13 gm per cigarette per day [27, 28].

Placenta

Long-term exposure to low levels of oxygen, CO, or maternal smoking may alter arterial linings, a possible explanation of the increased vascular complications observed among smoking gravidas. These changes may result in increased permeability of the endothelium and leakage of plasma and some red cells into the subendothelial space [29]. As a reaction to the smoke-induced injury of the placental vasculature, calcium deposition may occur at a more rapid rate, resulting in acceleration of placental maturation, which can be detected by ultrasound [30]. Recent investigations have demonstrated an acceleration of ultrasonically detectable changes in placental maturation in mothers who smoke [30] (Fig. 8-1). Premature aging of the placenta is associated with an increased risk of intrauterine growth retardation, fetal distress, and perinatal death [31–33]. The increased incidence of abruptio placentae and intrauterine growth retardation in pregnancies in which the mother smoked may be a result of accelerated placental aging [15, 16, 34–36].

Placental Ratio

As noted previously, the placental ratio increases in proportion to the smoking level [24]. This ratio is higher in pregnancies in which the mother smoked than in those in which she did not. Among smokers, the placental ratio is higher among heavy smokers (>20 cigarettes per day) [24]. As infant birthweight increases, the placental ratio decreases. The effects of high altitude on birthweight are also reflected in the placental ratio: Higher ratios are observed in births at high altitudes [23]. A high placental ratio has also been found in gravidas with severe anemia [37]. The finding of an increased placental ratio is independent of differences in maternal weight gain or length of gestation.

Hemorrhage

Antepartum hemorrhage, early and late bleeding, anemia, and placental complications are more frequent in pregnancies in which the gravida smoked [15, 30]. The incidence of bleeding and anemia among smokers is higher among blacks than whites [38]. Blacks may be more and differently affected than whites in that carbon monoxide may affect the carriers of sickle cell anemia and glucose 6-phosphate dehydrogenase deficiency anemia differently.

Nutrition-Related Effects

Nicotine, the component of tobacco that causes dependence, alters taste perception and, indirectly, body weight. Compared to nonsmokers, smokers have a decreased preference for sweet foods [39]. The weight gain commonly associated with the cessation of smoking (withdrawal from nicotine) may be due to an increased consumption of refined carbohydrates (sugar) [40]. Nicotine has been shown

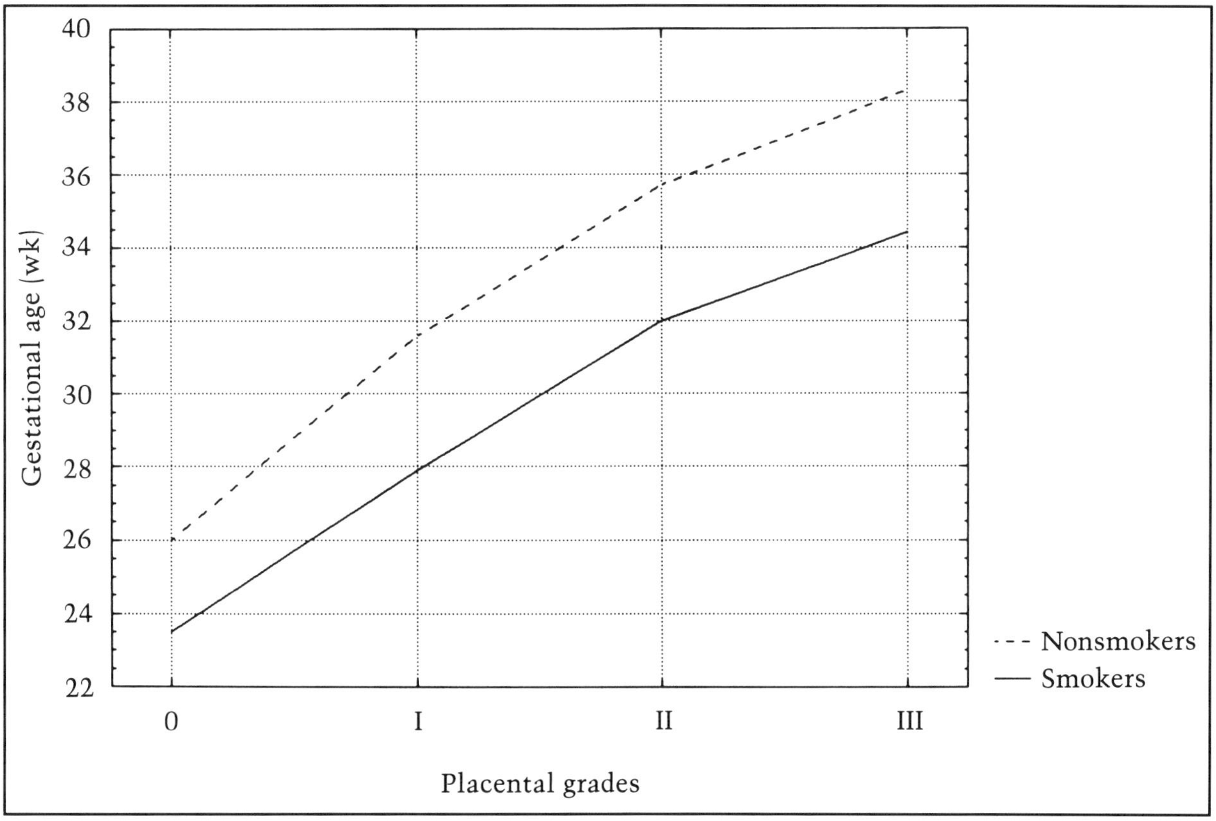

Fig. 8-1
Mean gestational age at appearance of placental grades 0, I, II, and III. (Adapted from MG Pinette et al., *Obstet. Gynecol.* 73:379–382, 1989.)

to increase basal metabolic rate at rest and during exercise, and the weight gain following smoking cessation may also be due to a lowering of the basal metabolic rate [41].

Cyanide, a component of cigarette smoke, is detoxified in the body in three ways or excreted unchanged by the lungs. The principal route of detoxification is by combination with thiosulfate, which requires the liver enzyme rhodanase; thiocyanate becomes the principal detoxification product. Cyanide can also combine with cystine and other amino acids; in cases of marginal dietary intake, however, this route competes with the fetus for available protein. In the last pathway, cyanide may combine with hydroxycobalamin to form physiologically inactive cyanocobalamin.

Under normal conditions, several factors affect the level of serum vitamin B_{12}. Pregnancy itself causes levels to drop. Low levels have been associated with premature delivery, intrauterine growth retardation, or both [42, 43]. The serum vitamin B_{12} level is lower in gravidas who smoke than in nonsmokers, and the level is also lower in women who are anemic and in those who are delivered of smaller babies [44]. These findings may reflect the combined effects of compromised oxygenation and nutritional state on the products of conception.

Other nutrients adversely affected by maternal smoking include vitamins A and C, zinc, and folate [45–47]. Both dietary intake and serum levels of ascorbic acid (vitamin C) have been shown to be lower in smokers than in nonsmokers [45, 48]. Smokers may require up to twice as much vitamin C to maintain a body pool of vitamin C comparable to that of nonsmokers.

Zinc is an essential element for many aspects of fetal growth and development [49]. It is required for the synthesis of nucleic acids and for protein synthesis. Interactions with cadmium, a toxic component of cigarette smoke, may partially explain the fetal growth retardation observed in infants of women who smoke [50]. In addition, cadmium may exert an adverse effect by competing with zinc in zinc-requiring metalloenzymes. Each cigarette smoked contains approximately 1 μg cadmium [51]. Cadmium in cigarette smoke may decrease placental transfer of zinc [50]. In addition, pregnant smokers have higher placental levels of cadmium and zinc, and their infants have lower red blood cell levels of zinc [50]. In pregnancies in which the mother smoked, increased maternal whole blood cadmium and decreased cord vein red blood cell zinc levels were both reported to be significantly related to decreased birthweight [52]. The infant of a smoking mother may therefore be marginally zinc deficient [53].

Studies of maternal plasma amino acids during pregnancy have also shown differences between nonsmokers and smokers suggestive of a relative malnutrition among the latter [54]. Crosby and associates [54] reported that all amino acids, including the eight essential amino acids that cannot be synthesized in vivo, were significantly lower in smokers than in nonsmokers.

Additional research indicates that smokers and nonsmokers differ in dietary habits, in contrast to the diets of ex-smokers, which are similar to those of people who never smoked [55, 56]. Smokers consume less cereals and fewer vegetables and fruits, but more meats, fats, alcohol, and coffee than people who never smoked. Other studies have reported that all nutrients are lower in the diets of smokers compared to nonsmokers [57].

Some investigators hypothesize a more direct agent as the cause of fetal growth retardation among infants of smoking gravidas. They suggest that a large part of the effect of maternal smoking is mediated through maternal weight gain, with a very small additional direct effect on the fetus [58, 59]. These investigators found that nonsmokers tended to gain more than heavy smokers (>15 cigarettes per day), with light to moderate smokers being intermediate. They hypothesize that smoking depresses fetal growth by suppressing caloric intake, as reflected by a lower maternal weight gain. Other investigators have shown that higher gestational weight gain, alone and in combination with higher pregravid weight, may counteract a considerable amount of the fetal growth-retarding effects of maternal smoking [60, 61]. Data from the 1980 National Natality Survey show that although mean infant birthweight parallels increases in maternal pregravid weight and weight gain, infants of smokers are lighter overall than those of nonsmokers [62] (Table 8-2). Meyer [63] reported a direct correlation between the number of cigarettes smoked during pregnancy and the percent of low-birthweight infants within each level of maternal weight gain. Luke and associates [60] reported that within maternal pregravid weight categories and weight gain groups, infants of smokers not only had lower birthweights, but also had smaller head circumferences and birthlengths compared to infants of nonsmokers (Fig. 8-2). D'Souza and colleagues [64] also reported lower birthweights, smaller head circumferences, and shorter birthlengths among infants of smokers, but in addition found skin-

Table 8-2
Mean birthweight (gm) of term infants by maternal pregravid weight, gestational weight gain, and smoking habits

Pregravid weight and smoking groups	*Gestational weight gain*				
	<16 lb	*16–20 lb*	*21–25 lb*	*26–35 lb*	*>36 lb*
Underweight					
Smoker	2631	2811	3069	3174	3314
Nonsmoker	2927	3100	3276	3374	3483
Normal weight					
Smoker	2918	3065	3135	3292	3398
Nonsmoker	3097	3231	3428	3471	3606
Overweight					
Smoker	3258	3365	3379	3384	3519
Nonsmoker	3330	3458	3526	3581	3665

Source: Adapted from the National Center for Health Statistics' 1980 National Natality Survey.

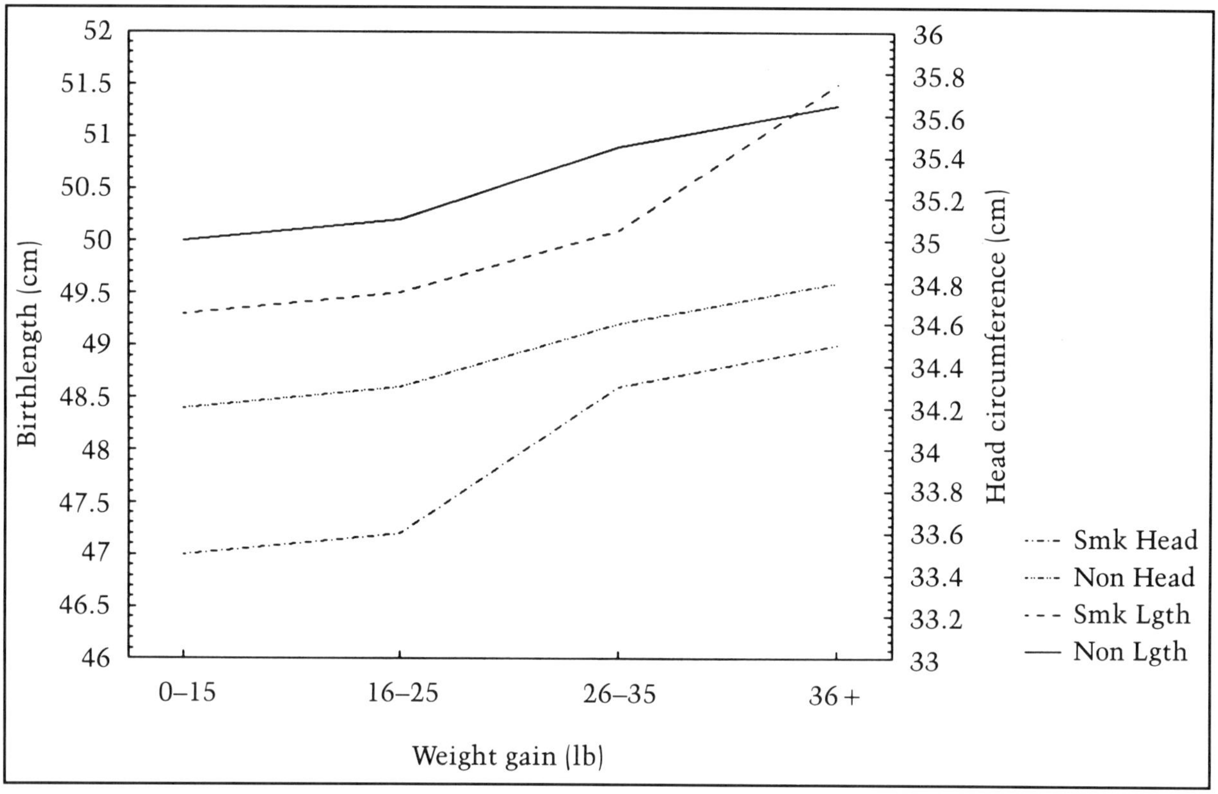

Fig. 8-2
Mean birthweight (lgth) and head circumference of term infants of smokers (smk) and nonsmokers (non) by gestational weight gain categories. (Adapted from B. Luke et al., *Am. J. Clin. Nutr.* 34:1410–1417, 1981.)

fold thicknesses of infants of smokers and nonsmokers to be comparable, suggesting that the growth retardation did not have a nutritional basis.

Influence on Infant Growth and Development

Davies and associates [58] noted that infants born to nonsmokers were heavier and longer with larger head circumferences than infants of smokers. These investigators described the second of two types of growth retardation previously documented by Gruenwald [65]. These are (1) the long, thin baby—the result of wasting during a period of days before birth, and (2) the small, proportionate baby—the result of a general cessation of fetal growth extending over a period of weeks, with resultant deficits in body weight and length at birth. Miller and colleagues [66] redefined these types of fetal growth retardation and applied them to the infants of smoking gravidas. The first type was shown to have an abnormally low ponderal index (PI) (birthweight/[length]^3). They suggested that the pathogenesis of this first type was due to an inadequate supply of nutrients in the latter part of pregnancy, and is most often observed in the infants of women with inadequate late gestational weight gain. During the postnatal period these infants show an increased appetite and accelerated growth, so that by 3 to 6 months of age they have caught up in weight to infants with normal prenatal growth. The authors concluded that infants with abnormally low PIs have a reversible type of growth retardation.

The second type of fetal growth retardation described by Miller and associates [66] was stunted in length, or short for dates. This type is most often seen among infants of smoking gravidas and was thought to be the result of some earlier event in pregnancy that led to reduced longitudinal skeletal growth. This retardation may be irreversible because during the postnatal period these infants have ordinary appetites and continue to grow on the same low percentiles for height and weight as they exhibited at birth. Other types of growth retardation where the fetus may not have low birthweight but is either very short (low crown-heel length) or very slim (low ponderal index) have also been suggested by Daikoku and colleagues [67]. The clinical implications of these non–low-birthweight intrauterine growth retardation (IUGR) patterns and their relation to intrauterine events have not been fully described [67].

The long-term effects of maternal smoking on infant growth and development are unclear. Russell and associates [68] state that at 1 year of age, infants of smokers and nonsmokers weigh almost the same [68]. Reports from the Johns Hopkins Child Development Study found that although average birthweight was 250 gm less and body length was 1.3 cm shorter in infants of smokers, when reexamined at 1, 4, and 7 years of age, these children were without differences in weight, and the difference in height was only present at 1 year of age [69]. All children were without neurologic or psychological differences. In contrast, British investigators found that 7-year-old children whose mothers had smoked during gestation were still short in stature and had a 3-month delay in acquiring reading skills compared with children of nonsmokers [70, 71].

Birth Defects

Smoking during pregnancy has been linked to increases in birth defects [72]. Based on an analysis of the Collaborative Perinatal

Project, Naeye [72] reported that cigarette smoking during gestation was teratogenic, in contrast to previous reports [73, 74]. Naeye concluded that because malformations that lead to perinatal death were commonly interrelated in repeating clusters, single factors were likely involved in their causation. Older studies had implied positive correlations between maternal smoking and malformations that were fatal to the newborn in the perinatal period [75–78]. Analyses of the 1984 data from the Maryland Birth Defects Reporting and Information System indicated that mothers of infants with oral clefts (cleft lip with and without cleft palate, and cleft palate) smoked more during pregnancy than mothers with infants with other defects [79]. There was a dose-response relation between the amount smoked and the risk of cleft formation, even after adjustment for confounding factors.

Sudden Infant Death Syndrome

Sudden infant death syndrome (SIDS) is the second leading cause of infant mortality in the United States [80]. Maternal smoking has been linked with SIDS [81–83]. In a population-based study in Sweden between 1983 and 1985, maternal smoking was associated with twice the risk of SIDS, and a clear dose-response relationship was observed [84]. A recent report for the Centers for Disease Control on smoking-attributable mortality in the United States estimated a relative risk (RR) of 1.5 for SIDS and 1.8 for respiratory distress syndrome for the infants of mothers who smoke [85].

Cancer

Prenatal exposure to maternal cigarette smoking also increases the child's subsequent risk of cancer. Associations with maternal smoking during pregnancy have been reported for all childhood cancers [86, 87], leukemia [88], and brain cancer [89]. Twofold higher risks of acute lymphocytic leukemia, non-Hodgkin's lymphoma, and Wilms' tumor have been reported with 10 or more cigarettes per day [90]. It is estimated that 6 percent of all childhood cancers and 17 percent of acute lymphocytic leukemia may be attributable to prenatal exposure to maternal smoking [86].

Psychological Development

The chronic prenatal hypoxia experienced by the child of a mother who smokes has been linked to long-term neurodevelopmental deficits. Such children have lower intelligence quotients, 4- to 5-month retardation in reading and mathematics skills, short attention spans, and hyperactive behavior [91–95] compared to children of nonsmokers. These differences were demonstrated even after controlling for potentially confounding factors such as socioeconomic class, maternal age, and parity.

Conclusions

Although the adverse effects of maternal smoking on reproduction and birthweight have been known empirically for decades, only recently have the metabolic and biochemical mechanisms of these associations been elucidated. Maternal smoking exerts a spectrum of adverse effects on the course and outcome of pregnancy. The increased mortality and morbidity linked to smoking is the result of acute and chronic hypoxia, the toxic effect of the components of smoke and their by-products, and the compensatory effects on the maternal-fetal-placental unit. Smoking also causes unique nutritional demands, including increases in vitamins B_{12} and C, folate, zinc, and selected amino acids. Although higher pregravid weight and increased gestational weight gain can partially offset fetal growth-retarding effects of maternal smoking, pregnant women should be encouraged to stop smoking to ensure the best health for themselves and their unborn children.

References

1. National Center for Health Statistics: *Health United States 1988*. DHHS Pub. No. (PHS) 89-1232. National Center for Health Statistics, Public Health Service, US Dept. of Health and Human Services, Hyattsville, MD, 1989. 208 pp.
2. Kleinman, JC, and Kopstein, A: Smoking during pregnancy, 1967–80. *Am. J. Public Health* 77:823–825, 1987.
3. Williamson, DF, Serdula, MK, Kendrick, JS, and Binkin, NJ: Comparing the prevalence of smoking in pregnant and nonpregnant women, 1985 to 1986. *J.A.M.A.* 261:70–74, 1989.
4. Simpson, WJ: A preliminary report on cigarette smoking and the incidence of prematurity. *Am. J. Obstet. Gynecol.* 73:808–815, 1957.
5. Frazier, TM, Davis, GH, Goldstein, H, and Goldberg, ID: Cigarette smoking and prematurity: A prospective study. *Am. J. Obstet. Gynecol.* 81:988–996, 1961.
6. Ravenholt, RT, Levinski, MJ, Nellist, DJ, and Takenaga, M: Effects of smoking upon reproduction. *Am. J. Obstet. Gynecol.* 96:267–281, 1966.

7. Lowe, CR: Effect of mothers' smoking habits on birth weight of their children. *Br. Med. J.* 2:673–676, 1959.
8. Herriot, A, Billewicz, WZ, and Hytten, FE: Cigarette smoking in pregnancy. *Lancet* 1:771–773, 1962.
9. Butler, NR, Goldstein, H, and Ross, EM: Cigarette smoking in pregnancy: Its influence on birthweight and perinatal mortality. *Br. Med. J.* 2:127–130, 1972.
10. Meyer, MB, and Comstock, GW: Maternal cigarette smoking and perinatal mortality. *Am. J. Epidemiol.* 96:1, 1972.
11. Comstock, GW, and Lundin, FE: Parental smoking and perinatal mortality. *Am. J. Obstet. Gynecol.* 98:708, 1967.
12. Meyer, MB, and Tonascia, JA: Maternal smoking, pregnancy complications, and perinatal mortality. *Am. J. Obstet. Gynecol.* 128:494–502, 1977.
13. Ahlborg, G, and Bodin, L: Tobacco smoke exposure and pregnancy outcome among working women. *Am. J. Epidemiol.* 133:338–347, 1991.
14. Meberg, A, Sande, H, Foss, OP, and Stenwig, JT: Smoking during pregnancy—Effects on the fetus and on thiocyanate levels in mother and baby. *Acta Paediatr. Scand.* 68:547–552, 1979.
15. Naeye, RL: The duration of maternal cigarette smoking, fetal and placental disorders. *Early Hum. Dev.* 3:229–237, 1979.
16. Meyer, MB, Jonas, BS, and Tonascia, JA: Perinatal events associated with maternal smoking during pregnancy. *Am. J. Epidemiol.* 103:464–476, 1976.
17. Stergachis, A, Scholes, D, Daling, JR, et al: Maternal cigarette smoking and the risk of tubal pregnancy. *Am. J. Epidemiol.* 133:332–337, 1991.
18. Coste, J, Job-Spira, N, and Fernandez, H: Increased risk of ectopic pregnancy with maternal cigarette smoking. *Am. J. Public Health* 81:199–201, 1991.
19. Handler, A, Davis, F, Ferre, C, and Yeko, T: The relationship of smoking and ectopic pregnancy. *Am. J. Public Health* 79:1239–1242, 1989.
20. Cole, PV, Hawkins, LH, and Roberts, D: Smoking during pregnancy and its effects on the fetus. *J. Obstet. Gynaecol. Br. Commonwlth.* 79:782, 1972.
21. Longo, L: Carbon monoxide: Effects on oxygenation of the fetus in utero. *Science* 194:523, 1976.
22. Centers for Disease Control criteria for anemia in children and childbearing-aged women. *MMWR* 38:400–404, 1989.
23. Kruger, H, and Arias-Stella, J: The placenta and infant at high altitudes. *Am. J. Obstet. Gynecol.* 106:586, 1970.
24. Wingerd, J, et al: Placental ratio in white and black women: Relation to smoking and anemia. *Am. J. Obstet. Gynecol.* 124:671, 1976.
25. Caton, D, Henderson, J, and Barron, DH: Relationship between oxygen consumption in utero and birthweight of lambs. Presented at the

American Physiological Society Satellite Symposium, Circulation in the Fetus and Newborn, August 11–13, 1976.

26. Garn, SM, Shaw, HA, and McCabe, KD: Effect of maternal smoking on hemoglobins and hematocrits of the newborn. *Am. J. Clin. Nutr.* 31:557–558, 1978.
27. Seidman, DS, Ever-Hadani, P, and Gale, R: The effect of maternal weight gain in pregnancy on birth weight. *Obstet. Gynecol.* 74:240–246, 1989.
28. Anderson, GD, Blidner, IN, McClemont, S, and Sinclair, JC: Determinants of size at birth in a Canadian population. *Am. J. Obstet. Gynecol.* 150:236–244, 1984.
29. Asmussen, I, and Ijeldsen, K: Intimal ultrastructure of human umbilical arteries. Observations on arteries from newborn children of smoking and nonsmoking mothers. *Circ. Res.* 36:579, 1975.
30. Pinette, MG, Loftus-Brault, K, Nardi, DA, and Rodis, JF: Maternal smoking and accelerated placental maturation. *Obstet. Gynecol.* 73:379–382, 1989.
31. Hopper, K, Komppa, GH, Bice, P, et al: A reevaluation of placental grading and its clinical significance. *J. Ultrasound Med.* 3:261–266, 1984.
32. Quinlan, RW, Cruz, AC, Buhi, WC, and Martin, M: Changes in placental appearance. II. Pathologic significance of grade III placental changes. *Am. J. Obstet. Gynecol.* 144:471–473, 1982.
33. Proud, J, and Grant, AM: Third trimester placental grading by ultrasonography as a test of fetal wellbeing. *Br. Med. J.* 294:1641–1644, 1987.
34. Meyer, MB, and Tonascia, JA: Maternal smoking, pregnancy complications, and perinatal mortality. *Am. J. Obstet. Gynecol.* 128:494–502, 1977.
35. Johnston, C: Cigarette smoking and the outcome of human pregnancies: A status report on the consequences. *Clin. Toxicol.* 18:189–209, 1981.
36. Goujard, J, Rumeau, C, and Schwartz, D: Smoking during pregnancy, stillbirth, and abruptio placentae. *Biomedicine* (Paris) 23:20–22, 1975.
37. Beischer, NA, et al: Placental hypertrophy in severe pregnancy anaemia. *J. Obstet. Gynaecol. Br. Commonwlth.* 77:398, 1970.
38. Lubs, MLE: Racial differences in maternal smoking effects on the newborn infant. *Am. J. Obstet. Gynecol.* 115:66, 1973.
39. Grunberg, NE: The effects of nicotine and cigarette smoking on food consumption and taste preferences. *Addict. Behav.* 7:317, 1982.
40. Rodin, J: Weight change following smoking cessation: The role of food intake and exercise. *Addict. Behav.* 12:303, 1987.
41. Perkins, KA, Epstein, LH, Marks, BL, et al: The effect of nicotine on energy expenditure during light physical activity. *N. Engl. J. Med.* 320:898–903, 1989.
42. Temperley, IJ, et al: Serum vitamin B-12 levels in pregnant women. *J. Obstet. Gynaecol. Br. Commonwlth.* 75:511, 1968.

43. Whiteside, MG, et al: Iron, folic acid and vitamin B-12 levels in normal pregnancy and their influence on birthweight and the duration of pregnancy. *Med. J. Austral.* 1:338, 1968.
44. McGarry, JM, and Andrews, J: Smoking in pregnancy and vitamin B-12 metabolism. *Br. Med. J.* 2:74, 1972.
45. Metcoff, J, Costiloe, P, Crosby, WM, et al: Smoking in pregnancy: Relation of birth weight to maternal plasma carotene and cholesterol levels. *Obstet. Gynecol.* 74:302–309, 1989.
46. Kallner, AB, Hartmann, D, and Hornig, DH: On the requirements of ascorbic acid in man: Steady-state turnover and body pool in smokers. *Am. J. Clin. Nutr.* 34:1347–1355, 1981.
47. Life Sciences Research Office: *Assessment of the Folate Nutritional Status of the U.S. Population Based on Data Collected in the Second National Health and Nutrition Examination Survey, 1976–1980.* Bethesda, MD: Federation of American Societies for Experimental Biology, 1984.
48. Keith, RE, and Mossholder, SB: Ascorbic acid status of smoking and nonsmoking adolescent females. *Intern. J. Vit. Nutr. Res.* 56:363–366, 1986.
49. Apgar, J: Zinc and reproduction. *Ann. Rev. Nutr.* 5:43–68, 1985.
50. Kuhnert, PM, Kuhnert, BR, Erhard, P, et al: The effect of smoking on placental and fetal zinc status. *Am. J. Obstet. Gynecol.* 157:1241–1246, 1987.
51. Menden, EE, Elia, VJ, Michael, LW, and Petering, HG: Distribution of cadmium and nickel of tobacco during cigarette smoking. *Environ. Sci. Technol.* 6:830–832, 1972.
52. Kuhnert, BR, Kuhnert, PM, Debanne, S, and Williams, TG: The relationship between cadmium, zinc, and birth weight in pregnant women who smoke. *Am. J. Obstet. Gynecol.* 157:1247–1251, 1987.
53. Kuhnert, BR, Kuhnert, PM, Lazebnik, N, and Erhard, P: The effect of maternal smoking on the relationship between maternal and fetal zinc status and infant birth weight. *J. Am. Coll. Nutr.* 7:309–316, 1988.
54. Crosby, WM, Metcoff, J, Costiloe, JP, et al: Fetal malnutrition: An appraisal of correlated factors. *Am. J. Obstet. Gynecol.* 128:22–31, 1977.
55. Morabia, A, and Wynder, EL: Dietary habits of smokers, people who never smoked, and exsmokers. *Am. J. Clin. Nutr.* 52:933–937, 1990.
56. Haworth, JC, Ellestad-Sayed, JJ, King, J, and Dilling, LA: Fetal growth retardation in cigarette-smoking mothers is not due to decreased maternal food intake. *Am. J. Obstet. Gynecol.* 137:719–723, 1980.
57. Haste, FM, Brooke, OG, Anderson, HR, et al: Nutrient intakes during pregnancy: Observations on the influence of smoking and social class. *Am. J. Clin. Nutr.* 51:29–36, 1990.
58. Davies, DP, Gray, OP, Ellwood, PC, and Abernathy, M: Cigarette smoking in pregnancy: Associations with maternal weight gain and fetal growth. *Lancet* 1:385–387, 1976.

59. Rush, D: Examination of the relationship between birthweight, cigarette smoking during pregnancy and maternal weight gain. *J. Obstet. Gynaecol. Br. Commwlth.* 81:746, 1974.
60. Luke, B, Hawkins, MM, and Petrie, RH: Influence of smoking, weight gain, and pregravid weight for height on intrauterine growth. *Am. J. Obstet. Gynecol.* 34:1410–1417, 1981.
61. Garn, SM, Hoff, K, and McCabe, KD: Is there a nutritional mediation of the "smoking effect" on the fetus? *Am. J. Clin. Nutr.* 32:1181–1187, 1979.
62. Taffel, S: Maternal weight gain and the outcome of pregnancy. *Vital and Health Statistics*, Series 21, No. 44, DHHS Pub. No. (PHS) 86-1922. Public Health Service. Washington, DC: US Govt. Printing Office, 1986.
63. Meyer, MB: How does maternal smoking affect birth weight and maternal weight gain? *Am. J. Obstet. Gynecol.* 131:888, 1978.
64. D'Souza, SW, Black, P, and Richards, B: Smoking in pregnancy: Associations with skinfold thickness, maternal weight gain, and fetal size at birth. *Br. Med. J.* 282:998–1000, 1981.
65. Gruenwald, P: Chronic fetal distress and placental insufficiency. *Biol. Neonate.* 5:215, 1963.
66. Miller, HC, Hassanein, K, and Hensleigh, PA: Fetal growth retardation in relation to maternal smoking and weight gain in pregnancy. *Am. J. Obstet. Gynecol.* 125:55, 1976.
67. Daikoku et al: Patterns of intrauterine growth retardation. *Obstet. Gynecol.* 54:211, 1979.
68. Russell, CS, Taylor, R, and Law, CE: Smoking in pregnancy, maternal blood pressure, pregnancy outcome, baby weight and growth and other related factors. *Br. J. Prev. Soc. Med.* 22:119, 1968.
69. Hardy, JB, and Mellits, ED: Does maternal smoking during pregnancy have a long-term effect on the child? *Lancet* 2:1332, 1972.
70. Davie, R, Butler, NR, and Goldstein, H: From birth to seven: The second report of the National Child Development Study. London: Longman and the National Children's Bureau, 1972.
71. Goldstein, H: Factors influencing the height of seven-year-old children—Results from the National Child Development Study. *Hum. Biol.* 43:92, 1971.
72. Naeye, RL: Relationship of cigarette smoking to congenital anomalies and perinatal death. *Am. J. Pathol.* 90:289, 1978.
73. Andrews, J, and McGarry, J: A community study of smoking in pregnancy. *Br. J. Obstet. Gynaecol.* 79:1057, 1972.
74. Comstock, GW, Shah, FK, Meyer, MB, and Abbey, H: Low birthweight and neonatal mortality rate related to maternal smoking and socioeconomic status. *Am. J. Obstet. Gynecol.* 111:53, 1971.
75. Butler, NR, and Alberman, ED (eds.): *Perinatal Problems: The Second Report of the 1958 British Perinatal Mortality Survey*. Edinburgh: Livingstone, 1969.

76. Lowe, CR: Effect of mother's smoking habits on birth weight of their children. *Br. Med. J.* 2:673–676, 1959.
77. Kullander, S, and Kallen, B: A prospective study of smoking and pregnancy. *Acta. Obstet. Gynecol. Scand.* 50:83, 1971.
78. Fedrick, J, Alberman, ED, and Goldstein, H: Possible teratogenic effect of cigarette smoking. *Nature* 231:529, 1971.
79. Khoury, MJ, Weinstein, A, Panny, S, et al: Maternal cigarette smoking and oral clefts: A population-based study. *Am. J. Public Health* 77:623–625, 1987.
80. Infant mortality—United States, 1988. *MMWR* 40:644–646, 1991.
81. Hoppenbrouwers, T, and Hodgman, JE: Sudden infant death syndrome (SIDS). *Neuropediatrics* 13(Suppl.):36–51, 1982.
82. Rintahaka, PJ, and Hirvonen, J: The epidemiology of sudden infant death syndrome in Finland in 1969–1980. *Forens. Sci. Int.* 30:219–233, 1986.
83. Peterson, DR, van Belle, G, and Chinn, NM: Epidemiologic comparisons of the sudden infant death syndrome with other major components of infant mortality. *Am. J. Epidemiol.* 110:699–707, 1979.
84. Haglund, B, and Cnattingius, S: Cigarette smoking as a risk factor for sudden infant death syndrome: A population-based study. *Am. J. Public Health* 80:29–32, 1990.
85. Smoking-attributable mortality and years of potential life—United States, 1988. *MMWR* 40:62–71, 1991.
86. John, EM, Savitz, DA, and Sandler, DP: Prenatal exposure to parent's smoking and childhood cancer. *Am. J. Epidemiol.* 133:123–132, 1991.
87. Stewart, A, Webb, J, and Hewitt, D: A survey of childhood malignancies. *Br. Med. J.* 1:1495–1508, 1958.
88. Neutel, CI, and Buck, C: Effect of smoking during pregnancy on the risk of cancer in children. *J. Natl. Cancer Inst.* 47:59–63, 1971.
89. Gold, E, Gordis, L, Tonascia, J, et al: Risk factors for brain tumors in children. *Am. J. Epidemiol.* 109:309–319, 1979.
90. Stjernfeldt, M, Berglund, K, Lindsten, J, et al: Maternal smoking during pregnancy and risk of childhood cancer. *Lancet* 1:1350–1352, 1986.
91. Naeye, RL, and Peters, EC: Mental development of children whose mothers smoked during pregnancy. *Obstet. Gynecol.* 64:601–607, 1984.
92. Butler, NR, and Goldstein, H: Smoking in pregnancy and subsequent child development. *Br. Med. J.* 4:573–575, 1973.
93. Rantakallio, P: A follow-up study up to the age of 14 of children whose mothers smoked during pregnancy. *Acta Paediatr. Scand.* 72:747–753, 1983.
94. Denson, R, Nanson, JL, and McWalters, MA: Hyperkinesis and maternal smoking. *Can. Psych. Assoc. J.* 20:183–187, 1975.

95. Dunn, HG, McBurney, AK, Ingram, S, and Hunter, CM: Maternal cigarette smoking during pregnancy and the child's subsequent development: II. Neurological and intellectual maturation to the age of 6½ years. *Can. J. Public Health* 68:43–50, 1977.

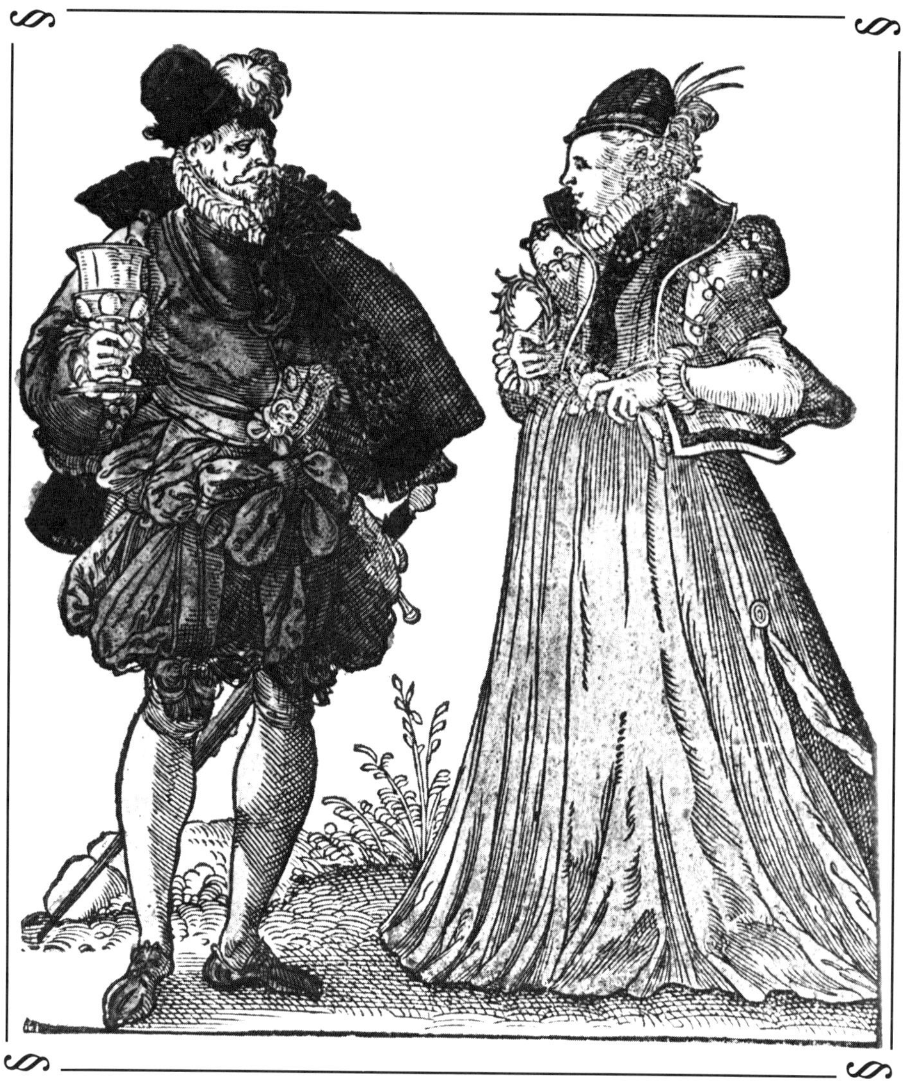

Illustration from *De Conceptu*. (From Jacobus Rueff. *De Conceptu*. Frankfurt: S. Feyerabendt, 1580.)

9 Alcohol

The per capita consumption of alcohol among the adult population 21 years of age and older in the United States rose to about 41 gal per year in 1985, up by more than one fourth from 1965 levels (Fig. 9-1). Consumption of alcohol peaks in the 20- to 40-year age group, and national statistics indicate that 70 percent of individuals between the ages of 20 and 34 consume alcohol [1]. In a 1985 survey, two thirds of high school seniors reported consuming alcohol during the past month, one third reported having five or more drinks on at least one occasion during the prior 2 weeks, and 5 percent described themselves as daily drinkers [2]. Although men are more likely to drink alcohol and to drink heavily than are women, the proportion of women who drink alcohol has increased during the past decade. The abuse of alcohol is a major social, economic, and public health problem throughout the world. In the United States, a recent estimate of the annual cost of alcohol-related loss of productivity and health expenses is $117 billion [2].

Alone and in combination with other factors, alcohol is potentially capable of producing a range of adverse perinatal outcomes. Alcohol is both embryotoxic and teratogenic. The adverse effects of maternal alcohol use on the developing fetus have been known empirically since ancient times. It was not until 1968, however, that a formal description of these effects appeared in the scientific literature, when Lemoine and associates [3] reported a constellation of abnormalities in children born to alcoholic women: **intrauterine growth retardation**, an **unusual facies**, **psychomotor retardation**, and a 25 percent incidence of **congenital anomalies** (especially cleft palate and cardiac malformations). This pattern of abnormalities was also described by other investigators, and, in 1973, Jones and colleagues [4] designated this pattern of altered growth and dysmorphogenesis as the **fetal alcohol syndrome (FAS)**. Many other investigators have subsequently described additional clinical findings (Table 9-1).

The diagnosis of FAS includes three criteria, as established by the Fetal Alcohol Study Group of the Research Society on Alcoholism [5]: (1) prenatal and/or postnatal growth retardation (weight, length, and/or head circumference below the 10th percentile when corrected for gestational age); (2) central nervous system involvement (signs of neurologic abnormality, developmental delay, or intellectual impairment); and (3) characteristic facial dysmorphology, with at least two of these three signs: (a) microcephaly (head circumference below the 3rd percentile), (b) microopthalmia and/or short palpebral fissures, (c) poorly developed philtrum, thin upper lip, and/or flattening of the maxillary area.

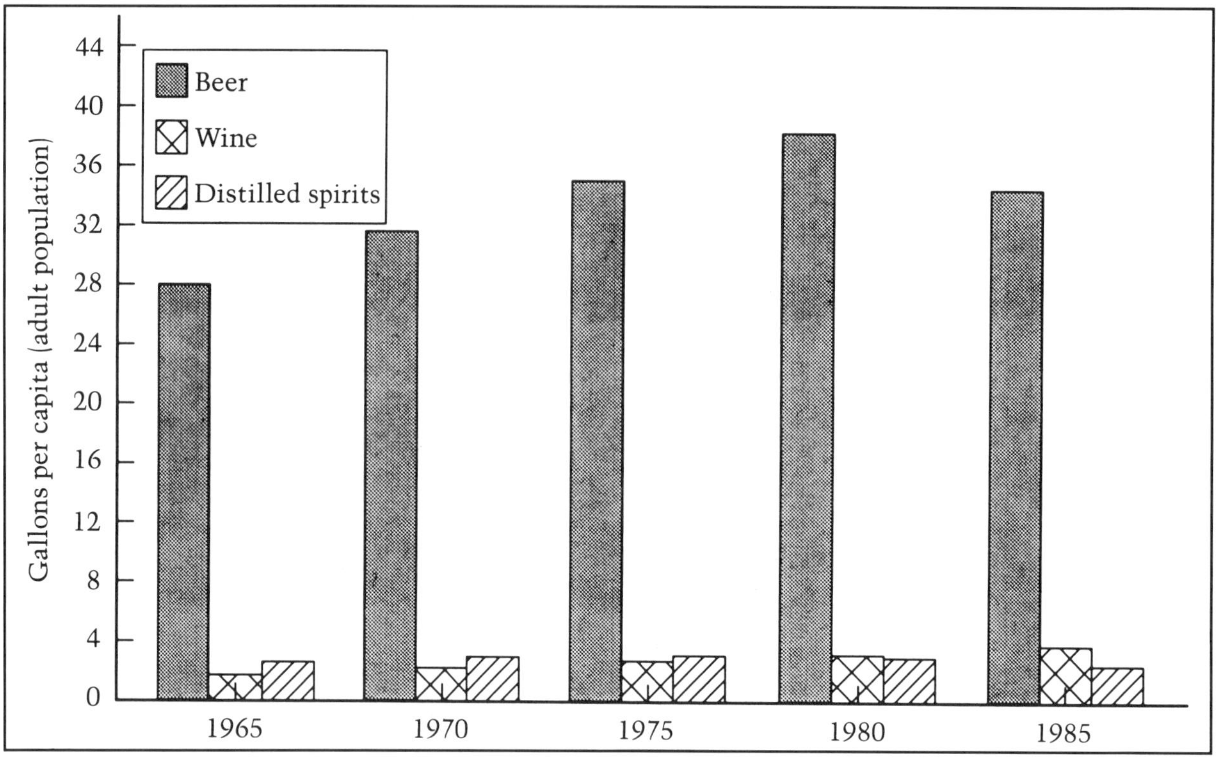

Fig. 9-1
Per capita consumption of alcoholic beverages, adult population, United States, 1965 to 1985. (Adapted from K Bunch, *Food Consumption, Prices, and Expenditures*, 1985 Statistical Bulletin 749, Economic Research Service, US Department of Agriculture. Washington, DC: US Govt. Printing Office, 1987.)

Children who do not have the full FAS but exhibit some components of the syndrome are classified as having **fetal alcohol effects**, or **FAE**. The most common sign of FAS and FAE is retarded growth in weight, length, and head circumference both pre- and postnatally. Prenatal growth retardation is independent of prematurity, with FAS neonates being small-for-gestational-age in weight, length, and head circumference. Postnatal growth deficits persist despite adequate nutrition and a stable home environment, except in children with milder forms of FAS. The severity of the neurodevelopmental pathology in FAS is related to the degree of facial dysmorphology [6–8]. Children with severe facial dysmorphology have shown little physical or developmental improvement over time, whereas those with milder facial abnormalities, as seen in FAE, responded more favorably to therapeutic interventions and training programs [9].

Table 9-1
Clinical symptoms of FAS and potential short- and long-term sequelae

Symptoms present at birth	*Short-term sequelae*	*Long-term sequelae*
Overall Growth [3, 4, 6, 12, 35, 40, 45, 56–58]		
Pre- and postnatal growth deficiency	Poor catch-up growth Failure to thrive	<2 SD length-for-weight Disproportionately diminished adipose tissue
Microcephaly Developmental delay Neurologic deficits	Poor suck, seizures Irritability, hypotonicity Hyperactivity	Intellectual impairment Mental retardation, attention deficit, epilepsy, language disability
Craniofacial abnormalities [3, 4, 6, 12, 40, 56]		
Ocular		
Short palpebral fissures Optic nerve hypoplasia Epicanthal folds Microphthalmia	Strabismus, ptosis	Exotropia and/or myopia
Maxillary hypoplasia	Eustachian tube dysfunction	Chronic serous otitis media, hearing loss
Cleft palate	Feeding difficulties	Surgical repair
Micrognathia	Retrognathia	Relative prognathism in adolescence; dental malignment, faulty enamel
Cardiac [4, 6, 12, 40, 59, 60]		
Ventricular septal defect Pulmonary artery dysplasia Pulmonary artery stenosis Patent ductus arteriosus Atrial septal defect Tetralogy of Fallot	Arrhythmias, congestive heart failure	Surgical repair
Renal [6, 40, 56, 61]		
Renal hypoplasia Labial hypoplasia Hydronephrosis Hypospadias	Fluid and electrolyte imbalance	Dialysis, surgical repair
Skeletal [62, 63]		
Hypoplastic toenails Camptodactyly of fingers Clinodactyly of toes, clubfoot Flexion contractures Spinal stenosis Congenital dislocation of hip	Limited movement	Surgical repair

The worldwide incidence of the full characteristics of FAS is estimated to be 1.9 per 1000 live births [10]; that of partial characteristics is 3 to 5 per 1000 live births [11, 12]. Among alcoholic women, the incidence of FAS (full characteristics) is estimated to be as high as 25 per 1000; in contrast, FAE (partial characteristics) is estimated to occur in as many as 90 per 1000 [12]. Some dysmorphic features of FAS and FAE recede with postnatal development [9]; however, hyperactivity and learning disabilities remain, and the more severe anomalies require surgical intervention (Table 9-1). FAS is the leading cause of mental retardation in the Western world, surpassing Down's syndrome and cerebral palsy [10]. In the United States, the annual cost for providing treatment to children with FAS has been conservatively estimated at about $321 million [10].

Alcohol and Reproduction

Most women report an aversion to alcohol during pregnancy and either decrease or eliminate their intake of alcoholic beverages. In a study of dietary cravings and aversions during pregnancy, Hook [13] reported that one fourth to one third of women who regularly drank alcohol before conception reduced their intake during the first half of pregnancy as a result of loss of taste for alcohol or nausea induced by these beverages. Little and co-workers [14] reported that two thirds of pregnant women in their study drank less alcohol during the first 4 months of pregnancy. However, an estimated 5 to 10 percent of pregnant women drink heavily, and this intake has serious consequences for their unborn children [15].

Alcohol alters the normal hormonal and metabolic balance of the reproductive system in both men and women. Heavy drinking in women can disrupt the menstrual cycle and decrease fertility [16, 17]. Among men, heavy drinking can result in impotence, decreased libido, testicular atrophy, and feminization, including proliferation of breast tissue and loss of body hair. Spermatogenesis requires retinal (vitamin A), which is generated from retinol by alcohol dehydrogenase. When ethanol diverts alcohol dehydrogenase, the testis becomes retinal-deficient and spermatogenesis decreases despite adequate dietary intake of vitamin A. Alcohol also impairs the functioning of the Leydig cells, which secrete testosterone.

Metabolism of Alcohol

Approximately one fourth to one third of ingested alcohol is rapidly absorbed through the stomach wall. The remainder mixes with gastric acids and mucus, and is absorbed through the small intestine. Alcohol diffuses from the stomach and intestine to the blood vessels and is transported by the portal vein to the liver. Because alcohol is soluble in both water and lipid, it diffuses through cell membranes and into all cells. Gastric absorption is increased by the presence of carbonated liquids and is delayed by a high sugar content, coldness, and the presence of food, especially proteins and fat. The bioavailability of alcohol resulting from gastric metabolism is termed **gastric first-pass metabolism**, and this process differs for men and women. Frezza and co-workers [18] have shown that the bioavailability of alcohol is much greater in women than in men, because women experience less gastric first-pass metabolism of alcohol. When alcohol passes into the duodenum and intestines, the intestinal mucosa absorbs it rapidly and completely, regardless of the presence of food.

More than 90 percent of ingested alcohol is oxidized by the liver; the remaining 10 percent is excreted unchanged through the lungs and kidneys. The amount in expired air and in the urine is directly proportional to blood alcohol concentrations (BAC). In most states, a BAC of 0.10 (100 mg%) is the legal definition of intoxication. Mild euphoria occurs at BAC of 30 mg percent, impaired coordination at 50 mg percent, ataxia at 100 mg percent, stupor at 300 mg percent, and narcosis and death at 400 mg percent. The oxidation of alcohol occurs in several steps. The first is the oxidation of alcohol to acetaldehyde, which is mainly catalyzed by the enzyme alcohol dehydrogenase. In the second step acetaldehyde is oxidized to acetate, which is catalyzed by the enzyme aldehyde dehydrogenase. Acetate is then oxidized to water and carbon dioxide through the Krebs cycle of intermediate metabolism. The BAC falls at approximately 15 mg percent per hour, regardless of the initial BAC. For example, after one drink, a 130-lb woman will have an initial BAC of about 43 mg percent. After 1 hour the BAC will fall to approximately 28 mg percent and by 3 hours will be close to zero.

Epidemiologic studies indicate that women are more susceptible than men to the adverse effects of alcohol [19, 20]. For instance, among women, liver damage occurs after alcohol is consumed in smaller quantities and for shorter periods than in men; this difference is due to higher initial BAC in women for the same quantity of alcohol [21]. Higher BAC in women results from a smaller volume of distribution, reflecting the lower total water content and larger lipid content of women's bodies. In addition, the higher BAC in women compared to men is also the result of a lower rate of alcohol dehydrogenase activity in the gastric mucosa, and a therefore higher bioavailability of alcohol in women after ingestion of similar quantities of alcohol.

Direct and Indirect Mechanisms of Action of Alcohol

The ethanol-related physical and metabolic disorders are caused by a combination of the toxic effects of ethanol and its derivatives, nutritional factors, and genetic predisposition. Ethanol and its oxidative metabolite acetaldehyde may directly damage the developing and mature nervous systems. Many experimental animal models (including primates) demonstrating the teratogenicity of alcohol have been developed; these have shown a clear dose-response effect between maternal alcohol consumption and fetal risk [12, 22]. For example, the characteristic midfacial abnormalities and many of the midline brain abnormalities can be produced in the mouse by one brief period of maternal alcohol intoxication during gastrulation [23, 24]. This effect has been confirmed in human studies [25]. Epidemiologic studies in humans have also demonstrated that risk increases with increasing alcohol intake [26–28]. Central to this risk is retarded and deviant growth, manifested in nearly every organ system in proportion to timing and amount of in utero alcohol exposure. For example, prenatal exposure to more than three drinks per day triples the risk of subsequent mental retardation (IQ <85) in the child at age four [29]. Such effects may be the result of direct or indirect consequences of alcohol metabolism. Both alcohol and its major metabolite, acetaldehyde, readily cross the placenta and both have been shown to be directly teratogenic [30]. Both also have been shown to impair nucleic acid and protein synthesis directly in vitro by inhibiting cell division and RNA synthesis [31]. Ethanol also disrupts protein synthesis by interfering with transmembrane signaling, a vital mediator of neural cell division, migration, differentiation, and synaptogenesis. In particular, the pharmacologic effects of ethyl alcohol are the result of cell membrane narcosis, leading to a general depression of cell function [30]. All cells are affected, but these effects are most pronounced in cells with excitable membranes [30].

Structural dysmorphogenesis of the brain in FAS and FAE includes aberrant neuronal and glial migration, including cerebellar dysplasia, leptomeningeal neuroglial heterotopias, and agenesis of the corpus callosum [12]. The pathogenesis of the mental retardation and learning disabilities characteristic of FAS and FAE includes these structural abnormalities as well as more subtle defects such as simplification of hippocampal dendrites [32].

The metabolism of alcohol is very different for the mother than it is for the developing fetus. Because alcohol is both water and lipid soluble, it passes readily through all biologic membranes, equilibrating rapidly throughout the entire water volume of the maternal-placental-fetal unit. The amniotic fluid thus acts as a reservoir for unchanged alcohol and acetaldehyde, and because the fetus lacks the necessary enzymes to degrade these substances [33], it is exposed to them long after they have been cleared from the maternal system [30, 34]. In addition, alcohol or acetaldehyde may be directly toxic to the placenta as well as to the fetus, and ethanol-associated placentotoxicity possibly results in "selective" fetal malnutrition, independent of maternal nutritional status [35].

Nutrition-Related Effects of Alcohol Exposure

Poor nutritional status of the mother, plus the toxic effects of alcohol, may be more detrimental to the developing fetus than either factor alone. In addition, decreased umbilical blood flow and impairment of placental transport of nutrients may result in intrauterine growth retardation, and potentially compound any toxic effects of ethanol on embryogenesis. Reduced placental transfer of zinc and folic acid has also been demonstrated in animal models of alcohol-induced teratogenesis [35, 36]. For example, protein malnutrition exacerbates alcohol's hepatotoxicity, and alcohol impairs the absorption, utilization, and metabolism of nutrients [37]. Although moderate to severe alcohol intake is often accompanied by some degree of undernutrition, current evidence strongly suggests that primary malnutrition is not solely responsible for the fetal alcohol syndrome [26, 38]. In studies of malnourished newborns born during the post–World War II famine in Holland, microcephaly at birth did not result in mental retardation in later development [39]. In contrast, among children with FAS, the severity of the physical abnormalities present at birth (including microcephaly) is highly predictive of intellectual development in later years [6, 40].

Among all nutrients investigated in association with FAS, zinc has emerged as central to both the characteristic patterns of growth retardation and the constellation of congenital malformations. Maternal zinc deficiency is known to be teratogenic [41]. Flynn and coworkers [42] reported lower plasma zinc levels in pregnant alcoholic women than in pregnant nonalcoholic women, and speculated that zinc may be a cofactor in the fetal dysmorphogenesis of FAS. Keppen and co-workers [43] compared the effects of alcohol and differing dietary zinc intakes on fetal development in rats and concluded that zinc deficiency acted as a coteratogen with alcohol. Zinc deficiency in FAS has also been related to increased urinary zinc excretion [44]. Ghishan and Greene [45] reported that neither physiologic nor pharmacologic doses of zinc could overcome the defect in placental transport of zinc caused by alcohol. Other studies have shown that increasing dietary protein levels did not attenuate the major adverse effects of alcohol on fetal development [46].

Alcohol can impair fetal development in a wide variety of indirect ways. Alcohol-related hypothermia, dehydration, fetal hypoxia and acidosis, placental pathology and dysfunction, and endocrine disturbances all have been shown to occur with increasing maternal alcohol intake [47–51]. Genetic factors, including individual variation in the metabolism of alcohol, and the possibility of paternal influences on the susceptibility of the fetus to alcohol's teratogenic actions, may also be important in the expression of the disease [4, 35, 52].

Cellular Mechanisms of Alcohol-Induced Growth Retardation

According to Kennedy [30], all alcohol-related developmental abnormalities result from derangements in protein synthesis that occur during periods of rapid organ growth. This hypothesis is based on three basic observations:

1. In both humans and nonhuman mammals, alcohol-related developmental abnormalities include a cluster of physical malformations involving many organ systems, which are highly variable in their frequency and severity of expression. This suggests that alcohol is a nonspecific teratogen that affects some developmental process common to all or most cell types.
2. The most common and consistent manifestation of gestational alcohol abuse is intrauterine growth impairment, apparent clinically as reductions in head circumference, body length, body weight, and (at autopsy) individual organ weights.

3. Normal growth and development are dependent on the accumulation and organization of protein. Alcohol directly and indirectly impairs protein synthesis in fetal and adult tissues [30, 31, 35]. Through reductions in RNA (transfer-, mitochondrial-, messenger-, ribosomal-) and DNA, as well as total and subcellular protein contents, alcohol impairs cellular processes that are fundamental to growth [30]. The suppression of cell division is proportional to ethanol dose and appears to be related to ethanol-induced changes in the metabolism of the prostaglandin hormones and resulting changes in the cyclic adenosine monophosphate (AMP) levels in the developing embryo [53].

Lesser Effects

The full features of FAS occur only in the children of women who drink heavily throughout pregnancy, although smaller and less frequent alcohol use during pregnancy may also adversely affect the fetus. Long-term neuropsychological studies of children of nonalcoholic mothers have established that prenatal ethanol exposure causes decreased habitation at birth [54], lower intelligence quotient at age four [55], and deficits in attention and reaction time at age seven [29]. These adverse effects correlate with self-estimates of alcohol intake during the first trimester and at 5 months' gestation, even after controlling for such confounding factors as maternal nutrition, education, smoking, and caffeine and aspirin use [29]. There is a linear relationship between the amount of prenatal ethanol exposure and subsequent behavioral and morphologic abnormalities, with no minimum threshold for adverse effects [25, 29].

Comments and Recommendations

In 1978, Clarren and Smith [56] summarized the prenatal risk of maternal alcohol intake. These comments are equally relevant today, more than a decade and a half later:

> The variability of the phenotype probably results from variable dose exposure at variable gestational timings offset by the genetic background of the individual fetus. Nearly all patients recognized as having the full fetal-alcohol-syndrome phenotype are born to daily heavy alcohol users or relatively frequent heavy intermittent users. Chronic consumption of 89 ml of absolute alcohol or more per day—the equivalent of about six hard drinks—constitutes a major risk to the fetus. Lower levels

of consumption or less frequent use of alcohol carries an unknown risk and may be shown to be associated with less seriously affected children. No absolutely safe level of ethanol consumption has yet been established.

Streissguth and co-workers [9], in their recent follow-up study of 61 adolescents and adults diagnosed as having FAS, concluded that "fetal alcohol syndrome is not just a childhood disorder. There is a predictable, long-term progression of the disorder into adulthood in which maladaptive behaviors present the greatest challenge to treatment. Gestational exposure to alcohol can cause a wide spectrum of disabilities that have lifelong physical, mental, and behavioral implications."

At present, there is no dietary therapy to overcome the metabolic imbalances caused by maternal alcohol ingestion. The optimal therapy is abstinence during pregnancy and moderation when not pregnant. Screening tools exist to identify those women who have been abusing alcohol during pregnancy. The most commonly used in clinical practice are the Michigan Alcohol Screening Test (MAST) and Cutdown, Annoyance, Guilt, and Eye-opener (CAGE) Questionnaires, although in obstetrics, the Tolerance, Annoyance, Cutdown, Eye-opener (TACE) screen has recently become popular [64, 65].

References

1. Schoenborn, CA, and Cohen, BH: Trends in smoking, alcohol consumption, and other health practices among U.S. adults, 1977 and 1983. DHHS Publication No. (PHS) 86-1250. Division of Health Interview Statistics, National Center for Health Statistics, Public Health Service, US Dept. of Health and Human Services, Hyattsville, MD, 1986.
2. National Institute on Alcohol Abuse and Alcoholism: *The Sixth Special Report to the U.S. Congress on Alcohol and Health from the Secretary of Health and Human Services*. DHHS Publication No. (ADM) 87-1519, National Institutes of Health, Public Health Service, USDHHS. Washington, DC: US Govt. Printing Office, 1987.
3. Lemoine, P, Harrousseau, H, Borteyru, JP, and Menuet, J: Les enfants de parents alcooliques: Anomalies observées. A propos de 127 cas. *Quest. Med.* 25:476–482, 1968.
4. Jones, KL, Smith, DW, Ulleland, CN, et al: Pattern of malformation in offspring of chronic alcoholic mothers. *Lancet* 1:1267–1271, 1973.
5. Rosett, HL: A clinical perspective of the fetal alcohol syndrome. *Alcohol. Clin. Exp. Res.* 4:119–122, 1980.
6. Streissguth, AP, Herman, CS, and Smith, DW: Intelligence, behavior and dysmorphogenesis in the fetal alcohol syndrome: A report on 20 patients. *J. Pediatr.* 92:363–367, 1978.

7. Dupuis, C, Dehaene, P, Deroubaix-Tella, P, et al: Les cardiopathies des enfants née de mère alcoolique. *Arch. Mal. Coeur* 71:565–572, 1978.
8. Majewski, F: Alcohol embryopathy: Some facts and speculations about pathogenesis. *Neurobehav. Toxicol. Teratol.* 3:129–144, 1981.
9. Streissguth, AP, Aase, JM, Clarren, SK, et al: Fetal alcohol syndrome in adolescents and adults. *J.A.M.A.* 265:1961–1967, 1991.
10. Streissguth, AP, Sampson, PD, Barr, HM, et al: Studying alcohol teratogenesis from the perspective of the fetal alcohol syndrome: Methodological and statistical issues. *Ann. N. Y. Acad. Sci.* 477:63–86, 1986.
11. Abel, EL, and Sokol, RJ: Incidence of fetal alcohol syndrome and economic impact of FAS-related anomalies. *Drug Alcohol Depend.* 19:51–70, 1987.
12. Streissguth, AP, Landesman-Dwyer, S, Martin, JC, and Smith, DW: Teratogenic effects of alcohol in humans and laboratory animals. *Science* 209:353–361, 1980.
13. Hook, EB: Dietary cravings and aversions during pregnancy. *Am. J. Clin. Nutr.* 31:1355–1362, 1978.
14. Little, RE, Schultz, FA, and Mandell, W: Drinking during pregnancy. *J. Stud. Alcohol.* 37:375, 1976.
15. Rosett, HL, and Weiner, L: *Alcohol and the Fetus.* New York: Oxford University Press, 1984.
16. Mello, NK: Some Behavioral and Biological Aspects of Alcohol Problems in Women. In OJ Kalant (ed.), *Alcohol and Drug Problems in Women.* New York: Plenum, 1980. Pp. 263–298.
17. Cicero, TJ: Sex Differences in the Effects of Alcohol and Other Psychoactive Drugs on Endocrine Function: Clinical and Experimental Evidence. In OJ Kalant (ed.), *Alcohol and Drug Problems in Women.* New York: Plenum, 1980. Pp. 545–593.
18. Frezza, M, di Padova, C, Pozzato, G, et al: High blood alcohol levels in women: The role of decreased gastric alcohol dehydrogenase activity and first-pass metabolism. *N. Engl. J. Med.* 322:95–99, 1990.
19. Ashley, MJ, Olin, JS, le Riche, WH, et al: Morbidity in alcoholics: Evidence for accelerated development of physical disease in women. *Arch. Intern. Med.* 137:883–887, 1977.
20. Saunders, JB, Davis, M, and Williams, R: Do women develop alcoholic liver disease more readily than men? *Br. Med. J.* 282:1140–1143, 1981.
21. Norton, R, Batey, R, Dwyer, T, and MacMahon, S: Alcohol consumption and the risk of alcohol related cirrhosis in women. *Br. Med. J.* 295:80–82, 1987.
22. Clarren, SK, and Bowden, DM: Fetal alcohol syndrome: A new primate model for binge drinking and its relevance to human ethanol teratogenesis. *J. Pediatr.* 101:819–824, 1982.
23. Sulik, KK, Johnston, MC, and Webb, MA: Fetal alcohol syndrome: Embryogenesis in a mouse model. *Science* 214:936–938, 1981.

24. Sulik, KK, and Lauder, JM: Brain malformations in fetal mice resulting from acute maternal alcohol exposure during the gastrulation stage of embryogenesis (abstract). *Int. J. Dev. Neurosci.* 1:(3), 1983.
25. Ernhart, CB, Sokol, RJ, Martier, S, et al: Alcohol teratogenicity in the human: A detailed assessment of specificity, critical period, and threshold. *Am. J. Obstet. Gynecol.* 156:33–39, 1987.
26. Kaminsky, M, Rumeau, C, and Schwartz, D: Alcohol consumption in pregnant women and the outcome of pregnancy. *Alcoholism: Clin. Exp. Res.* 2:155–163, 1978.
27. Sokol, RJ, Miller, SI, and Reed, G: Alcohol abuse during pregnancy: An epidemiological study. *Alcoholism: Clin. Exp. Res.* 4:135–145, 1980.
28. Smith, DW: The fetal alcohol syndrome. *Hosp. Prac.* Oct: 121–129, 1979.
29. Streissguth, AP, Barr, HM, Sampson, PD, et al: IQ at age 4 in relation to maternal alcohol use and smoking during pregnancy. *Dev. Psychol.* 25:3–11, 1989.
30. Kennedy, LA: The pathogenesis of brain abnormalities in the fetal alcohol syndrome: An integrating hypothesis. *Teratology* 29:363–368, 1984.
31. Dreosti, IV, Ballard, J, Belling, B, et al: The effect of ethanol and acetaldehyde on DNA synthesis in growing cells and on fetal development in the rat. *Alcoholism: Clin. Exp. Res.* 5:362–375, 1981.
32. Davies, DL, and Smith, DE: A Golgi study of mouse hippocampal CA1 pyramidal neurons following perinatal ethanol exposure. *Neurosci. Lett.* 26:49–54, 1981.
33. Pikkarainen, PH, and Raiha, NC: Development of alcohol dehydrogenase activity in the human liver. *Pediatr. Res.* 1:165–168, 1967.
34. Brien, JF, Loomis, CW, Tranmer, J, and McGrath, H: Disposition of ethanol in human maternal venous blood and amniotic fluid. *Am. J. Obstet. Gynecol.* 146:181–186, 1983.
35. Fisher, SE: Ethanol: Effect on Fetal Brain Growth and Development. In RE Tarter and DH Van Thiel (eds.), *Alcohol and the Brain: Chronic Effects*. New York: Plenum, 1985. Pp. 265–281.
36. Ghishan, FK, Patwardhan, R, and Greene, HL: Fetal alcohol syndrome: Failure of zinc supplementation to reverse the effect of ethanol on placental transport of zinc. *Pediatr. Res.* 17:529–531, 1983.
37. Shaw, S, and Lieber, CS: Effects of Ethanol on Nutritional Status. In RE Hodges (ed.), *Human Nutrition: Metabolic and Clinical Applications*. New York: Plenum, 1979. Pp. 223–298.
38. Weiner, SG, Shoemaker, WJ, Koda, LY, and Bloom, FE: Interaction of ethanol and nutrition during gestation: Influence on maternal and offspring development in the rat. *J. Pharmacol. Exp. Ther.* 216:572–579, 1981.
39. Stein, Z, Susser, M, Saenger, G, and Marolla, F: *Famine and Human Development: The Dutch Hunger Winter of 1944/45*, New York: Oxford University Press, 1975. Pp. 197–214.

40. Streissguth, AP, Clarren, SK, and Jones, KL: Natural history of the fetal alcohol syndrome: A 10-year follow-up of eleven patients. *Lancet* 2:85–91, 1985.
41. Hurley, LS, Gowan, J, and Swenerton, H: Teratogenic effects of short-term and transitory zinc deficiency in rats. *Teratology* 4:199–204, 1971.
42. Flynn, A, Martier, SS, Sokol, RJ, et al: Zinc status of pregnant alcoholic women: A determinant of fetal outcome. *Lancet* 1:572–574, 1981.
43. Keppen, LD, Pysher, T, and Rennert, OM: Zinc deficiency acts as a co-teratogen with alcohol in fetal alcohol syndrome. *Pediatr. Res.* 19:944–947, 1985.
44. Assadi, FK, and Ziai, M: Zinc status of infants with fetal alcohol syndrome. *Pediatr. Res.* 20:551–554, 1986.
45. Ghishan, FK, and Greene, HL: Fetal alcohol syndrome: Failure of zinc supplementation to reverse the effect of ethanol on placental transport of zinc. *Pediatr. Res.* 17:529–531, 1983.
46. Weinberg, J: Effects of ethanol and maternal nutritional status on fetal development. *Alcoholism: Clin. Exp. Res.* 9:49–55, 1985.
47. Henderson, GI, Hoyumpa, AM, and Schenker, S: Effect of Chronic and Acute Maternal Alcohol Consumption on Fetal Growth Parameters and Protein Synthesis in Fetal Tissues. In EL Abel (ed.) *Fetal Alcohol Syndrome: Animal Studies*, Vol. 3. Boca Raton, Fla: CRC Press, 1982. Pp. 151–158.
48. Henderson, GI, Turner, D, Patwardhan, RV, et al: Inhibition of placental valine uptake after acute and chronic maternal alcohol ingestion. *J. Pharmacol. Exp. Ther.* 216:465–472, 1981.
49. Mukherjee, AB, and Hodgen, GD: Maternal ethanol exposure induces transient impairment of umbilical circulation and fetal hypoxia in monkeys. *Science* 218:700–702, 1982.
50. Wunderlich, SM, Boliga, S, and Munro, HN: Rat placental protein synthesis and peptide secretion in relation to malnutrition from protein deficiency in alcohol administration. *J. Nutr.* 109:1534–1541, 1979.
51. Clarren, SK, Alvord, CA, Jr., Sumi, SM, et al: Brain malformations related to prenatal exposure to ethanol. *J. Pediatr.* 92:64–67, 1978.
52. Chernoff, GF: The fetal alcohol syndrome in mice: Maternal variables. *Teratology* 22:71–75, 1980.
53. Pennington, SN, Boyd, JW, Kalmus, GW, and Wilson, RW: The molecular mechanism of fetal alcohol syndrome (FAS) I. Ethanol-induced growth suppression. *Neurobehav. Toxicol. Teratol.* 5:259–262, 1983.
54. Streissguth, AP, Barr, HM, and Martin, DC: Maternal alcohol use and neonatal habituation assessed with Brazelton scale. *Child Dev.* 54:1109–1118, 1983.
55. Streissguth, AP, Barr, HM, Sampson, PD, et al: Attention, distraction and reaction time at age 7 years and prenatal alcohol exposure. *Neurobehav. Toxicol. Teratol.* 8:717–725, 1986.

56. Clarren, SK, and Smith, DW: The fetal alcohol syndrome. *N. Engl. J. Med.* 298:1063–1067, 1978.
57. Shaywitz, SE, Caparulo, BK, and Hodgson, ES: Developmental language disability as a consequence of prenatal exposure to ethanol. *Pediatrics* 68:850–855, 1981.
58. Marcus, JC: Neurological findings in the fetal alcohol syndrome. *Neuropediatrics* 18:158–160, 1987.
59. Steeg, CN, and Woolf, P: Cardiovascular malformations in the fetal alcohol syndrome. *Am. Heart J.* 98:635–637, 1979.
60. Sandor, GGS, Smith, DF, and MacLeod, PM: Cardiac malformations in the fetal alcohol syndrome. *J. Pediatr.* 98:771–773, 1981.
61. Qazi, QA, Masakawa, A, Milman, D, et al: Renal anomalies in fetal alcohol syndrome. *Pediatrics* 63:886–889, 1979.
62. Herrmann, J, Pallister, PD, and Opitz, JM: Tetraectrodactyly and other skeletal manifestations in the fetal alcohol syndrome. *Eur. J. Pediatr.* 133:221–226, 1980.
63. Spiegel, PG, Pekman, WM, Rich, BH, et al: The orthopedic aspects of the fetal alcohol syndrome. *Clin. Orthop.* 139:58–63, 1979.
64. Ewing, JA: Detecting alcoholism: The CAGE questionnaire. *J.A.M.A.* 252:1905–1909, 1984.
65. Sokol, RJ, Martier, SS, and Ager, JW: The TACE questions: Practical prenatal detection of risk drinking. *Am. J. Obst. Gynecol.* 160:863–870, 1989.

Advertisement in *Practical Dietetics with Reference to Diet in Disease.* (From AF Pattee. *Practical Dietetics with Reference to Diet in Disease.* [5th ed.]. New York: Pattee, 1905.)

HALL'S WINE.

THE MARVELLOUS RESTORATIVE.

More than 100,000 persons in Great Britain are at present suffering from the effects of recent illness or from Neuralgia, Sleeplessness, Nervous Depression, or Weakness. Yet, if facts have any value, arguments any cogency, testimony any merit, all this suffering might be immediately relieved and a speedy recovery assured if Hall's Wine were taken.

So many remedies are advertised to cure every ill that it is well nigh impossible o convince the reading public of the genuineness of a simple remedy that does not profess to cure "all the ills that flesh is heir to."

It is only claimed for

HALL'S WINE

THAT IT

CURES EXTREME WEAKNESS FOLLOWING ILLNESS, NEURALGIA, SLEEPLESSNESS, ANÆMIA, NERVOUS & PHYSICAL BREAKDOWN,

but it does this so rapidly that those who use it describe it as marvellous. In cases of weakness its good effect is apparent after taking one bottle, but neuralgia is often cured within an hour. These statements are not made haphazard. For over a decade Hall's Wine has been before the public.

Hall's Wine has been favourably reported on by most of the leading medical authorities, including "The Lancet," "The British Medical Journal," "The Hospital,' &c. It has been extensively prescribed by physicians. It is used in many of the leading nursing institutions, and to-day has a larger sale than ever.

UNSOLICITED TESTIMONY is received from doctors, nurses, public speakers barristers, actors—in fact, by every class of society, all praising its wonderful restorative and sustaining qualities.

Its action on the throat is immediate and effective. What is commonly called "speaker's throat" disappears at once, and the stimulating and sustaining properties give confidence when it is needed most.

HALL'S WINE IS EXTREMELY PALATABLE,

being undistinguishable from Port; and is economical, because a little goes a long way. It is the most satisfactory pick-me-up in the world.

To give those who have not tried it an opportunity of testing its value,

A Sample Bottle will be sent on receipt of Six Penny Stamps

To cover cost of postage and packing.

Sold by Grocers, Chemists and Wine Merchants.

3/- and 1/9 per Bottle.

SIXPENNY SAMPLES FROM

STEPHEN SMITH & Co., Ltd.,

BOW, LONDON.

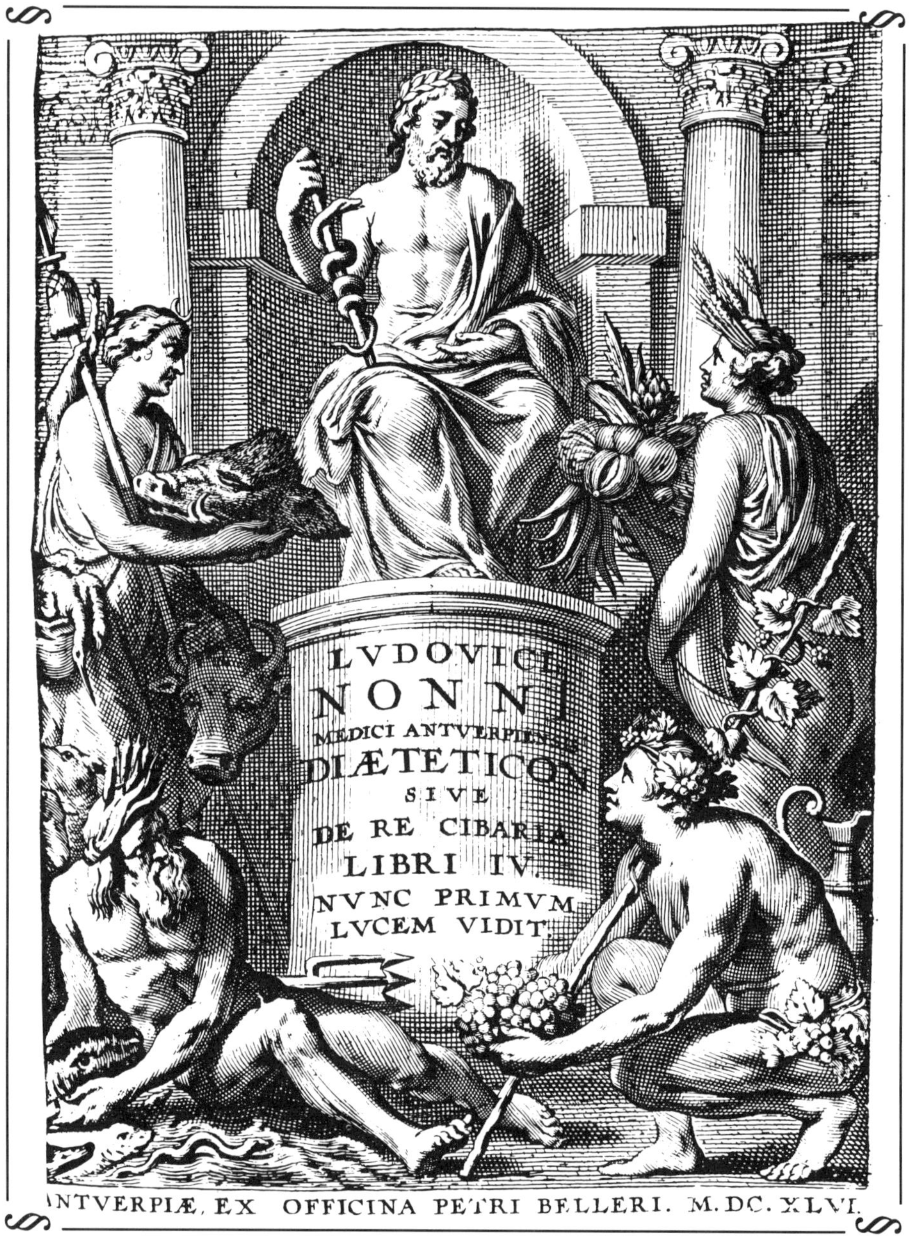

LVDOVICI
NONNI
MEDICI ANTVERPIENSIS
DIÆTETICON
SIVE
DE RE CIBARIA
LIBRI IV.
NVNC PRIMVM
LVCEM VIDIT.

ANTVERPIÆ, EX OFFICINA PETRI BELLERI. M.DC.XLVI.

Seventeenth-century nutrition book. (From Ludovicus Nonnis. *Diaeteticon Sive De Re Cibaria*. Italy: P. Belleri, 1646.)

10 Diabetes Mellitus

Historical Perspective

The association between diabetes mellitus and pregnancy was almost nonexistent before the discovery of insulin by Banting and Best in 1921. Untreated female diabetics had irregular ovulatory cycles and rarely conceived. When they did become pregnant, the perinatal mortality for their infants was greater than 42 percent [1]. The diabetic diets that antedated insulin therapy included such regimens as 85 percent of calories from fat (Naunyn, 1898–1914), oatmeal and fat alternating with days restricted to only vegetables (von Noorden, 1903), fasting and severe caloric restriction (Allen, 1914–1921), and low carbohydrate and high fat (Newburgh and Marsh, 1923). Joslin was the first physician of the preinsulin era who focused specifically on the diets of pregnant diabetics. Joslin recommended a diet consisting of low carbohydrate and moderate fat and protein; fasting was advised when excessive glycosuria was present [2].

During the early years of insulin use, treatment with starvation therapy, and its resulting general malnutrition, was followed by delayed puberty, anovulation, and reduced fertility in many diabetic women [3]. When insulin therapy was combined with a more liberal diet, fertility rose dramatically. Even after long-acting protamine insulin became available in 1937, however, fetal loss remained at 50 percent, the stillbirth rate was 30 percent, and maternal mortality was 10 percent [4]. By 1950, the calculation and planning of diabetic diets was simplified by the publication of exchange lists by the American Diabetes Association [5], although the prevailing philosophy for pregnant diabetics limited sodium intake and restricted weight gain to 12 lb or less [6].

Both the metabolic management and the diet therapy of pregnant diabetics have improved during the past decades, so that the perinatal mortality of 1.6 to 2.0 percent currently achieved by some centers approaches that of the nondiabetic general population [7]. This chapter discusses the metabolic alterations of pregnancy, the pathophysiology of diabetes during gestation, and the most recent insulin and diet therapy recommendations for the clinical management of these pregnancies.

Metabolic Alterations During Pregnancy

During pregnancy amino acids and glucose are siphoned from the maternal to the fetal compartments, causing maternal hypoglycemia, decreased gluconeogenesis, and corresponding hypoinsulinemia. As a result of insufficient insulin and elevated levels of maternal plasma human somatomammotropin, particularly after prolonged fasting, lipolysis and hyperketonemia occur at an accelerated rate. These metabolic changes are exaggerated in the third trimester and have been characterized as "accelerated starvation" [7]. After a 12- to 14-hour fast, pregnant women have lower levels of plasma glucose and plasma alanine (an important precursor of hepatic gluconeogenesis), and higher levels of plasma free fatty acids and beta-hydroxybutyrate compared to nonpregnant women [8, 9].

The most potent diabetogenic insulin antagonists—estrogen, prolactin, progesterone, cortisol, and human placental lactogen—all increase with advancing pregnancy. These hormones alter the effects of insulin and result in the ketosis-prone tendency associated with fasting during pregnancy despite an increase in insulin secretion. The five hormones cited are at their highest concentration at 24 to 28 weeks of gestation, at which time gestational diabetes most commonly occurs. Because of this, all pregnant women should be screened at 24 to 28 weeks' gestation using a 50-gm oral glucose load followed by a plasma glucose determination one hour later [10–13]. If the initial screening is negative but the woman is still thought to be at risk for development of gestational diabetes, this test should be repeated at 32 weeks.

Pathophysiology of Diabetes During Pregnancy

Depending on the screening and diagnostic criteria used, the incidence of gestational diabetes is about 3 to 12 percent, and the incidence of pregestational or insulin-dependent diabetes is about 0.1 to 0.5 percent in American obstetric patients [10, 14]. The increased perinatal morbidity and mortality traditionally characterizing pregnancies complicated by diabetes during pregnancy are attributed to the altered metabolic environment to which the fetus is exposed. If maternal diabetes is not well controlled (maintenance of normoglycemia), then the fetus will be exposed to either intermittent or constant levels of hyperglycemia, both of which stimulate fetal insulin secretion. Pedersen and Pedersen [15] hypothesize that maternal hyperglycemia-induced fetal hyperinsulinemia may result in (1) increased fetal body fat (macrosomia) and, therefore, a difficult vaginal delivery; (2) inhibition of pulmonary maturation of surfactant; (3) decreased serum potassium, which results in muscle weakness or cardiac arrhythmias; and (4) neonatal hypoglycemia, which may result in permanent neurologic damage. Further, impaired maternal glucose metabolism during early embryogenesis has been linked to subsequent early intrauterine growth retardation as well as an increase in birth defects [16–19]. Preconception control of diabetes has been shown to decrease the incidence of congenital malformations and to be cost-effective [20]. Using the glycosylated hemoglobin (HbA_{1c}) as the measure of antecedent diabetic control, it has been shown that elevated blood sugars before pregnancy are related to an increased incidence of birth defects and that adequate control before conception can reverse this effect [21]. In addition, the severity and duration of pregestational diabetes, as indicated by the classification (see Appendix A), also influence pregnancy outcome.

Management of Diabetes During Pregnancy

The primary goal of the management of diabetes during pregnancy is strict metabolic control throughout the entire gestation, but especially during the critical period of embryogenesis. Maintenance of normoglycemia is of paramount importance. Appropriate levels for fasting blood glucose range between 55 and 65 mg/100 ml and one-hour postprandial blood glucose levels range between 120 and 140 mg/100 ml [10, 22]. Insulin-dependent patients should be normoglycemic at the time of conception and throughout the first trimester [23]. Preconceptional counseling of all known diabetics should stress the importance of these precepts and prepare the patient to perform regular self-monitoring of her glucose levels if this had not been routine before the onset of pregnancy.

Insulin

Insulin is an essential component of the therapy for pregestational diabetics and for gestational diabetics for whom plasma glucose levels cannot be controlled with diet alone. There are three major categories of insulin: short-acting (regular and semilente); intermediate-acting (neutral protamine Hagedorn [NPH] and lente); and long-acting (protamine zinc insulin [PZI] and ultralente) (Table 10-1). Individual patients vary with regard to the time of onset and duration of action irrespective of the type of insulin used because of differences in subcutaneous absorption, metabolism, and the presence or absence of antibodies to exogenous insulin.

During pregnancy insulin requirements depend on maternal body weight, degree of maternal obesity, and whether the mother has a singleton or multiple gestation. Jovanovic and co-workers [24–26] suggest that the insulin requirements at the beginning of pregnancy

Table 10-1
Insulin preparations and durations of action

Type of insulin	*Peak action (hr)*	*Duration of action (hr)*
Rapid acting		
Crystalline zinc, regular	2	5–7
Semilente	2	8–16
Intermediate acting		
NPH	6–12	18–24
Lente	6–12	18–24
Long acting		
Protamine zinc	8–14	24–36
Ultralente	12–16	24–36

Table 10-2
*Calculation and distribution of insulin dosage**

	Time		
Insulin type	*7:30 AM*	*4:30 PM*	*10 PM*
NPH	8/18		3/18
Regular	4/18	3/18	
Total	12/18	3/18	3/18

*Total insulin requirement calculated as:
0.7 units/kg/day for weeks 6–18
0.8 units/kg/day for weeks 18–26
0.9 units/kg/day for weeks 26–36
1.0 units/kg/day for weeks 36–40.
The total dose is divided into eighteenths and administered in two or three daily injections.

Source: Adapted from L Jovanovic and CM Peterson, Optimal insulin delivery for the pregnant diabetic patient. *Diabetes Care* 5 (Suppl. 1):24–37, 1982.

are 0.7 units/kg body weight per day, increasing to 0.8 units/kg/day at about 26 weeks' gestation, 0.9 units/kg/day by 32 weeks, and 1.0 units/kg/day by 36 weeks of gestation. Higher dosages are required in cases of maternal obesity and in multiple gestations [24]. Intermediate-acting insulin is given to cover metabolic needs and rapid-acting insulin (crystalline zinc, regular) to cover meals. The total dose of insulin is divided into eighteenths and administered in two or three daily injections as described in Table 10-2.

It is mandatory that the patient self-monitor plasma glucose levels with the home glucose meter in order to achieve optimal "tight" control [27]. In addition, periodic evaluation of the glycosylated hemoglobin (HbA_{1c}) level, which reflects the level of maternal plasma glucose for the previous 6 to 10 weeks, aids in judging overall plasma glucose control [28]. Infant birthweight has been correlated with both the postprandial glucose level [29] and the level of HbA_{1c} [30]. When the plasma glucose levels were higher, so was the incidence of macrosomia.

Diet Therapy

The diet prescribed for pregestational or gestational diabetes has changed dramatically in recent decades and is much more like the diet of the general, nondiabetic population. The current dietary prescription for diabetic patients includes a caloric allowance sufficient to achieve and maintain a desired body weight distributed as 40 percent carbohydrate, 20 percent protein, and 40 percent lipids, with a reduction in saturated fats and cholesterol and an increase in fiber [31].

Caloric Requirement

For the normal-weight woman, the caloric requirement during pregnancy is calculated as 36 kcal/kg/day (2200 kcal/day) for the first trimester, increasing to 40 kcal/kg/day (2500 kcal/day) during the second and third trimesters [32]. Jovanovic-Peterson and Peterson [28] recommend a lower caloric intake based on the concept of sustaining women above the ketonuric threshold while preventing postprandial hyperglycemia. These investigators propose 30 kcal/kg/day for normal-weight women (80–120% of ideal body weight), 40 kcal/kg/day for underweight women (<80% ideal body weight), and 24 kcal/kg/day for overweight women (>120% ideal body weight). The caloric prescription by maternal pregravid weight and the distribution of carbohydrates are given in Fig. 10-1. The distribution of diet exchanges by maternal pregravid weight is given in Fig. 10-2. A worksheet for calculating the diabetic diet is given in Fig. 10-3.

The caloric requirement, and subsequent weight gain, in overweight nondiabetic and diabetic women during pregnancy is controversial. Recent recommendations from the National Academy of Sciences suggest a range of weight gain of 15 to 25 lb for women over 120 percent ideal body weight [33]. Although there is concern regarding the potential adverse fetal effect of maternal ketonuria with insufficient caloric intake, studies of overweight pregnant diabetics have shown improved pregnancy outcomes with moderate caloric restriction (25 kcal/kg/day or 1800–2000 kcal/day) [34, 35]. Severe maternal ketosis, which would affect maternal acid-base balance, should be avoided because it would adversely affect both the mother and her fetus. With severe caloric restriction (<1200 kcal/day), ketonuria and acetonuria result, and both have been associated with neurodevelopmental damage and lowered intelligence in the child [36].

Weight Pounds	Weight Kg	Kcal 30/kg	20% PRO△	40% CHO@	40% FAT		Bkft 8A 2/18	Snack 1030A 1/18	Lunch 12N 5/18	Snack 3PM 2/18	Dinner 5PM 5/18	Snack 8PM 2/18	Snack 11PM 1/18
							Kcal-CHO	Kcal-CHO	Kcal-CHO	Kcal-CHO	Kcal-CHO	Kcal-CHO	Kcal-CHO
100	45.5	1365	68	137	61		150-15	75-7.5	375-38	150-15	375-38	150-15	75-7.5
105	47.7	1431	72	143	64		157-16	79-8	394-39	157-16	394-39	157-16	79-8
110	50	1500	75	150	67		165-17	83-8	413-41	165-17	413-41	165-17	83-8
115	52.3	1569	78	157	70		173-17	86-9	431-43	173-17	431-43	173-17	86-9
120	54.5	1635	82	164	73		180-18	90-9	450-45	180-18	450-45	180-18	90-9
125	56.8	1704	85	170	76		187-19	94-9	469-46	187-19	469-46	187-19	94-9
130	59	1770	89	177	79		195-20	97-10	487-49	195-20	487-49	195-20	97-10
135	61.4	1842	92	184	82		203-20	101-10	507-51	203-20	507-51	203-20	101-10
140	63.6	1908	95	191	85		210-21	105-11	525-53	210-21	525-53	210-21	105-11
145	66	1980	99	198	88		218-22	109-11	545-54	218-22	545-54	218-22	109-11
150	68.2	2046	102	205	91		225-23	113-11	563-56	225-23	563-56	225-23	113-11
155	70.5	2115	106	212	94		233-23	116-12	582-58	233-23	582-58	233-23	116-12
160	72.7	2181	109	218	97		240-24	120-12	600-60	240-24	600-60	240-24	120-12
165	75	2250	113	225	100		248-25	124-12	619-62	248-25	619-62	248-25	124-12
170	77.3	2319	116	232	103		255-26	128-13	638-64	255-26	638-64	255-26	128-13
175	80	2400	120	240	107		264-26	132-13	660-66	264-26	660-66	264-26	132-13
180	81.8	2454	123	245	109		270-27	135-14	675-67	270-27	675-67	270-27	135-14
185	84.1	2523	126	252	112		278-28	139-14	694-69	278-28	694-69	278-28	139-14
190	86.4	2592	130	259	115		285-29	143-14	713-71	285-29	713-71	285-29	143-14
195	88.6	2658	133	266	118		292-29	146-15	731-73	292-29	731-73	292-29	146-15
200	90.9	*2727	136	273	121		300-30	150-15	750-75	300-30	750-75	300-30	150-15
205	93.2	2796	140	280	124		308-31	154-15	769-77	308-31	769-77	308-31	154-15
210	95.5	2865	143	287	127		315-32	158-16	789-79	315-32	789-79	315-32	158-16
215	97.7	2931	147	293	130		322-32	161-16	806-81	322-32	806-81	322-32	161-16
220	100	**3000	150	300	133		330-33	165-17	825-83	330-33	825-83	330-33	165-17
225	102.3	3069	153	307	136		338-34	169-17	844-84	338-34	844-84	338-34	169-17
230	104.5	3135	157	314	139		345-35	173-17	862-86	345-35	862-86	345-35	173-17
235	106.8	3204	160	320	142		352-35	176-18	881-88	352-35	881-88	352-35	176-18
240	109.1	3273	164	327	145		360-36	180-18	900-90	360-36	900-90	360-36	180-18

*26-28 Kcal/kg   **24-26 Kcal/kg   △PRO = Protein   @CHO = Carbohydrate

Fig. 10-1
Diabetic diet prescriptions and carbohydrate distribution by maternal pregravid weight.

Weight Pounds/Kilograms	130/ 59	135/ 61.4	140/ 63.6	145/ 66	150/ 68.2	155/ 70.5	160/ 72.7	165/ 75	170/ 77.3	175/ 80	180/ 81.8	185/ 84.1	190/ 86.4
Exchanges:													
Milk													
2%	4	4	4	4	4								
Whole						4	4	5	4	5	5	6	5
Vegetables	2	3	2	2	3	3	4	4	3	2	3	3	3
Fruit	4½	4½	5	5	6½	6	6	6	5	5	5	5	5
Bread	5	5	5½	6	6	6	6	6	8	8	8	8	9
Meat	6	6	7	7	7½	8	8	9	8	8	9	9	9
Fat	5	6	7	7	7	6	6½	6½	4	4	3	4	3
Prescription:													
CHO	178	184	191	198	208	213	218	225	233	240	245	252	260
PRO	88	92	96	101	102	106	108	113	117	116	125	125	127
FAT	78	83	86	85	90	94	97	100	104	114	107	112	115
Calories	1766	1851	1980	1961	2046	2122	2177	2250	2336	2450	2443	2516	2583

Fig. 10-2
Diabetic diet exchange for gestational diabetes.

Food	Bkft	Snack	Lunch	Snack	Dinner	Snack	Snack	Total	Carbohydrate	Protein	Fat
Milk (skim) (1%) (2%) (whole)									12 12 12 12	8 8 8 8	tr. 2.5 5 10
Vegetables									5	2	–
Fruit									10	–	–
Bread									15	2	–
Meat (lean) (medium) (high)									– – –	7 7 7	3 5.5 8
Fat									–	–	5
Prescription: CHO PRO FAT											
Calories									×4 =	×4 =	×9 =

Maternal Weight: ________________

Date: ________________

Weeks' Gestation: ________________

Fig. 10-3
Pregnancy diabetic diet prescription.

Carbohydrates

The recommended carbohydrate content of the diabetic diet has risen steadily from 35 percent in the early insulin years (1922–1940) [37], to 45 percent by 1971 [38], to the current levels of 50 to 60 percent by 1979 [39]. Higher carbohydrate recommendations have been used by various investigators, including 60, 65, and 85 percent, resulting in improved glycemic control and lowered exogenous insulin requirements [40–44].

Traditionally, diet therapy for diabetes has been based on the concept that there are two major classes of carbohydrates: **simple** or **refined** (glucose, sucrose, and fructose), which are rapidly absorbed and cause a relatively large rise in blood glucose, and **complex** or **starches** (such as rice, potatoes, and legumes), which are digested and absorbed more slowly, resulting in a smaller rise in blood glucose.

Diabetics have traditionally been counseled to avoid simple sugars in the belief that these specific carbohydrates would result in hyperglycemia and poor metabolic control of the disease. Recent studies, however, have shown that the glycemic response of a specific carbohydrate food, whether simple or complex, is influenced by three factors: (1) the form of the food (cooked or uncooked), (2) the amount and type of dietary fiber also in the food, and (3) the nature of the carbohydrate itself. For example, studies have shown that glucose, potatoes, and honey produce similar postprandial glucose responses, whereas rice, beans, and fructose yield similar but lower glycemic responses [45, 46]. Different glycemic responses have been observed even when a single food is prepared in different ways: Ingestion of whole rice results in a flatter glycemic response curve than does ingestion of rice flour, and wheat in pasta produces a lower blood glucose than does wheat in bread [47, 48]. Jenkins and co-workers [45] have suggested the use of a glycemic index to characterize foods, based on the blood glucose response to a food in comparison with the response to an equivalent amount of glucose (Table 10-3). Using this standard of evaluation, legumes, peas, and soybeans produce the lowest glycemic response, while potatoes and carrots elicit the highest. In addition, the incorporation of simple sugars into processed foods [49] or meals [50] does not aggravate postprandial hyperglycemia. To date, evaluations of the glycemic index and the effect of incorporating simple sugars into the diet have been evaluated only in nonpregnant diabetics; their utility in diabetic pregnancies remains to be determined.

Fiber

Although dietary fiber was effectively used to control hyperglycemia with the inclusion of oatmeal in the diabetic diet by von

Table 10-3
*The glycemic index of selected foods**

100%	*50–59%*	*30–39%*
Glucose	Buckwheat	Butter beans
	Spaghetti	Black-eyed peas
80–99%	Sweet corn	Chick peas
Cornflakes	All-Bran cereal	Apples (Golden Delicious)
Carrots	Frozen peas	Ice cream
Potatoes (instant)	Yams	Milk (skim or whole)
Maltose	Sucrose	Yogurt
Honey	Potato chips	Tomato soup
70–79%	*40–49%*	*20–29%*
Bread (whole grain)	Porridge oats	Kidney beans
Rice (white)	Sweet potatoes	Lentils
New potatoes	Oranges	Fructose
	Sponge cake	
	Peaches	
	Pears	
60–69%		*10–19%*
Bread (white)		Soybeans
Brown rice		Peanuts
Shredded wheat		
Bananas		
Raisins		

*The glycemic index is the area under the blood glucose response curve for each food, expressed as the area after taking the same amount of carbohydrate as glucose.

Noorden in 1903 [51], not until 1976 were the therapeutic effects of dietary fiber on postprandial glycemic and serum insulin responses in diabetics clinically demonstrated [52, 53]. Studies with nonpregnant diabetics show beneficial effects of high-carbohydrate, high-fiber, low-fat diets, including decreased postprandial hyperglycemia, mean plasma glucose, glycosuria, and insulin requirement [54–57]. Current research shows that high-carbohydrate (65% of calories), high-fiber diets (60–70 gm/day) result in lower insulin requirements and better glycemic control of diabetes during pregnancy [43]. High-fiber diet has been suggested as a method of managing the gestational diabetic without the need for insulin therapy.

Conclusions

The current prognosis for pregnancies complicated by diabetes is excellent and differs little from that of the general population if the diabetes is known to the treatment team. Pregestational diabetics should receive counseling about the benefit of "tight" metabolic control in the first trimester. All women, regardless of personal or family history, should be screened for diabetes, using appropriate techniques, between the 24th and 28th weeks of gestation. Regardless of whether insulin is required, diet therapy provides the cornerstone of modern clinical management.

Gestational diabetes or chemical diabetes identified during pregnancy remains a controversial area. Gestational diabetes is determined on the basis of an abnormal glucose tolerance test performed during pregnancy in the absence of overt symptoms of diabetes. Two abnormal values in the oral glucose tolerance test lead to a diagnosis of gestational diabetes, and control is usually with diet therapy [58]. Failure to control the fasting blood sugar can lead to the institution of insulin therapy. It has been suggested that empiric insulin therapy in women with abnormal glucose tolerance tests during pregnancy can decrease the incidence of macrosomia and other complications, although routine insulin therapy remains controversial [59].

Screening for gestational diabetes also remains controversial, the issue being whether women should be screened only because of risk factors such as previous macrosomia, obesity, history of stillbirth, or family history of diabetes, or whether routine screening should be undertaken, since 50 percent of women who have an abnormal glucose tolerance test and are given a diagnosis of gestational diabetes have no associated risk factors.

References

1. Williams, JW: The clinical significance of glycosuria in pregnant women. *Am. J. Med. Sci.* 137:1, 1909.
2. Joslin, EP: *The Treatment of Diabetes Mellitus With Observations Upon the Disease Based Upon One Thousand Cases* (1st ed.). Philadelphia: Lea & Febiger, 1916. Pp. 342–354.
3. Parson, E, Randall, LM, and Wilder, RM: Pregnancy and diabetes. *Med. Clin. North Am.* 10:679–688, 1926.
4. White, P: Pregnancy Complicating Diabetes. In EP Joslin, HF Root, P White, and A Marble (eds.), *The Treatment of Diabetes Mellitus* (6th ed.). Philadelphia: Lea & Febiger, 1937. Pp. 618–637.
5. *Meal Planning With Exchange Lists*. New York: American Diabetes Association, Inc., and the American Dietetic Association, 1949.
6. Ney, D, and Hollingsworth, DR: Nutritional management of pregnancy complicated by diabetes: Historical perspective. *Diabetes Care* 4:647–655, 1981.

7. Freinkel, N, Dooley, SL, and Mtezger, BE: Care of the pregnant woman with insulin-dependent diabetes mellitus. *N. Engl. J. Med.* 313:96–101, 1985.
8. Ravnikar, V, Metzger, BE, and Freinkel, N: Is there a risk of "accelerated starvation" in normal human pregnancy? *Diabetes* 27:463, 1978.
9. Cousins, L, Rigg, L, Hollingsworth, D, et al: The 24-hour excursion and diurnal rhythm of glucose, insulin, and C-peptide in normal pregnancy. *Am. J. Obstet. Gynecol.* 136:483, 1980.
10. Gabbe, S: Management of diabetes mellitus in pregnancy. *Am. J. Obstet. Gynecol.* 153:824–828, 1985.
11. Freinkel, N, and Josimovich, J: Conference Planning Committee. American Diabetes Workshop: Conference on Gestational Diabetes. *Diabetes Care* 3:499, 1980.
12. Marquette, GP, Klein, VR, and Niebyl, JR: Efficacy of screening for gestational diabetes. *Am. J. Perinatol.* 2:7, 1985.
13. O'Sullivan, JB, Mahan, CM, Charles, D, and Dandrow, RV: Screening criteria for high-risk gestational diabetic patients. *Am. J. Obstet. Gynecol.* 116:895, 1973.
14. Hadden, DR: Geographic, ethnic, and racial variations on the incidence of gestational diabetes mellitus. *Diabetes* 34 (Suppl. 2):8–12, 1985.
15. Pedersen, J, and Pedersen, LM: Diabetes Mellitus and Pregnancy. The Hyperglycemia, Hyperinsulinemia Theory and the Weight of the Newborn Baby. In RR Rodriguez and J Vallance-Owen (eds.): *Proceedings of the 7th Congress of the International Diabetes Federation.* Amsterdam: Excerta Medica, 1971. Pp. 678–685.
16. Pedersen, JF, and Molsted-Pedersen, L: Early growth retardation in diabetic pregnancy. *Br. Med. J.* 1:18–19, 1979.
17. Pedersen, JF, and Molsted-Pedersen, L: Early fetal growth delay detected by ultrasound marks increased risk of congenital malformations in diabetic pregnancy. *Br. Med. J.* 283:269–271, 1981.
18. Leslie, RDG, John, PN, Pyke, DA, and White, JM: Haemoglobin A_1 in diabetic pregnancy. *Lancet* 2:958–959, 1978.
19. Miller, E, Hare, JW, Clogerty, JP, et al: Elevated maternal hemoglobin A_{1c} in early pregnancy and major congenital anomalies in infants of diabetic mothers. *N. Engl. J. Med.* 304:1331–1334, 1981.
20. Scheffler, RN, Feuchtbaum, LB, and Phibbs, CS: Prevention: The cost-effectiveness of the California diabetes and pregnancy program. *Am. J. Public Health* 82:168, 1992.
21. Kitzmiller, JL, et al: Preconception care of diabetes: Glycemic control prevents congenital anomalies. *J.A.M.A.* 265:731, 1991.
22. Gillmer, MDG, Beard, RW, Brooke, RW, and Oakley, NWE: Carbohydrate metabolism in pregnancy. I. Diurnal plasma glucose profile in normal and diabetic women. *Br. Med. J.* 3:339, 1975.
23. Fuhrmann, K, Reiher, H, Semmler, K, et al: Prevention of congenital malformations in infants of insulin-dependent diabetic mothers. *Diabetes Care* 6:219, 1983.

24. Jovanovic, L, Druzin, M, and Peterson, CM: Effect of euglycemia on the outcome of pregnancy in insulin-dependent diabetic women compared with normal control subjects. *Am. J. Med.* 71:921–927, 1981.
25. Jovanovic, L, Peterson, CM, Saxena, BB, et al: Feasibility of maintaining normal glucose profiles in insulin-dependent pregnant women. *Am. J. Med.* 68:105–112, 1980.
26. Jovanovic, L, and Peterson, CM: Optimal insulin delivery for the pregnant diabetic patient. *Diabetes Care* 5(Suppl. 1):24–37, 1982.
27. Varner, MW: Efficacy of home glucose monitoring in diabetic pregnancy. *Am. J. Med.* 75:592, 1983.
28. Jovanovic-Peterson, L, and Peterson, CM: Dietary manipulation as a primary treatment strategy for pregnancies complicated by diabetes. *J. Am. Coll. Nutr.* 9:320–325, 1990.
29. Jovanovic-Peterson, L: The relationship between glucose levels and macrosomia: The diabetes in early pregnancy study. *Diabetes* 38(Suppl. 2):129, 1989.
30. Jovanovic, L, and Peterson, CM: Intensified treatment of pregnant insulin-dependent diabetic women. *Acta Endocrinol.* 277(Suppl.): 77–80, 1986.
31. American Diabetes Association: Nutritional recommendations and principles for individuals with diabetes mellitus. *Diabetes Care* 10:126, 1987.
32. National Academy of Sciences: *Recommended Dietary Allowances* (10th ed.). Washington, DC: National Academy Press, 1989.
33. National Academy of Sciences: *Nutrition During Pregnancy*. Washington, DC: National Academy Press, 1990.
34. Algert, S, Shragg, P, and Hollingsworth, DR: Moderate caloric restriction in obese women with gestational diabetes. *Obstet. Gynecol.* 65:487–491, 1985.
35. Boberg, C, Gillmer, MDG, Brunner, EJ, et al: Obesity in pregnancy: The effect of dietary advice. *Diabetes Care* 3:476, 1980.
36. Churchill, JA, Berendes, HW, and Nemore, J: Neuropsychological deficits in children of diabetic mothers. *Am. J. Obstet. Gynecol.* 105:257–268, 1969.
37. White, P: Pregnancy Complicating Diabetes. In EP Joslin, HF Root, P White, and A Marble (eds.), *The Treatment of Diabetes Mellitus* (7th ed.). Philadelphia: Lea & Febiger, 1940. Pp. 693–709.
38. Committee on Food and Nutrition, American Diabetes Association and American Dietetic Association: Principles of nutrition and dietary recommendations for patients with diabetes mellitus: 1971. *Diabetes* 29:633–634, 1971.
39. American Diabetes Association: Principles of nutrition and dietary recommendations for individuals with diabetes mellitus. *Diabetes Care* 2:520–523, 1979.
40. Weinsier, RL, Seeman, A, Herrera, G, et al: High- and low-carbohydrate diets in diabetes mellitus. *Ann. Intern. Med.* 80:332, 1974.

41. Stone, DB, and Connor, WE: The prolonged effects of a low cholesterol, high carbohydrate diet on the serum lipids in diabetic patients. *Diabetes* 12:127, 1963.
42. Brunzell, JD, Lerner, RL, Hazzard, WR, et al: Improved glucose tolerance with high carbohydrate feeding in mild diabetes. *N. Engl. J. Med.* 284:521–524, 1971.
43. Ney, D, Hollingsworth, DR, and Cousins, L: Decreased insulin requirement and improved control of diabetes in pregnant women given a high-carbohydrate, high-fiber, low-fat diet. *Diabetes Care* 5:529–533, 1982.
44. Garg, A, Bonanome, A, Grundy, SM, et al: Comparison of a high-carbohydrate diet with a high-monounsaturated-fat diet in patients with non–insulin-dependent diabetes mellitus. *N. Engl. J. Med.* 319:829–834, 1988.
45. Jenkins, DJA, Wolever, TMS, Taylor, RH, et al: Glycemic index of foods: A physiological basis for carbohydrate exchange. *Am. J. Clin. Nutr.* 34:362–366, 1981.
46. Crapo, PA, Insel, J, Sperling, M, and Kolterman, OG: Comparison of serum glucose, insulin, and glucagon responses to different types of complex carbohydrate in noninsulin-dependent diabetic patients. *Am. J. Clin. Nutr.* 34:184–190, 1981.
47. O'Dea, K, Nestel, PJ, and Antonoff, L: Physical factors influencing postprandial glucose and insulin responses to starch. *Am. J. Clin. Nutr.* 33:760–765, 1980.
48. Jenkins, DJA, Wolever, TMS, Jenkins, AL, et al: Glycemic response to wheat products: Reduced response to pasta but no effect of fiber. *Diabetes Care* 6:155–159, 1983.
49. Crapo, PA, Scarlett, JA, and Kolterman, OG: Comparison of the metabolic responses to fructose and sucrose sweetened foods. *Am. J. Clin. Nutr.* 36:256–261, 1982.
50. Bantle, JP, Laine, DC, Castle, GW, et al: Postprandial glucose and insulin responses to meals containing different carbohydrates in normal and diabetic subjects. *N. Engl. J. Med.* 309:7–12, 1983.
51. von Noorden, C: Veber Hafercuren ber schwerem diabetes mellitus. *Berliner Klin. Wochenschr.* 40:817–821, 1903.
52. Jenkins, DJA, Leeds, AR, Gassull, MA, et al: Unabsorbable carbohydrate and diabetes: Decreased postprandial hyperglycemia. *Lancet* 2:172, 1976.
53. Kiehm, TG, Anderson, JW, and Ward, K: Beneficial effects of a high carbohydrate, high fiber diet on hyperglycemic diabetic men. *Am. J. Clin. Nutr.* 29:895, 1976.
54. Miranda, PM, and Horwitz, DL: High-fiber diets in the treatment of diabetes mellitus. *Ann. Intern. Med.* 88:482, 1978.
55. Jenkins, DJA, Leeds, AR, Gassull, MA, et al: Decrease in postprandial insulin and glucose concentrations by guar and pectin. *Ann. Intern. Med.* 86:20, 1977.
56. Anderson, JW, and Ward, K: High-carbohydrate, high-fiber diets for

insulin treated men with diabetes mellitus. *Am. J. Clin. Nutr.* 32:2312, 1979.

57. Christiansen, JS, Bonnevie-Nielsen, V, Svendsen, PA, et al: Effect of guar gum on 24-hour insulin requirements of insulin-dependent diabetic subjects as assessed by an artificial pancreas. *Diabetes Care* 3:659, 1980.
58. Summary and Recommendations of the 2nd International Workshop/Conference on Gestational Diabetes. *Diabetes* 34 (Suppl. 2):123, 1985.
59. Coustan, DR, and Imarag, HJ: Prophylactic insulin treatment of gestational diabetes reduced the incidence of macrosomia, operative delivery, and birth trauma. *Am. J. Obstet. Gynecol.* 150:836, 1984.

Appendix A: Classification of Pregnant Diabetic Patients

Joslin Clinic (Boston)		*Rigshospitalet (Copenhagen): Prognostically bad signs in pregnancy (PBSP)*	*Johns Hopkins (Baltimore)*
Class	*Criterion*		
A	Chemical diabetes	*Clinical pyelonephritis:* Urinary tract infection with an acute elevation of temperature exceeding 39°C, confirmed by culture of the urine	*Gestational diabetes* A. Dietary control B. Exogenous insulin and dietary control
B	Maturity onset (age >20 yr), duration <10 yr, no vascular lesions		
C_1	Age 10–19 yr at onset	*Precoma:* Diabetic acidosis with a venous standard bicarbonate <10 mEq/liter	*Pregestational diabetes* A. Without related complications B. With related complications 1. Renovascular 2. Retinal
C_2	10–19 yr duration	*Severe acidosis:* Venous standard bicarbonate 10–17 mEq/liter	
D_1	<10 yr at onset		
D_2	>20 yr duration	*Severe toxemia:* Two of the following three signs present: (1) blood pressure >150/100 for at least 5 days before delivery, (2) >0.1% albuminuria for at least 24 hr before delivery, (3) severe edema or a weight gain >20 kg	
D_3	Benign retinopathy		
D_4	Calcified vessels of legs		
D_5	Hypertension	*Mild toxemia:* Two of the following signs present: (1) blood pressure 140/90 for at least 3 days before delivery, (2) >0.05% albuminuria for at least 24 hr before delivery, (3) moderate edema or weight gain >15 kg	
E	No longer sought		
F	Nephropathy		
G	Many failures	*Neglect:* Failure to follow the recommended regimen, irrespective of cause, e.g., "psychopathy," low intelligence, first attendance late in pregnancy (at delivery), poor social circumstances, and lack of proper information	
H	Cardiopathy		
R	Proliferating retinopathy		
T	Renal transplant by Tagatz and colleagues of the University of Minnesota		

Source: Adapted from SG Gabbe, Definition, detection, and management of gestational diabetes. *Obstet. Gynecol.* 67:121, 1986; JE Tyson and RA Hock, Gestational and pregestational diabetes: An approach to therapy. *Am. J. Obstet. Gynecol.* 125:1009, 1976; and P White, Classification of obstetric diabetes. *Am. J. Obstet. Gynecol.* 130:228, 1978.

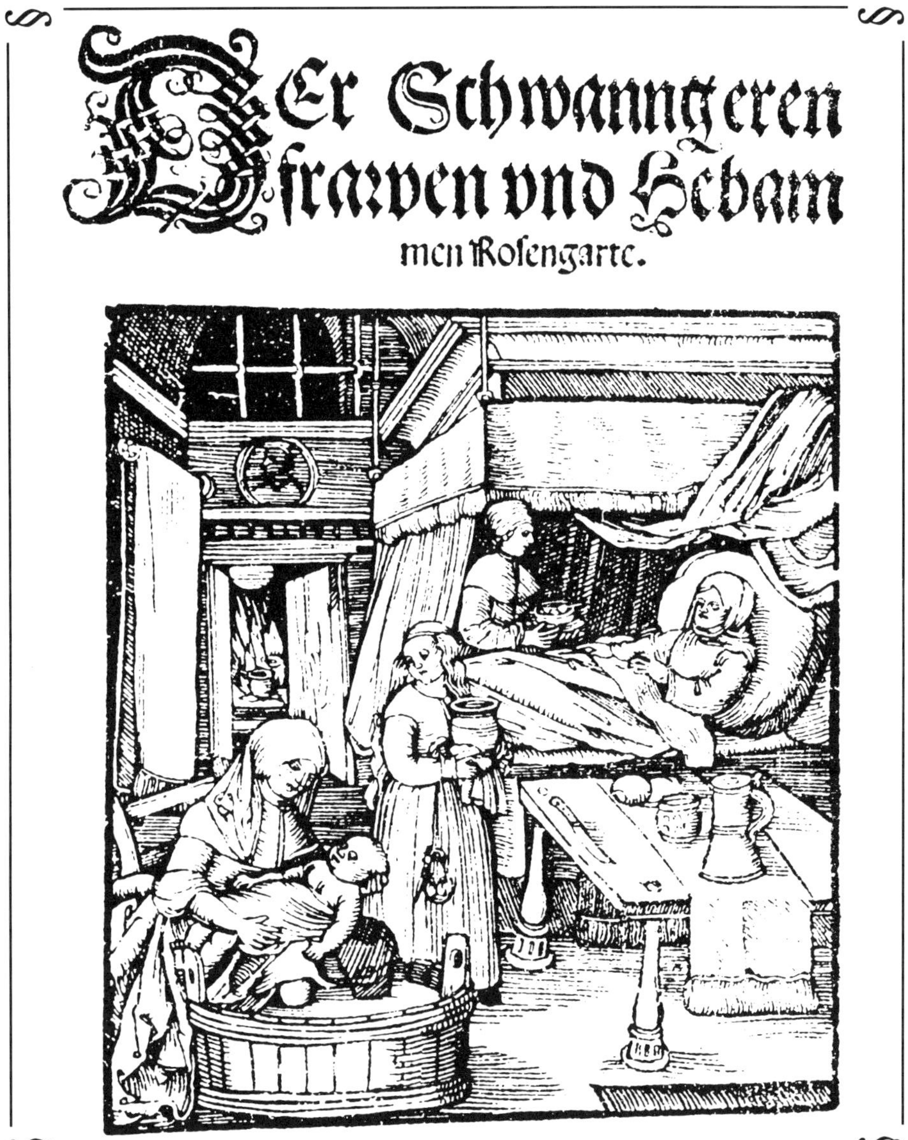

Birth at home. (From Eucharis Roeslin. *Rosengarten*. Frankfurt: Christian Egenolph, 1526.)

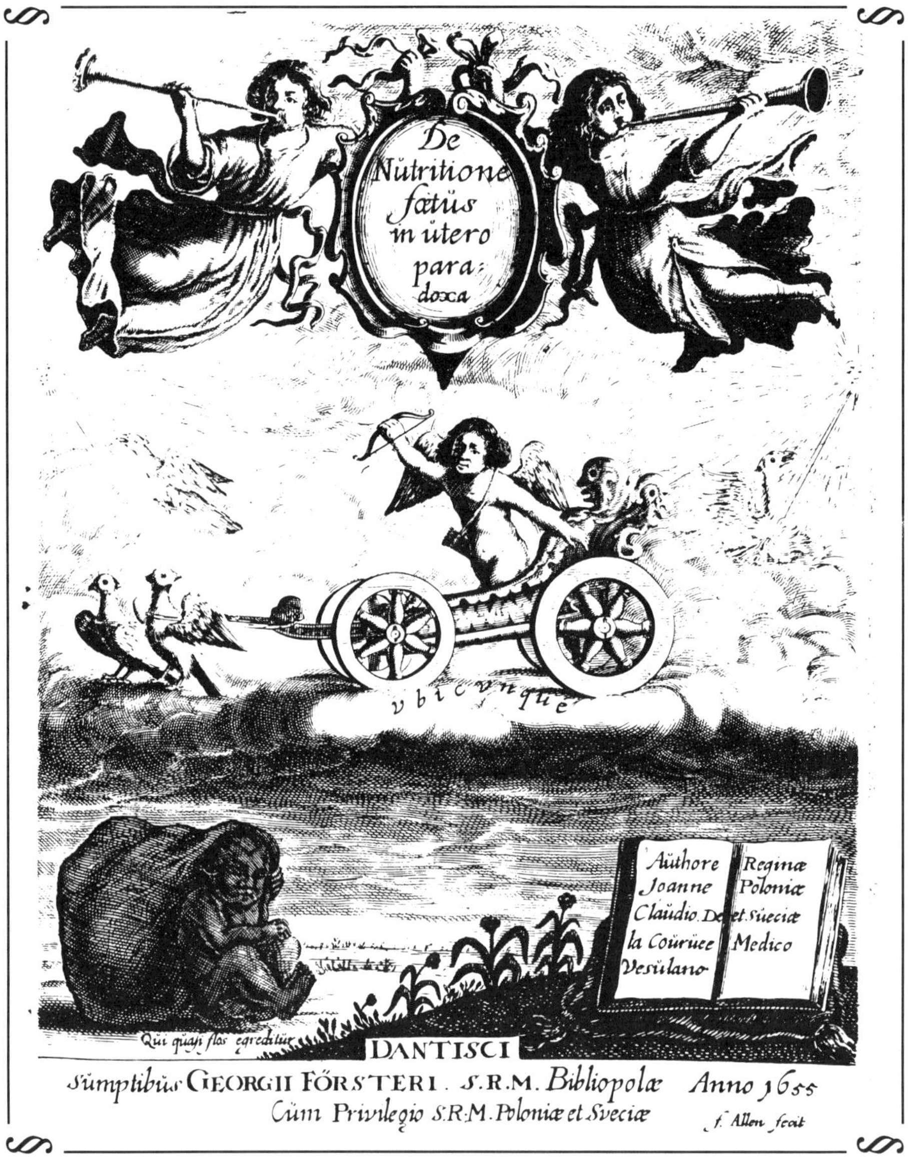

Prenatal nutrition book from the 17th century. (From Jean Claude de la Courvée. *De Nutritione Foetus in Utero Paradoxa*. Italy: G. Försteri, 1655.)

11

Maternal Phenylketonuria

Phenylketonuria (PKU) is a genetic disorder of amino acid metabolism that cannot be cured. Its adverse effects can be minimized by appropriate diet therapy. If untreated, PKU results in mental retardation. Since 1961, all newborn infants in the United States have been screened for this disorder. Once detected, a phenylalanine-restricted diet is prescribed until the child is about 6 years of age. After the diet is discontinued, many patients are lost to medical follow-up study. The first cohort of patients treated with phenylalanine-restricted diets reached reproductive age in 1975, and each year new members enter the cohort. A minimum of 5500 women of childbearing age in the United States are presently estimated to be at risk for having a PKU-affected infant [1].

Women who were treated for PKU during their infancy and childhood pose a special problem when they conceive because untreated PKU in the mother results in mental retardation of the unborn child. It has been suggested that if each woman with untreated PKU were to have two affected children, within one generation the prevalence of mental retardation related to PKU could rebound to the level present before the advent of mass screening and treatment [2].

The challenge to obstetricians is to screen women of childbearing age for PKU and effectively treat those who are detected before irreversible damage has been done to the developing infant. This chapter presents the metabolic and clinical aspects of PKU and the diet therapy to treat maternal PKU.

The Genetic Basis of PKU

Phenylketonuria was originally described more than half a century ago. This disorder illustrates three principles of human genetics [3]. First, it is inherited as an autosomal recessive trait according to Mendel's law of segregation. Second, as an inborn error of metabolism, it illustrates Garrod's cardinal principal of gene action: Genetic factors specify chemical reactions and human biochemical individuality [4]. Third, it illustrates the fact that phenotypes are determined by both genetic constitution and environmental influences. Specifically, hyperphenylalaninemia is a phenotype only when the mutant allele is expressed in an obligatory environment containing an abundance of L-phenylalanine.

Phenylketonuria and mild hyperphenylalaninemia result from mutations in the gene for the phenylalanine hydroxylase apoenzyme and are inherited as autosomal recessive. The severity of the disease induced by the phenotype is a result of the combined effects of two mutant phenylalanine hydroxylase alleles and other combinations of alleles, which can contain mutations with different levels of severity [5].

The Chemical Basis of PKU

Classic PKU occurs in the absence or inactivity of the enzyme phenylalanine hydroxylase. As a consequence, phenylalanine is not converted to tyrosine and a number of alternative metabolites, such as phenylpyruvic acid (the product of deamination of phenylalanine), phenyllactic acid (the reduction product of phenylpyruvic acid), and phenylacetic acid (produced by decarboxylation and oxidation of phenylpyruvic acid), are formed. Most phenylacetate is conjugated in the liver with glutamine and excreted in the urine as the conjugate phenylacetylglutamine. The presence of the keto acid phenylpyruvate in the urine gives this disease its name (Table 11-1).

The Types of PKU

The major metabolic disorders associated with impaired ability to convert phenylalanine to tyrosine are classified into three broad categories: defects in phenylalanine hydroxylase (hyperphenylalaninemia, type I, or classic PKU), dihydrobiopterin reductase (hyper-

Table 11-1
Metabolites of phenylalanine in the plasma and urine of patients with phenylketonuria

Metabolites of phenylalanine	*Plasma levels (mg/100 ml)*		*Urinary levels (mg/100 ml)*	
	Normal	*PKU*	*Normal*	*PKU*
Phenylalanine	1–2	15–63	30	300–1000
Phenylpyruvate	–	0.3–1.8	–	300–2000
Phenyllactate	–	–	–	290–550
Phenylacetate	–	–	–	Increased
Phenylacetylglutamine	–	–	200–300	2400

Source: Adapted from Chap. 22, Catabolism of the Carbon Skeletons of Amino Acids. In DW Martin, PA Mayes, VW Rodwell, and DK Granner (eds.), *Harper's Review of Biochemistry* (12th ed.). Los Altos, CA: Lange Medical Publications, 1985. P. 307.

phenylalaninemia, types II and III), and dihydrobiopterin biosynthesis (hyperphenylalaninemia, types IV and V). In addition, other variants of this disease are listed in Table 11-2.

Clinical Manifestations of PKU

The major consequence of untreated PKU is mental retardation. An intelligence quotient of less than 70 is noted by late childhood in an estimated 96 to 98 percent of patients [6]. Additional clinical signs include seizures, psychoses, eczema, and a distinctive "mousy" odor. If diagnosis and treatment are timely, however, these symptoms can be avoided.

The cornerstone of treatment for PKU is a diet containing very low levels of phenylalanine from birth to age 6 or older [7]. If adherence to the diet is strict, blood phenylalanine levels return to normal, and the excretion of alternative metabolites is reduced. The phenylala-

Table 11-2
The hyperphenylalaninemias

Type	*Condition*	*Defect*	*Treatment*
I	Phenylketonuria	Phenylalanine hydroxylase absent	Low-phenylalanine diet
II	Persistent hyperphenylalaninemia	Decreased phenylalanine hydroxylase	None or temporary low-phenylalanine diet
III	Transient mild hyperphenylalaninemia	Maturational delay of phenylalanine hydroxylase	Same as for type II
IV	Dehydropteridine	Deficient or absent dehydropteridine reductase	Dopa, 5-OH-tryptophan, carbidopa
V	Abnormal dihydrobiopterin function	Dihydrobiopterin synthesis defect	Dopa, 5-OH-tryptophan, carbidopa
VI	Persistent hyperphenylalaninemia	Catabolism of tyrosine	Reduced phenylalanine intake
VII	Transient neonatal tyrosinemia	*p*-hydroxyphenylpyruvic oxidase inhibition	Vitamin C
VIII	Hereditary tyrosinemia	Deficiency in P-OH phenylpyruvate deoxygenase	Low-tyrosine diet
		Cytoplasmic tyrosine aminotransferase	Low-tyrosine diet
		Fumarylacetoacetate	Low-tyrosine diet plus glutathione injections

nine-restricted diet is usually terminated after age 6, when high concentrations of phenylalanine and its derivatives are no longer injurious to the brain; some investigators, however, recommend that the phenylalanine-restricted diet be maintained indefinitely [8]. Phenylketonuria exists in a spectrum of milder forms in which developmental delay is more variable (Table 11-2). Some of these milder forms do not result in mental retardation and do not require treatment, although their existence may pose special problems for affected female children during subsequent pregnancies.

Extent of the Problem

In the United States, national screening of newborn infants for PKU began in 1961. This condition is estimated to occur in about 1 in 10,000 to 15,000 infants [9]. Between the years 1961 and 1985, approximately 90 million newborn infants could have been tested for PKU [10]. Of this number, about 60 percent (55 million) were born between 1961 and 1975, and now are in their childbearing years, between ages 16 and 30. Assuming that half of all infants are female, an estimated 27 million girls born between 1961 and 1975 are potentially fecund at present. Applying the conservative estimate of 1 in 10,000 incidence of PKU, about 2700 women who are currently of reproductive age are potentially at risk of delivering infants adversely affected by maternal PKU.

None of the estimated 57 million children born between 1945 and 1960 were tested for the presence of PKU [10]. Again, assuming that half of those infants were female and that 1 in 10,000 were PKU positive, an additional 2800 women between the ages of 29 and 44 are also at risk of giving birth to a PKU-affected infant. Many of these women may themselves be severely mentally retarded and/or may have suffered increased morbidity (and possibly reduced fecundability) and mortality because of unrecognized and untreated prenatal PKU. Thus, a minimum of 5500 women in the United States who are currently between the ages of 14 and 44 years are at risk of delivering a PKU-affected infant.

Pathophysiology of Maternal PKU

For about two decades, it has been recognized that excess maternal phenylalanine levels exert a teratogenic effect on the developing fetus [11–15]. A positive gradient of phenylalanine exists from mother to fetus during pregnancy. Maternal blood phenylalanine levels greater than 20 mg/100 ml (1200 μmole/liter) during pregnancy are associated with increased intrauterine mortality. Among surviving infants, there is a 90 percent incidence of mental retardation associated with various degrees of microcephaly, congenital cardiac anomalies, and low birthweight. Maternal blood phenylalanine levels less than 16 mg/100 ml (970 μmole/liter) result in a 20 percent incidence of these adverse outcomes among the survivors [11–15]. Women with PKU more commonly experience spontaneous abortion, possibly from the toxic effects of high levels of phenylalanine or its related metabolites, or both [12, 13, 16, 17].

Clinical Studies

In a 10-year study (1971–1981) evaluating 92 percent of all births in Massachusetts, 22 maternal cases of PKU or hyperphenylalaninemia were identified from an analysis of 725,197 cord blood specimens [18]. Nine of the 22 women (41% of the sample) had a second delivery during the screening period, resulting in an estimated 1 : 20,000 incidence of maternal PKU. Maternal parameters, including intelligence quotient and blood phenylalanine and tyrosine levels, were correlated with the child's head circumference and weight at birth and later intelligence quotient. It was shown that substantial fetal damage occurred not only when the maternal blood phenylalanine level was greater than 1200 μmole (20 mg/100 ml), but also when the level was 1000 to 1200 μmole per liter (18–20 mg/100 ml). The authors concluded that the classic and severe atypical forms of maternal PKU had a substantial adverse effect on the fetus and that women with these disorders should be treated with a low-phenylalanine diet during pregnancy, preferably initiated before conception.

In 1987, the Medical Research Council, Department of Health and Social Security of the United Kingdom, published the results of a prospective study of the outcome of pregnancy in women with blood phenylalanine levels greater than 240 μmole per liter (4 mg/100 ml) [19]. Between 1978 and 1986, 48 women with PKU had 64 pregnancies resulting in live births. The infants were categorized according to the mother's dietary treatment during pregnancy. Mothers who maintained a strict (low) phenylalanine diet and had blood phenylalanine levels less than 600 μmole per liter (10 mg/100 ml) at the time of conception delivered infants who had normal birthweights and head circumferences and did not exhibit any malformations. In contrast, the 29 infants whose mothers had either a relaxed or normal diet at the time of conception and initiated a strict diet only after conception had birthweights and head circumferences below those of the healthy infants. Moreover, the incidence of malformations was increased among these infants. These findings closely resemble those observed in the 18 infants whose mothers received no dietary treatment whatsoever during pregnancy. In this study, birthweight and head circumference were inversely related to maternal phenylalanine levels around the time of conception; only when a strict diet was initiated before conception was fetal damage prevented.

Screening Programs

A variety of solutions to the problem of preconceptional or early prenatal identification of maternal PKU have been proposed. In 1972, MacCready and Levy [15] suggested that physicians screen women during premarital examinations or at the first prenatal visit using reagent strips (Phenistix) to test for the presence of high levels of phenylpyruvate. In Canada, a national attempt to address this problem led to the development of the Register of the Quebec Network of Genetic Medicine [2]. This genetic registry, which functions as a part of the area's central laboratory for neonatal screening, also provides continuous surveillance of affected individuals, personal notification when young women reach age 12, and counseling about the consequences of maternal hyperphenylalaninemia and the options to prevent these adverse effects.

A decade ago it was suggested that the United States follow Canada's lead in developing a national register to provide appropriate follow-up study for women with PKU when they reach adolescence [20]. Unfortunately, this suggestion has gone unheeded. Nonetheless, the critical importance of initiating dietary therapy in women in their childbearing years before conception and the need to organize programs that include young men are clearly evident [21].

Diet Therapy

The initiation of diet therapy before conception results in the most favorable pregnancy outcomes [22]. Specific dietary guidelines have been published to assist patients in achieving adequate prenatal nutrition while sufficiently restricting dietary phenylalanine to lower levels and maintaining blood phenylalanine levels in the range of 120 to 580 μmole per liter (2–8 mg/100 ml) [23] (Tables 11-3 and 11-4). Consultation with a dietitian is strongly advised, so that patients receive instruction, full dietary lists, and appropriate dietary support before and during pregnancy. It is also recommended that L-tyrosine be added as a supplement to maintain blood tyrosine levels of 30 μmole per liter (0.5 mg/100 ml) or greater.

In cases of classic phenylketonuria, the phenylalanine content of the diet is restricted to between 250 and 500 mg per day. This diet is composed of foods naturally low in phenylalanine and special dietary products. The latter include such products as Lofenalac (Mead Johnson and Co., Evansville, IN), a casein hydrolysate from which over 95 percent of the pheynlalanine has been removed; PKU-Aid (Milner Scientific and Medical Research Co., Liverpool, England, and Ross Laboratories, Columbus, OH [US distributor]), a hydrolysate of beef serum from which phenylalanine has been removed; and Phenyl Free (Mead Johnson and Co.), a phenylalanine free formula. Food sources of phenylalanine are given in Table 11-5.

Table 11-3
Recommendations for the evaluation of nutritional status of a pregnant woman with phenylketonuria

1. Determination of serum phenylalanine, tyrosine, and all other plasma amino acid levels before institution of the diet
2. Evaluation of diet (phenylalanine, tyrosine, protein, energy, vitamins, minerals) before initiation of therapy
3. Monitoring weekly serum phenylalanine and tyrosine levels; these tests should be accompanied by a prior 3-day diet record that is evaluated for phenylalanine, tyrosine, protein, energy, vitamins, and minerals
4. Monthly plasma amino acid profiles
5. Measurement of total serum protein and albumin during each trimester
6. Determination of hemoglobin and hematocrit during each trimester
7. Evaluation of plasma vitamins A, C, and B_6; folate; erythrocyte glutathione reductase; and transketolase each trimester
8. Determination of serum iron, copper, zinc, magnesium, and manganese during each trimester
9. Measurement of initial height and monthly weights of mother with estimates of growth of fetus

Source: Adapted from P Acosta, M Blaskovics, H Cloud, et al, Nutrition in pregnancy of women with hyperphenylalaninemia. *J. Am. Diet. Assoc.* 80:443–450, 1982.

Table 11-4
Suggested protocol for dietary management of maternal phenylketonuria

I. Establish diet prescription
  A. Phenylalanine
    1. 250–600 mg per day. After targeted blood phenylalanine level of 2–6 mg/100 ml is attained, dietary phenylalanine can be prescribed based on the patient's individual tolerance.
  B. L-Tyrosine supplement[a]
    1. First half of gestation
      a. 1 gm tyrosine daily if patient's phenylalanine tolerance is greater than 1000 mg daily.
      b. 1.5 gm tyrosine daily if patient's phenylalanine tolerance is 500–1000 mg daily.
      c. 2 gm tyrosine daily if patient's phenylalanine tolerance is less than 500 mg daily.
    2. Second half of gestation
      a. 2 gm tyrosine daily if patient's phenylalanine tolerance is greater than 1000 mg daily.
      b. 3 gm tyrosine daily if patient's phenylalanine tolerance is 500–1000 mg daily.
      c. 4–5 gm tyrosine daily if patient's phenylalanine tolerance is less than 500 mg daily.
  C. Protein
    1. First half of gestation, 50 gm daily.
    2. Second half of gestation, 100 gm daily.
  D. Energy
    1. First half of gestation
      a. Adequate to provide for appropriate weight gain
      b. Never less than 1800 kcal daily
    2. Second half of gestation
      a. Adequate to provide for appropriate weight gain
      b. Probably no less than 2000 kcal daily; more may be required depending on age and physical activity.

II. Meeting the diet prescription
  A. Phenylalanine. Use solid food serving lists to fill phenylalanine prescription.

List	*Phenylalanine (mg)*	*Protein (gm)*	*Energy (kcal)*
Bread/cereal	30	0.6	30
Fats	5	0.1	60
Fruits	15	0.6	60
Fruits	15	0.5	20

  B. L-Tyrosine. Make a suspension of L-tyrosine in water. Mix so that there is a known amount of L-tyrosine per milliliter.

Table 11-4 (continued)
Suggested protocol for dietary management of maternal phenylketonuria

C. Protein
   1. Determine amount of protein in solid foods used to meet phenylalanine prescription.
   2. Subtract from protein prescription.
   3. Fill remainder of protein prescription with Phenyl-Free.[b] One unpacked tablespoon of Phenyl-Free weighs 9.8 gm and provides 2 gm protein.
   4. Phenyl-Free should be mixed to a volume the patient will take in 6–8 feedings.
      a. L-tyrosine suspension in the appropriate amount should be mixed with the Phenyl-Free.
      b. A source of phenylalanine should be ingested if Phenyl-Free is not taken with meals.

D. Energy
   1. Determine amount of energy in solid foods used to meet phenylalanine prescription and that in Phenyl-Free used to meet protein requirements.
   2. Subtract from energy prescription.
   3. Supply remaining energy need with free foods (see Table 11-5).

E. Minerals and vitamins
   1. Minerals
      a. Evaluate diet for calcium, phosphorus, magnesium, iron, and zinc.
      b. Magnesium and zinc are likely to be low; provide supplements.
   2. Vitamins
      a. Evaluate diet for all major vitamins.
      b. Folate likely to be low; provide supplement.

[a]Ajinomto Co., Inc., New York, NY.
[b]Mead Johnson and Co., Evansville, IN.

Source: Adapted from P Acosta, M Blaskovics, H Cloud, et al: Nutrition in pregnancy of women with hyperphenylalaninemia. *J. Am. Dietet. Assoc.* 80:443–450, 1982.

Recommendations

The effectiveness of neonatal screening for PKU has relegated this disorder to the category of a rare cause of mental retardation. Metabolic screening for the presence of PKU in newborn infants has resulted in a generation of fertile, healthy, intelligent women in whom timely diet therapy has prevented disease or death. Because their diet therapy did not have to be continued indefinitely, many of

Table 11-5
Phenylalanine content of selected foods

Food	Amount	Phenylalanine (mg)	Protein (gm)	Energy (kcal)
Vegetables				
Each serving in the amount specified contains about 15–18 mg phenylalanine.				
Asparagus	1½ stalks	17	0.6	5
Beans, green, cooked	3 tbsp	14	0.4	6
Beans, yellow, cooked	¼ cup	16	0.4	7
Bean sprouts, cooked	1 tbsp	16	0.3	3
Beets, cooked	⅔ cup	16	1.2	34
Beet greens, cooked	3 tbsp	15	0.6	6
Broccoli, chopped, cooked	1 tbsp	14	0.4	3
Brussels sprouts, cooked	1 medium	13	0.4	4
Cabbage, raw, shredded	½ cup	15	0.6	12
Cabbage, cooked	⅓ cup	14	0.6	11
Carrot, raw	½ large	18	0.6	21
Carrots, cooked	⅓ cup	15	0.5	16
Cauliflower, cooked	3 tbsp	17	0.5	5
Celery, raw	2 stalks	15	0.3	6
Collards, cooked	1 tbsp	13	0.4	4
Cucumber, pared, raw	1 whole	14	0.6	14
Eggplant, cooked	3 tbsp	17	0.4	7
Lettuce	2 leaves	14	0.4	5
Mushrooms, raw	3 small	17	0.8	8
Mushrooms, canned	3 tbsp	16	0.7	7
Mustard greens, cooked	2 tbsp	16	0.5	5
Onion, raw, chopped	¼ cup	15	0.6	15
Peppers, raw, chopped	3 tbsp	17	0.4	7
Pickles, dill	1 large	16	0.7	11
Pumpkin, cooked	4 tbsp	16	0.6	18
Sauerkraut	¼ cup	15	0.6	11
Spinach, cooked	1 tbsp	15	0.3	3
Squash, winter, cooked	¼ cup	16	0.6	20
Tomato, raw	½ small	14	0.6	11
Tomato catsup	2 tbsp	17	0.7	36
Soups (Campbell's, prepared with equal amounts of water)				
Each serving in the amount specified contains about 75–80 mg phenylalanine.				
Asparagus	1 cup	80	2.7	64
Beef Broth	½ cup	68	2.4	16
Celery	1 cup	80	1.6	85
Minestrone	¾ cup	71	3.2	68
Mushroom	⅔ cup	79	1.6	59
Onion	¾ cup	76	3.6	44
Tomato	1 cup	90	2.1	85

Table 11-5 (continued)
Phenylalanine content of selected foods

Food	*Amount*	*Phenylalanine (mg)*	*Protein (gm)*	*Energy (kcal)*
Vegetarian Vegetable	1 cup	74	1.6	64
Vegetable and Beef Broth	1¼ cup	80	2.5	75
Chicken Gumbo	⅔ cup	74	2.1	37
Cream of Chicken	⅔ cup	79	2.1	63
Beef Noodle	½ cup	76	2.0	32
Fruits				
Each serving in the amount specified contains about 14–18 mg phenylalanine.				
Apple, raw	2½ small	15	0.5	145
Applesauce	¾ cup	14	0.5	207
Apricots, raw	1½ medium	14	0.6	31
Apricots, canned	3 halves	14	0.6	31
Apricots, dried	2 halves	14	0.6	31
Avocado, cubed or mashed	3 tbsp	14	0.6	48
Banana, raw sliced	½ small	17	0.6	48
Blackberries, raw	6 tbsp	17	0.6	31
Blueberries, raw	10 tbsp	16	0.6	55
Cantaloupe, raw, diced	5 tbsp	16	0.5	23
Cherries, sour	4 tbsp	16	0.6	30
Cranberry sauce	1⅔ cups	16	0.5	780
Dates	2 tbsp	15	0.6	69
Fig, raw	1 large	15	0.6	40
Fig, dried	1 small	16	0.6	41
Fruit cocktail	¾ cup	16	0.6	119
Grapefruit, raw	½ large	14	0.7	59
Honeydew, raw, diced	5 tbsp	16	0.5	21
Mango, raw	½ medium	18	0.7	66
Orange, raw	1 medium	18	1.5	74
Peach, raw	1 large	16	0.8	50
Pear, raw	½ medium	17	0.7	61
Pineapple, raw	1 cup diced	14	0.5	67
Pineapple, canned in syrup	2 large slices	16	0.6	148
Plums, damson, raw	2 whole	13	0.5	66
Prunes, dried, medium	3 whole	18	0.4	54
Raisins, dried, seedless	2 tbsp	15	0.5	58
Raspberries, red, raw	6 tbsp	15	0.6	27
Strawberries, raw	10 large	17	0.7	37
Watermelon	⅔ cup	17	0.7	36
Prepared cereals				
Each serving in the amount specified contains about 27–32 mg phenylalanine.				
Cheerios	2 tbsp	27	0.5	15
Corn Chex	½ cup	29	0.6	30

Table 11-5 (continued)
Phenylalanine content of selected foods

Food	*Amount*	*Phenylalanine (mg)*	*Protein (gm)*	*Energy (kcal)*
Cornflakes	¼ cup	28	0.6	31
Kix	½ cup	28	0.6	32
Puffed rice	10 tbsp	31	0.6	40
Puffed wheat	¼ cup	32	0.9	12
Rice Chex	6 tbsp	31	0.6	44
Rice Krispies	¼ cup	28	0.5	30
Shredded Wheat	¼ biscuit	29	0.6	21
Trix	6 tbsp	30	0.7	47
Wheaties	¼ cup	31	0.7	25
Wheat Chex	7 biscuits	31	0.7	25
Quaker Life	1 tbsp	30	0.6	12
Special K	2 tbsp	29	0.6	11
Granola	1 tbsp	32	0.6	19
Cooked cereals				
Each serving in the amount specified contains about 28–31 mg phenylalanine.				
Cornmeal	4 tbsp	29	0.7	30
Cream of Rice	5 tbsp	31	0.6	38
Cream of Wheat	2 tbsp	28	0.6	17
Farina	3 tbsp	31	0.6	19
Oatmeal	2 tbsp	33	0.6	17
Rice, white	3 tbsp	28	0.5	29
Rice, brown	2 tbsp	28	0.5	25
Wheatena	2 tbsp	31	0.6	22
Crackers				
Each serving in the amount specified contains about 27–33 mg phenylalanine.				
Animal crackers	5	33	0.7	43
Arrowroot Cookies	2	30	0.6	45
Graham cracker	1	28	0.6	21
Ritz Crackers	3	35	0.7	45
Saltines	2	27	0.5	26
Wheat Thins	4	34	0.7	32
Miscellaneous				
1. Each serving in the amount specified contains about 28–32 mg phenylalanine.				
Corn, cooked	2 tbsp	29	0.5	17
Macaroni, cooked	2 tbsp	32	0.6	20
Noodles, cooked	2 tbsp	32	0.7	20
Potato chips	6 (2-in. diameter)	29	0.6	68
Potatoes, French fried	3 (½ × ½ × 2 in.)	30	0.6	41
Popcorn, popped, plain	5 tbsp	33	0.7	36
Spaghetti, cooked	2 tbsp	32	0.6	20
Sweet potatoes, cooked	3 tbsp	28	0.6	38

Table 11-5 (continued)
Phenylalanine content of selected foods

Food	*Amount*	*Phenylalanine (mg)*	*Protein (gm)*	*Energy (kcal)*
2. Each serving in the amount specified contains about 1–6 mg phenylalanine.				
Butter	1 tbsp	4	0.1	100
French dressing	5 tbsp	5	0.2	442
Margarine	1 tbsp	5	0.1	108
Miracle Whip	1 tbsp	5	0.1	68
Mayonnaise	2 tbsp	5	0.1	72
Fruit pie filling	¼ cup	4	0.2	80
Corn starch	1 tbsp	1	Trace	29
Cool Whip	1 tbsp	2	Trace	14
Olives, green	2 tbsp	5	0.2	16
Free Foods				
Apple juice	6 oz			85
Candies:				
Butterscotch	1 piece			20
Cream mint	1 piece			7
Fondant, patty or mint	1 piece			40
Gum drop	1 large			35
Hard candies	2 pieces			39
Jellybeans	10			110
Lollipop	1 medium (2½ in.)			108
Carbonated beverages	6 oz			78
Corn syrup	1 tbsp			58
Fruit butter	1 tbsp			37
Fruit ices	½ cup			69
Jelly	1 tbsp			55
Kool-Aid	4 oz			48
Lemonade	4 oz			53
Maple syrup	1 tbsp			50
Molasses	1 tbsp			46
Popsicle	1 twin bar			95
Sugar, brown	1 tbsp			43
Sugar, white	1 tbsp			59
Tang liquid	4 oz			59

Source: Adapted from American Dietetic Association, *Handbook of Clinical Dietetics*. New Haven: Yale University Press, 1981. Pp. C36–C40.

these women may not remember ever having had PKU. An equal number may have had a lesser form of PKU that was never detected or treated during the neonatal period. This generation of healthy women is now entering their childbearing years. Unless properly screened and treated with phenylalanine-restricted diets before conception, these women will cause irreparable damage to their children. The adverse neonatal effects of maternal PKU can be completely prevented with early and comprehensive diet therapy.

References

1. Luke, B, and Keith, LG: The challenge of maternal phenylketonuria screening and treatment. *J. Reprod. Med.* 35:667–673, 1990.
2. Cartier, L, Clow, CL, Lippman-Hand, A, et al: Prevention of mental retardation in offspring of hyperphenylalaninemic mothers. *Am. J. Public Health* 72:1386–1390, 1982.
3. Scriver, CR, and Clow, CL: Phenylketonuria: Epitome of human biochemical genetics. *N. Engl. J. Med.* 303:1336–1342, 1980.
4. Garrod, AE: The incidence of alkaptonuria: A study in chemical individuality. *Lancet* 2:1616–1620, 1902.
5. Ledley, FD, Levy, HL, and Woo, SLC: Molecular analysis of the inheritance of phenylketonuria and mild hyperphenylalaninemia in families with both disorders. *N. Engl. J. Med.* 314:1276–1280, 1986.
6. Tourian, A, and Sidbury, J: Phenylketonuria and hyperphenylalaninemia. In JB Stanbury, JB Wyngaarden, and DS Frederickson (eds.), *The Metabolic Basis of Inherited Disease.* New York: McGraw-Hill, 1985. Pp. 270–286.
7. American Dietetic Association: *Handbook of Clinical Dietetics.* New Haven: Yale University Press, 1981. Pp. C29–C44.
8. Schuett, V, Gurda, R, and Brown, E: Diet discontinuation policies and practices of PKU clinics in the United States. *Am. J. Public Health* 70:498–503, 1980.
9. United States Congress, Office of Technology Assessment: *Healthy Children: Investing in the Future.* OTA-H-345. Washington, DC: US Govt. Printing Office, 1988.
10. National Center for Health Statistics: Advance Report of Final Natality Statistics, 1985. *Vital and Health Statistics* 36 (Suppl.):1, 1987.
11. Fisch, R, Doeden, D, Lancky, et al: Maternal phenylketonuria: Detrimental effects on embryogenesis and fetal development. *Am. J. Dis. Child.* 118:847–858, 1969.
12. Stevenson, RE, and Huntley, CC: Congenital malformations in offspring of phenylketonuria mothers. *Pediatrics* 40:33–45, 1967.
13. Lenke, R, and Levy, H: Maternal phenylketonuria and hyperphenylalaninemia: An international survey of the outcome of untreated and treated pregnancies. *N. Engl. J. Med.* 303:1202–1208, 1980.

14. Koch, R, Friedman, E, Wenz, E, et al: The maternal PKU collaborative study. *J. Inherit. Metab. Dis.* 9 (Suppl. 2):159–168, 1986.
15. MacCready, R, and Levy, H: The problem of maternal phenylketonuria. *Am. J. Obstet. Gynecol.* 113:121–128, 1972.
16. Kerr, G, Chamove, A, Harlow, H, et al: "Fetal PKU": The effect of maternal hyperphenylalaninemia during pregnancy in the rhesus monkey (Macaca mulatta). *Pediatrics* 42:27–36, 1968.
17. Menkes, J, and Aeberhard, E: Maternal phenylketonuria: The composition of cerebral lipids in an affected offspring. *J. Pediatr.* 74:924–931, 1969.
18. Levy, HL, and Waisbren, SE: Effect of untreated maternal phenylketonuria and hyperphenylalaninemia on the fetus. *N. Engl. J. Med.* 309:1269–1274, 1983.
19. Drogari, E, Beasley, M, Smith, I, et al: Timing of strict diet in relation to fetal damage in maternal phenylketonuria: An international collaborative study by the MRC/DHSS phenylketonuria register. *Lancet* 2:927–930, 1987.
20. Levy, H: Maternal PKU: Control of an emerging problem. *Am. J. Public Health* 72:1320–1321, 1982.
21. Guthrie, R: Maternal PKU: A continuing problem. *Am. J. Public Health* 78:771, 1988.
22. Lenke, R, and Levy, H: Maternal phenylketonuria: Results of dietary therapy. *Am. J. Obstet. Gynecol.* 142:548–553, 1982.
23. Acosta, P, Blaskovics, M, Cloud, H, et al: Nutrition in pregnancy of women with hyperphenylalaninemia. *J. Am. Dietet. Assoc.* 80:443–450, 1982.

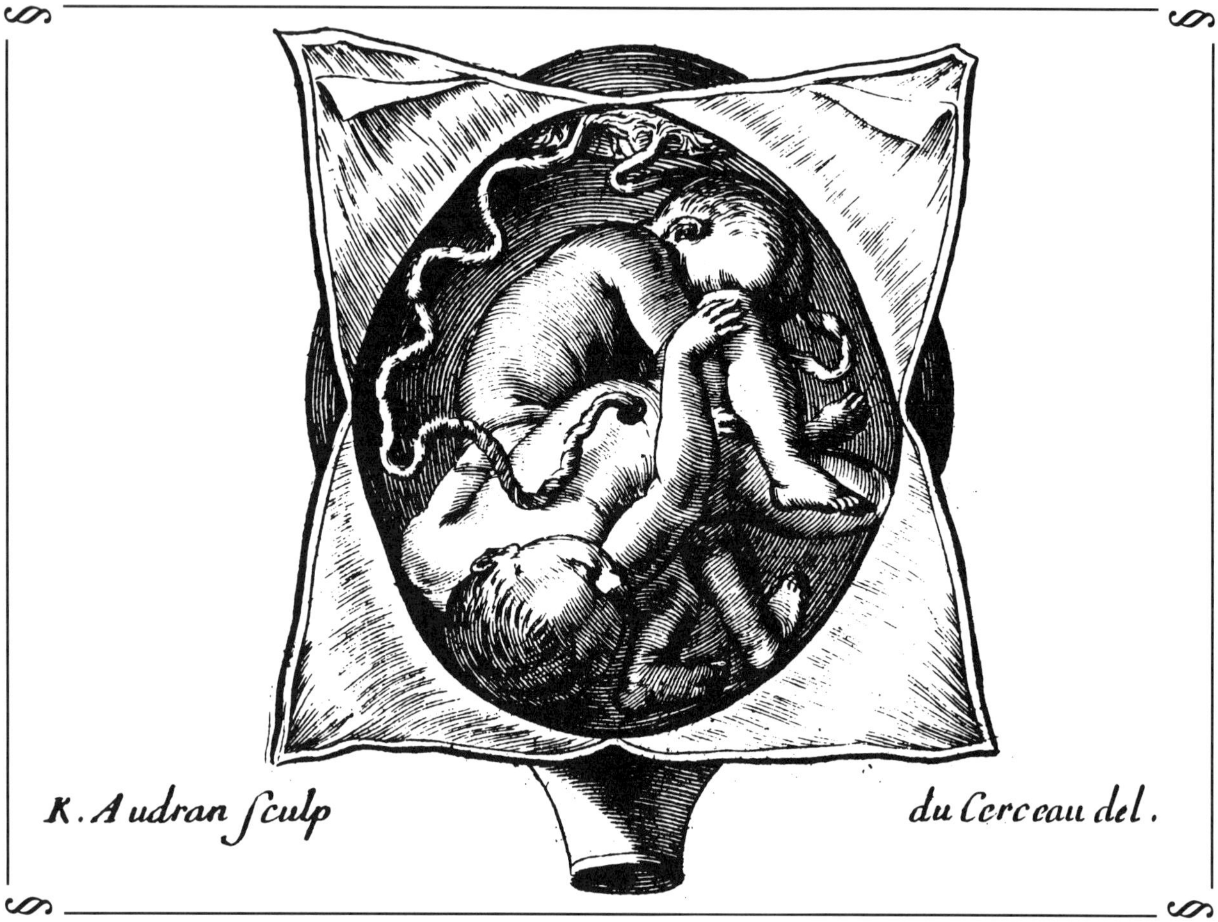

Engraving of twins in utero. (From Françoise Mauriceau. *Traite des Maladies des Femmes Grosses*. Paris: Charles Coignard, 1668.)

12 Multiple Gestation

Scope and Incidence

Multiple births in the United States have been steadily increasing, both in absolute number and in proportion to total births (Table 12-1). In the decade between 1979 and 1989, the number of singleton live births increased by 15 percent, twins by 35 percent, and triplets and higher-order multiples by 133 percent [1, 2]. The increase in multiple births has been attributed in part to a trend in delaying childbirth, with multiple births occurring with a greater natural frequency among older mothers. For example, mothers 30 years of age and older accounted for 20 percent of all births in 1980, compared to 29 percent in 1989 [2, 3]. In addition, the increased use of fertility-enhancing agents and in vitro fertilization has also contributed to the increase in multiple births, particularly among women over age 35, although it is not possible to assess from vital records the relative contribution of natural versus induced multiple gestations to the overall incidence [4].

This chapter focuses on twin gestations, since they comprise more than 97 percent of all multiple births in the United States; information on triplets and other higher-order multiples is included whenever possible. Birthweight and length of gestation, zygosity and placental considerations on fetal growth, perinatal effects of growth discordancy, perinatal morbidity and mortality, and maternal factors are discussed.

Birthweight and Length of Gestation

Among twins, lower birthweight and shorter gestation are more often the rule than the exception. As shown in Tables 12-2 and 12-3, twins are five times as likely to be born preterm (<37 wk) as singletons and are 8.5 times as likely to have low birthweight (<2500 gm). Among all preterm births, more than three fourths of twin births are also low birthweight, twice as many as singletons (Table 12-4). The intrauterine growth of singletons and twins, as measured by birthweight, diverges from about 30 weeks of gestation [5–8]. Significant differences increase from the 35th week of gestation to delivery [7] (Fig. 12-1). Leroy and associates [6] reported differences of 150 gm at 31 weeks' gestation, increasing to 420 gm at 35 weeks and 610 gm by 40 weeks. According to Wilson [8], after 31 weeks of gestation twin birthweight fell progressively behind that of singletons such that by 38 weeks the singleton 10th percentile was equivalent to the twin 50th percentile, and the singleton 50th

Table 12-1
Trends in live births in the United States: all births, multiple births, and twins, 1950–1989

Year	*Total live births*	*Multiple births*	*Total MBR*	*White MBR*	*Black MBR*
1989	4,040,958	92,916	23.0	22.5	26.9
1988	3,909,510	87,700	22.4	22.0	25.8
1987	3,809,394	81,778	22.0	21.6	25.4
1986	3,756,547	79,485	21.6	21.2	24.9
1985	3,760,561	77,102	21.0	20.4	25.3
1984	3,669,141	72,949	20.3	19.8	24.2
1983	3,638,933	72,287	20.3	19.6	24.5
1982	3,680,537	71,631	19.9	19.2	24.1
1981	3,629,238	70,049	19.7	18.8	24.7
1980	3,612,258	68,339	19.3	18.5	24.1
1979	3,494,398	66,858	19.5	18.6	24.2
1978	3,333,279	64,163	19.6	18.8	24.2
1977	3,326,632	62,880	19.2	18.5	23.3
1976	3,167,788	60,664	19.2	18.5	22.9
1975	3,144,198	59,192	18.8	18.1	22.8
1974	3,159,958	57,836	18.3	17.7	21.8
1973	3,136,965	56,777	18.1	17.4	21.9
1972	3,258,411	59,122	18.1	17.4	22.0
1971	3,555,970	63,298	17.8	17.0	22.4
1970	3,731,386	–	–	–	–
1969	3,600,206	–	–	–	–
1968	3,501,564	69,300	19.8	19.0	–
1967	3,520,959	68,336	19.4	18.5	–
1966	3,606,274	70,340	19.5	18.5	–
1965	3,670,358	74,594	20.3	18.7	–
1964	4,027,490	78,954	19.6	18.4	–
1963	4,098,020	80,044	19.5	18.4	–
1962	4,167,363	80,180	19.2	18.2	–
1961	4,268,326	84,926	19.9	18.7	–
1960	4,257,850	85,440	20.1	19.0	–
1959	4,244,796	86,426	20.4	19.2	–
1958	4,203,812	84,934	20.2	19.1	26.9
1957	4,254,784	85,196	20.0	19.0	26.5
1956	4,163,090	84,765	20.4	19.4	26.5
1955	4,047,295	84,394	20.9	20.0	26.5
1954	4,017,362	82,626	20.6	19.7	26.6
1953	3,902,120	81,000	20.8	19.8	27.0
1952	3,846,986	78,457	20.4	19.6	25.7
1951	3,750,850	75,335	20.1	19.4	24.8
1950	3,554,149	73,499	20.7	20.0	25.3

MBR, multiple birth ratio.

Source: Adapted from birth certificate data from the National Center for Health Statistics. Dashes indicate that data were not specifically coded or collected for that category for that year.

Table 12-2
Percent distribution of twin and singleton live births by period of gestation, United States, 1987

Period of gestation (wk)	*Twins*	*Singletons*
Total	100.0	100.0
<28	4.7	0.7
28–31	6.3	1.0
32–35	22.3	4.5
36	11.3	3.2
37–39	41.4	40.0
40	7.1	22.1
41	3.1	14.8
≥42	3.8	13.7
Percent <37 wk	44.5	9.4

Source: Adapted from unpublished data from Selma Taffel, National Center for Health Statistics, Hyattsville, MD, 1990.

Table 12-3
Percent distribution of twin and singleton live births of all gestations by birthweight, United States, 1987

Birthweight (gm)	*Twins*	*Singletons*
Total	100.0	100.0
<1000	4.8	0.5
1000–1499	5.1	0.5
1500–1999	12.5	1.0
2000–2499	27.9	3.8
2500–2999	31.4	15.7
3000–3499	15.2	37.1
≥3500	3.1	41.3
Percent <2500 gm	50.3	5.9

Source: Adapted from USDHHS, NCHS: *Vital Statistics of the United States, 1987*, Vol. 1, *Natality*. Washington, DC: US Govt. Printing Office, 1989. P. 240.

percentile was equivalent to the twin 90th percentile. Kiely [5] reported that twins born in New York City between 1978 and 1984 at 40 weeks' gestation and later were actually lighter than those born at 38 to 39 weeks, suggesting that intrauterine growth for twins stops after 39 weeks. Williams and colleagues [9] concluded that the peak growth rate in weight was about 250 gm per week at 33 weeks for singletons compared to 175 gm per week at 31 weeks for multiples.

Table 12-4
Percent distribution of twin and singleton live births of less than 37 weeks' gestation by birthweight, United States, 1987

Birthweight (gm)	*Twins*	*Singletons*
Total	100.0	100.0
<1000	9.8	4.7
1000–1499	10.3	4.6
1500–1999	21.9	8.1
2000–2499	34.2	17.4
2500–2999	19.4	26.8
3000–3499	3.9	24.6
≥3500	0.5	13.8
Percent <2500 gm	76.2	34.8

Source: Adapted from USDHHS, NCHS: *Vital Statistics of the United States, 1987*, Vol. 1, *Natality*. Washington, DC: US Govt. Printing Office, 1989. P. 240.

Zygosity and Placental Considerations

Much of the variation in intrauterine growth in twins results from differences in zygosity and placental factors. Monozygotic (MZ) twins account for about 25 to 35 percent of all twins and develop from a single fertilized ovum (zygote) after splitting of the cell mass at various stages of development. If the separation occurs very early, such as at the two-cell stage, two separate blastocysts develop. Each blastocyst then implants separately and each embryo develops its own chorionic sac and placenta (**diamniotic, dichorionic placenta**). In most cases, however, the zygote splits at the early blastocyst stage. The inner cell mass divides into two separate groups of cells within the same blastocyst cavity, and the resulting two embryos have a common chorionic cavity and placenta but separate amnionic sacs (**diamniotic, monochorionic placenta**). The least common type of division occurs at the stage of the bilaminar germ disk just before the appearance of the primitive streak. The resulting two embryos have one chorion and one amnion, as well as a common placenta (**mono-amniotic, monochorionic placenta**). These variations are shown in Fig. 12-2.

In contrast, dizygotic (DZ) twins, which account for the remaining 65 to 75 percent of all twins, result from the release of two oocytes and their subsequent fertilization by two different spermatozoa. Both zygotes implant separately in the uterus and each develops its own amnion, chorion, and placenta (**diamniotic, dichorionic placen-**

Fig. 12-1
Birthweights of twins versus singletons. (Adapted from B Luke et al, Gestational age-specific birthweights of twins versus singletons. *Acta Genet. Med. Gemellol.* 40:69–76, 1991.)

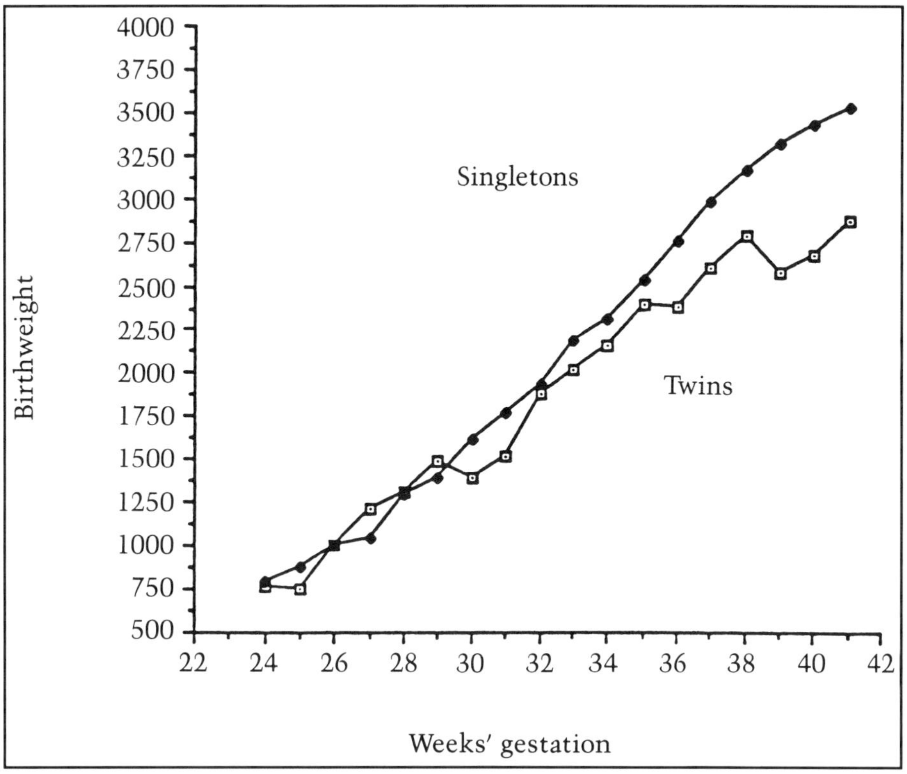

tas). Based on infant sex and the relationship of the chorions, Gruenwald [10] estimated that 37 percent of all same-sex dichorionic twins should be monozygotic. According to these calculations, 44 percent of all twin pairs are presumed to be monozygotic.

Fujikura and Froehlich [11] evaluated 569 pairs of twin infants from the Collaborative Perinatal Project and concluded that placentation was a principal factor determining the rate of fetal growth. Bleker and associates [12], in a comparison of birthweights and placental weights of 3000 singletons, 1500 twin pairs, and 67 triplets, reported that from 24 weeks' gestation onward the placental weights of multiples were smaller than those of singletons. Bleker and colleagues [13] also reported that multiparas had heavier placentas than primiparas, in both singleton and twin pregnancies. Such a finding may in part account for the association between higher birthweight and greater parity [13].

Congenital anomalies of the placenta are more common in twin pregnancies, with marginal or velamentous insertions of the umbilical cord occurring twice as frequently in monochorionic as in dichorionic placentas [13, 14]. Ultrasound studies [15] have shown that twin placentas mature more quickly than singleton placentas. This

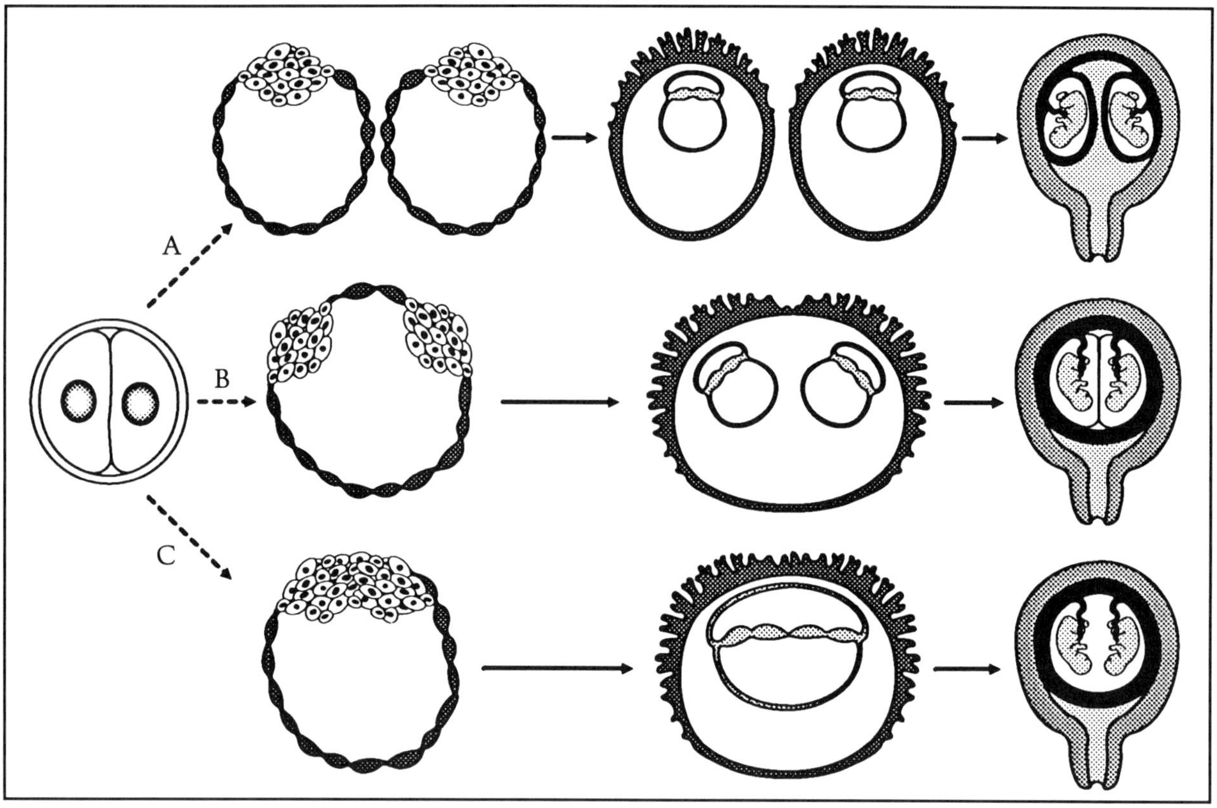

Fig. 12-2
Variations of uterine growth of monozygotic twins. A. Diamniotic, dichorionic placenta. B. Diamniotic, monochorionic placenta. C. Monoamniotic, monochorionic placenta.

observation may also explain part of the variation in birthweights of twins compared to singletons.

Perinatal Effects of Growth Discordancy

Intertwin birthweight differences, also known as discordancy, are expressed as a percentage of the weight of the larger twin [16]. Although intertwin birthweight differences greater than 20 percent occur in fewer than 10 percent of all twin pregnancies, half of these cases also exhibit intrauterine growth retardation (IUGR, weight-for-gestation ≤10th percentile) [16]. However, growth discordancy is not a risk factor for increased perinatal morbidity or mortality when the twin pair has reached term and the lighter twin weighs at least 2500 gm [17]. In one study of 194 twin pairs, Guaschino and associates [18] found the relative risk of perinatal mortality to be 5.4 when intertwin birthweight differences were more than 20 percent and 7.2

when differences were greater than 25 percent. Other studies have also reported an increase in perinatal mortality, especially intrauterine mortality, when growth discordancy exceeded 25 percent [19].

Growth discordancy can result from differences in the genetic growth potential of each fetus, variations in the placental implantation sites, or the twin transfusion syndrome. This latter process may occur when the arteries or veins of the placentas of both twins are connected by surface or deep anastomoses. Such connections result in the transfer of blood from one twin (the donor) to the other (the recipient) and occur only in monochorionic twin gestations. Based on pathologic examinations, it has been estimated that one third of monochorionic placentas have some interconnection between fetal circulations [20].

Both acute and chronic variations of the twin transfusion syndrome have been identified [21]. The chronic type results in greater intertwin birthweight disparities (>20%), whereas the acute type leads to greater differences in hemoglobin levels [22]. In severe cases, these anastomoses can lead to significant differences in hemoglobin levels at birth, reflecting the anemia of the donor twin and the plethora of the recipient twin. Depending on severity, the imbalance in placental blood supply between twins can result in significant birthweight differences. The donor twin may be smaller in weight and length, or even die before birth, while the recipient is larger and may even have symptoms of acute hydramnios. The disparity in cardiac size, cardiac fiber size, and muscle mass of the pulmonary and systemic arteries characteristic of this syndrome reflects the adaptations to chronic hypertension in utero in the recipient and the relative or absolute hypotension in the donor [23].

The diagnosis of twin transfusion syndrome is not precise and depends on a combination of clinical, anatomic, and hematologic criteria. It has been suggested that a birthweight difference of 500 gm or more or intertwin discordancy greater than 20 percent [22], or a hemoglobin difference of 5 gm/100 ml [24] is diagnostic of this syndrome. When this syndrome develops before 28 weeks' gestation, the prognosis is very poor, and survival rates of about 21 percent are common [25]. In contrast, when it develops later in gestation the outlook is better, with survival rates ranging between 40 and 50 percent [26].

Perinatal Morbidity and Mortality Among Twins

The mortality for twin births is four to eight times higher than for singletons, and most of this excess has been attributed to low birthweight, secondary to prematurity, and to IUGR, secondary to monozygosity and inadequate maternal nutrition [27–30]. Data from linked birth and death certificates in California showed that multiples have a fetal mortality 3.7 times higher than for singletons, a perinatal mortality 5.4 times higher, and a neonatal mortality 7.3 times higher [9]. Among twins, boys have higher mortality than girls [9], and monozygotic twins have higher mortality than dizygotic twins [28, 30, 31].

Birthweight-specific mortality, however, varies considerably between singletons and multiples. Williams and associates [9] found that for birthweights between 1251 and 2500 gm, the perinatal mortality for multiples was two to three times lower than for singletons, reversing above 2750 gm. Kiely [5] reported that for birthweights between 1001 and 2500 gm, twins had birthweight-specific mortality equivalent to or substantially lower than that of singletons, even after adjusting for gestational age. Among all twins in this study [5], perinatal mortality was 70 percent higher for infants with birthweights above 3000 gm than for infants with birthweights between 2500 and 3000 gm.

Improvements in birthweight-specific neonatal mortality have occurred for both singletons and twins. Data from linked birth and death certificates from 1950, 1960, and 1983 indicate that below 2500 gm twins have lower neonatal mortality, between 2501 and 3000 gm the rates are comparable, and above 3000 gm singletons have the survival advantage. These data are shown in Table 12-5.

Table 12-5
Neonatal mortality by birthweight (gm) and plurality, United States, 1950, 1960, and 1983*

	Year	*<500*	*501–1000*	*1001–1500*	*1501–2000*	*2001–2500*	*2501–3000*	*3001–3500*	*3501–4000*	*4001–4500*	*>4501*
Singletons	1950	— 871.7 —		562.3	228.9	52.8	12.6	6.7	5.6	7.4	14.2
	1960	996.1	993.5	577.4	220.4	48.2	10.2	4.4	3.3	3.6	7.6
	1983	994.9	538.8	154.1	52.2	15.4	3.9	1.5	1.1	1.1	2.7
Twins	1950	— 871.5 —		503.7	145.4	32.9	11.3	10.4	18.7	38.1	N/A
	1960	997.1	996.3	538.5	119.3	22.5	7.4	6.5	— 8.1 —		
	1983	994.1	612.1	117.6	16.3	5.5	3.1	2.4	— 10.2 —		

N/A, data not reported for this weight category during this year.

*Neonatal mortality is defined as deaths under 28 days per 1000 live births. Data presented are based on matched infant birth and death certificates.

Source: Adapted from Neonatal mortality rates by birthweight, race, sex, and plurality of birth: United States, January 1 to March 31, 1950. In *Vital Statistics of the United States, 1950*, Vol. 1, *Natality*. Washington, DC: USDHEW, 1954. P. 106; and JC Kleinman, MG Fowler, and SS Kessel, Comparison of infant mortality among twins and singletons: United States, 1960 and 1983. *Am. J. Epidemiol.* 133:133–143, 1991.

Other investigators have reported similar results. In the British study of 38,413 multiple births (of which 25,515 were twins), Botting and associates [32] reported that for birthweights under 2500 gm twins had significantly lower perinatal mortality than singletons, between 2500 and 3499 gm the rates were comparable, and for birthweights of 3500 gm and above singletons had the survival advantage. Fabre and colleagues [33], in their analysis of the Spanish Perinatal Mortality National Survey, which included 1956 twin births, also found lower perinatal mortality for twins compared to singletons at birthweights below 2500 gm.

Less research has been conducted evaluating the association between twin birthweight, birthweight for gestational age, and perinatal morbidity. Bronsteen and coworkers [34] compared the prognostic value of IUGR versus discordancy in neonatal morbidity and mortality in 142 sets of twins. These investigators found that preterm birth accounted for almost half of all variance in neonatal outcome, and that birthweight percentile based on singleton norms proved to be more effective than discordancy in representing the relationship of intrauterine growth to neonatal outcome. Birthweight percentile accounted for almost three times as much variance in morbidity as did discordancy. In this study [34] birthweight below the 10th percentile was significantly correlated with neonatal morbidity. In another recent study, the role of IUGR in newborn length of stay (LOS) was evaluated in twins versus singletons [35]. Below 37 weeks of gestation, LOS was 1.5 to 2.0 times greater for twins with IUGR compared to non-IUGR twins, whereas no significant differences were found between non-IUGR twins and singletons (Fig. 12-3). Below 2500 gm, IUGR twins had significantly higher LOS compared to non-IUGR twins, whereas non-IUGR twins actually had lower LOS compared to singletons (Fig. 12-4). Specifically, for non-IUGR twins compared to singletons, LOS was nearly 50 percent shorter and 30 percent shorter, respectively, for birthweights between 1000 and 1499 gm and 1500 and 1999 gm. Both of these studies [34, 35] suggest that a substantial portion of neonatal morbidity in newborn twins is secondary to IUGR.

The lower birthweight-specific morbidity and mortality of twins with birthweights below 2500 gm, even after adjustment for gestational age, may be due to their greater maturity compared to singletons at equivalent weight. Two recent studies, one evaluating fetal lung maturity [36] and the other placental aging [15], suggest that the maturation process in twins is triggered earlier than in singletons. Using the lecithin/sphingomyelin (L/S) ratio, Leveno

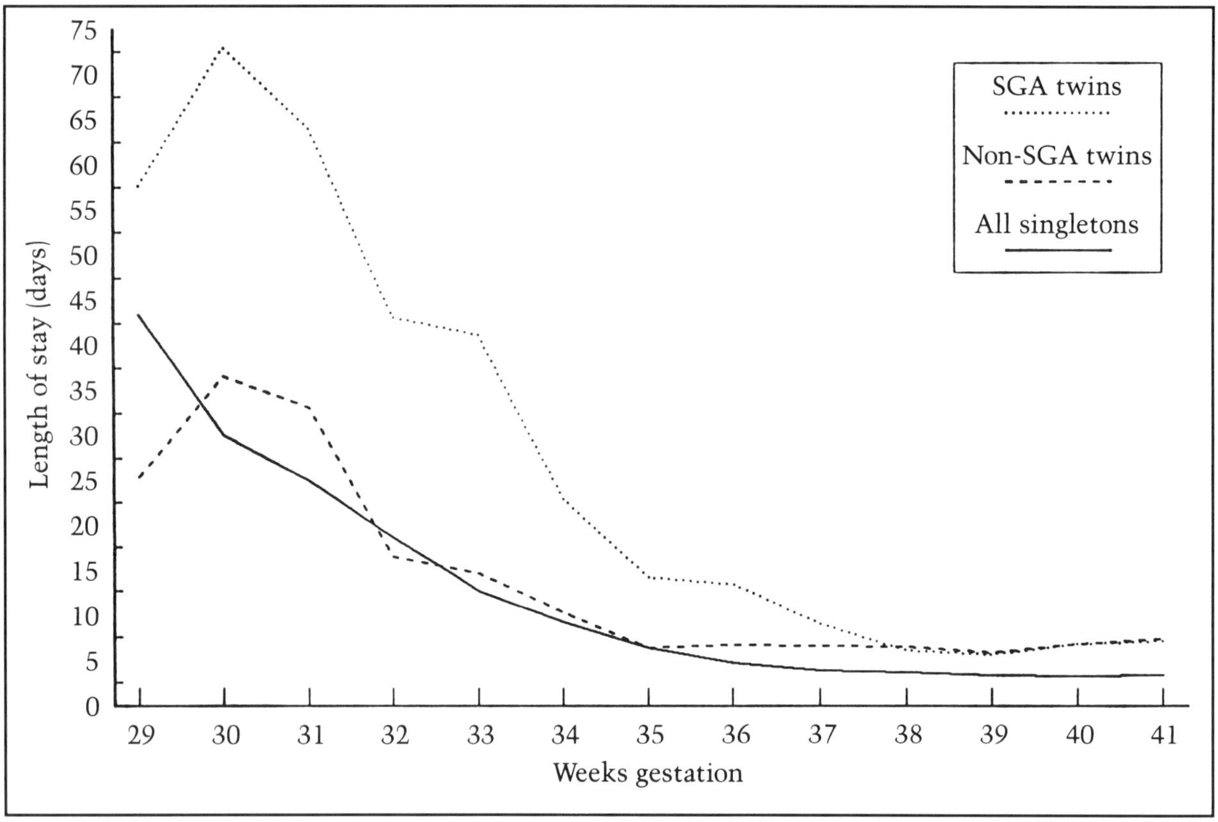

Fig. 12-3
Mean length of stay by gestational age, plurality, and birthweight percentile. SGA, small-for-gestational-age. (Adapted from B Luke, FR Witter, and TRB Johnson, The effect of higher birthweights for gestational age on length of stay of newborn twins. Presented at the XIII World Congress of Gynaecology and Obstetrics, Singapore, Sept. 1991.)

and associates [36] evaluated fetal lung maturation in 84 twin and 137 singleton neonates. An L/S ratio that exceeds 2, indicating maturity, was achieved between 34 and 36 weeks in singletons, compared to 31 to 32 weeks in twins. Ohel and colleagues [15] compared sonographically determined placental gradings of 158 twin and 474 singleton pregnancies at different gestational ages. Using a grading classification of I to III, these investigators found that at each gestational age from 29 weeks and later, the proportion of grade III placentas was significantly greater in twins, suggesting different rates of maturation in these two groups.

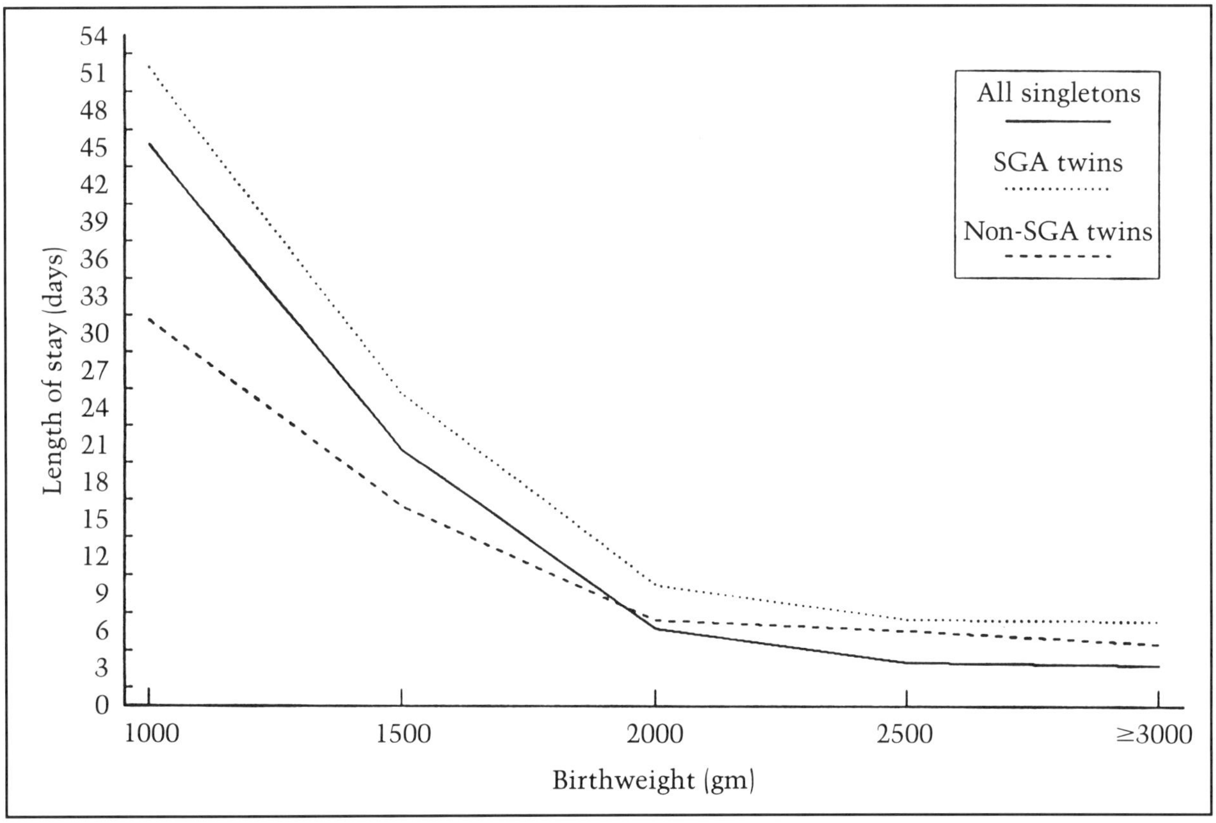

Fig. 12-4
Mean length of stay by birthweight, birthweight percentile, and plurality. SGA, small-for-gestational-age. (Adapted from B Luke, FR Witter, and TRB Johnson, The effect of higher birthweights for gestational age on length of stay of newborn twins. Presented at the XIII World Congress of Gynaecology and Obstetrics, Singapore, Sept. 1991.)

Neonatal Complications

In addition to the complications commonly associated with low birthweight, IUGR, and preterm birth, twins have a higher incidence of other complications [37]. They have a higher frequency of hyaline membrane disease, retinopathy of prematurity, group B streptococcal disease, and necrotizing enterocolitis.

Twins also have a higher incidence of congenital anomalies compared to singletons. Overall, the rates of congenital anomalies are higher among whites compared to blacks, boys compared to girls, and multiples compared to singletons [38]. Schinzel and associates [39] proposed three etiologies for the congenital anomalies observed in twins: restricted intrauterine environment imposed late in gestation, alteration of normal blood flow due to placental vascular communications, and defects in morphogenesis in early gestation. Congenital anomalies observed more often in twins as a result of the restricted intrauterine environment include positional foot defects and hip contractures. Alteration in blood flow can result in acardia, cardiomegaly and other cardiac defects, and micro- or macroencephaly. Defects in morphogenesis early in gestation are closely related to the twinning process itself, particularly monozygotic twinning in which one fertilized egg splits before implantation. The most extreme example of this phenomenon is seen in conjoined twins, a congenital anomaly that results from the incomplete division of the blastocyst [40]. The incidence of structural anomalies is extremely high among conjoined twins, providing further evidence of an association between the twinning process and defective morphogenesis, particularly among monozygotic twin pregnancies [41].

Maternal Factors

Prenatal

The incidence and type of twinning worldwide varies by a number of maternal characteristics, including age and race. Monozygotic twinning rates are remarkably constant at about 3 to 4 per 1000 live births, while the rate for dizygotic twinning has been shown to vary by racial groups and with maternal age. As shown in Table 12-6, the DZ twinning rate ranges from 1.3 per 1000 live births in Japan to 37 per 1000 live births in Nigeria. Within racial groups, there is evidence that DZ twinning is at least partially related to a maternal recessive trait [42]. An estimated 11 to 27 percent of white women (more than the proportion who actually bear twins) may be twin prone [42]. In the United States, the multiple birth ratio (MBR), an indicator of the overall rate of twinning, varies widely between ethnic and racial groups, ranging from a high of 25.8 for blacks and 24.9 for Alaskan natives, 19.6 for whites, 18.8 for American Indians, to 17.0 for Japanese, 15.3 for Hawaiian, 13.2 for Filipino, and 11.2 for Chinese women [43, 44]. Increases in the MBR parallel increasing maternal age and are differentially higher for blacks compared to whites (see Table 12-1). For example, among whites, the MBR for women aged 30 to 34 years is more than twice that of women under 20 years; a similar pattern is seen among blacks.

Physical Differences

There appear to be no particular maternal physical characteristics associated with MZ twinning, but women who conceive DZ twins are different from women who conceive singletons or MZ twins in

Table 12-6
International incidence of twinning by zygosity

Country	*Dizygotic*	*Monozygotic*
Japan (Hiroshima)	1.3	3.0
Spain	5.9	3.2
Portugal	6.5	3.6
United States (whites)	7.1	4.2
France	7.1	3.7
Belgium	7.3	3.6
Austria	7.5	3.4
India and Pakistan	7.8	4.3
Luxembourg	7.9	3.5
Switzerland	8.1	3.6
Holland	8.1	3.7
West Germany	8.2	3.3
Norway	8.3	3.8
Sweden	8.6	3.2
Italy	8.6	3.2
England and Wales	8.9	3.6
East Germany	9.1	3.3
United States (blacks)	11.1	4.7
Congo	18.7	3.1
Nigeria	37.0	3.0

that they are older, of higher parity, taller, and heavier. For example, several studies have reported that twinning rates are higher among overweight and obese women [45–47]. This increased rate may be due to the accompanying greater age and parity.

Maternal height has also been positively correlated with the rate of twinning [48], and therefore may partially explain the mechanism by which zygosity influences birthweight. In addition, it has been shown that mothers of DZ twins are taller than mothers of MZ twins and mothers of singletons [49]. Heights of mothers of MZ twins and singletons were not found to differ.

Menstrual and Hormonal Differences

The physical differences just noted may reflect underlying hormonal differences between women who conceive twins versus those who conceive singletons. For example, in a study of reproductive and menstrual characteristics, mothers of multiples were found to have an earlier age at menarche and shorter menstrual cycles than mothers of singletons [47]. Mothers of like-sexed twins experience an earlier menopause than mothers of singletons [50]. The earlier the twin birth, the shorter the menstrual life thereafter [50]. Women who have twins have a higher level of follicle-stimulating hormone (FSH) compared to women who have singletons. Mothers of DZ twins have an earlier age of menarche and a lower frequency of menstrual irregularities than mothers of singletons [51]. Obese women have elevated levels of circulating estrogens, and presumably this circumstance is associated with higher levels of FSH [52]. FSH levels increase with age [53] and may account in part for the effect of maternal age on DZ twinning rates [49]. The increased height among mothers of DZ twins may also reflect a further manifestation of anterior pituitary activity, namely growth hormone secretion.

Physiologic Changes and Adaptations to Multiple Gestation

Endocrine and Metabolism

Adaptation to multiple pregnancy is in many ways an exaggerated version of the maternal response to a singleton pregnancy. The trigger to the physiologic response is hormonal, with increased production of both steroid and protein hormones from the fetoplacental unit during multiple pregnancy, primarily due to an increase in placental mass. Urinary and plasma estriol levels increase in twin pregnancies to more than double the singleton mean by term [54]. Progesterone is also increased during twin pregnancies above that observed in singleton pregnancies [55]. Other hormones that increase above singleton pregnancy levels include human placental lactogen (HPL) and Schwangerschafts protein (SP_1) [56, 57]. Alpha-fetoprotein levels are also elevated in multiple pregnancy, although elevated values are also indicative of fetal abnormalities in singleton pregnancies. There is a difference in the production of alpha-fetoprotein levels in MZ versus DZ twin pregnancies, which may be related to differences in placentation [58].

The hormonal changes in multiple pregnancy additionally result in alterations in metabolism. Women with twin pregnancies have significantly lower blood glucose and insulin levels [59, 60]. Despite these differences, women with twin pregnancies do not have an increased frequency of gestational diabetes [61].

Uterine Changes

At the beginning of the second trimester, the total intrauterine volume in twin pregnancy is similar to that of singleton pregnancy; by 18 weeks' gestation the uterus of a twin pregnancy is twice as large as that of a singleton pregnancy [62]. By 25 weeks of gestation, the uterus of a twin gestation is equivalent to a singleton uterus at term. By term, the uterus with a singleton pregnancy has a total intrauterine volume of about 5000 ml, compared to nearly 10,000 ml in a twin pregnancy [62].

Weight Gain

A major physiologic response to pregnancy is gestational weight gain, and generally the weight gain with multiple pregnancy is greater and of a different pattern than in singleton pregnancies. MacGillivray and Campbell [45] reported that weight gain in the first trimester was much higher among mothers with twins compared to mothers of singletons, and was greater than expected. Campbell and associates [63] reported that women with twin pregnancies tend to gain more weight and in a different pattern than women with singleton pregnancies. In a study of 378 primiparas who delivered twins between 1950 and 1969, Campbell found the mean total weight gain for women with twins to be 14.6 kg (32.1 lb) compared to 11.1 kg (24.4 lb) for singletons. Campbell noted that the maximum rate of gain in twin pregnancies occurs during the early and late weeks of gestation, compared to midgestation for singletons. Mean rates of gain for twins compared to singletons for gestational weeks 13 to 20 were 0.60 versus 0.42 kg per week; for weeks 20 to 30, 0.55 versus 0.47 kg per week; and for weeks 30 to 36, 0.64 versus 0.40 kg per week.

In a more recent study, Campbell [54] evaluated the influence of infant zygosity and maternal parity on weight gain in twin pregnancies. Primiparas tended to gain more rapidly from midgestation to delivery; however, no significant differences were noted by zygosity. Mean rates of gain for primigravidas compared to multigravidas for gestational weeks 12 to 20 were 0.50 versus 0.52 kg per week; for weeks 20 to 30, 0.63 versus 0.55 kg per week; and for weeks 30 to 36, 0.67 versus 0.55 kg per week.

In a recent study of weight gain patterns in twin pregnancies, Pederson and associates [64] reported that optimum pregnancy outcome (≥37 weeks' gestation, both infants ≥2500 gm each with Apgar scores ≥7) was associated with gestational weight gains of 20 kg (44 lb) versus 16.8 kg (37 lb) for women with less-than-optimum outcomes. These investigators also found that the weight gain patterns of both groups were parallel until 30 weeks' gestation, at which time weight gain slowed in the less-than-optimum group.

Konwinski and associates [65] reported that among twin gestations, the rate of preterm delivery was higher among women with pregravid weights less than 136 lb who had inadequate gestational weight gain: less than 6 kg (13.2 lb) by 28 weeks, or less than 8 kg (17.6 lb) by 36 weeks.

Using linked birth and death certificates from Kansas between 1980 and 1986, Brown and Schloesser [46] investigated the relationships between pregravid weight, gestational weight gain, and outcome in 922 twin births delivered at term. These investigators found a positive linear relationship between gestational weight gain and infant birthweights in women who were underweight or of normal weight before conception, but not for those who were overweight or obese. The proportion of low-birthweight infants declined as pregravid weight increased. The mean gestational weight gain of underweight women who were delivered of twin infants at term with birthweights in the range of the lowest perinatal mortality (3001–3500 gm) [9] was 44.2 lb; for women of normal pregravid weight, the corresponding figure was 40.9 lb.

A recent study of 163 twin pregnancies at the Johns Hopkins Hospital examined the association between maternal pregravid weight, weight gain to selected weeks of gestation, and average birthweight as the mean of the twin pair and as a ratio derived by dividing the average birthweight by the 50th percentile weight-for-gestation [66]. This study reported that, regardless of maternal pregravid weight, twin birthweight greater than 2500 gm was associated with higher maternal weight gain to 24 weeks of gestation, higher rate of gain and total gain, shorter newborn length of stay, and higher birthweight ratios. Total weight gain of 40 to 45 lb and a rate of gain of 1.25 lb per week were significantly associated with higher twin birthweights and better intrauterine growth for gestational age.

Cardiovascular and Hematologic

Other adaptations made to a greater degree in twin compared to singleton pregnancy include cardiovascular and hematologic changes. One of the earliest adaptations in pregnant women is cardiovascular change. Total peripheral resistance is lowered even further in a twin pregnancy because of the greater production of progesterone and prostaglandins, resulting in vasodilation and a lowering of diastolic blood pressure.

Other related changes include the plasma volume and constituents of the blood. From about 20 weeks of gestation onward, the plasma volume in twin gestations is approximately 20 percent greater than in singleton gestations [54]. Total red cell volume also increases above singleton levels in twin pregnancy by about 25 percent [54]. This is indicative of a markedly increased oxygen-carrying capacity required for the oxygen transfer for two fetuses. The increase in red cell volume is not as great as that of the plasma, resulting in a more exaggerated hemodilution. The hemoglobin concentration for women with twins averaged 10 gm/100 ml from 20 weeks' gestation onward, and supplementation with iron or folic acid, or both, did not alter the hemoglobin concentration or mean cell volume [67].

Dietary Recommendations

At present there are no dietary recommendations for women pregnant with twins, triplets, or higher-order multiples. The most current guidelines on gestational weight gain from the National Academy of Sciences [68] suggest a range of gain of 25 to 35 lb for a singleton gestation, depending on the mother's pregravid weight. Current research suggests optimal weight gain for twin gestations to be 40 to 45 lb, with 24 lb by 24 weeks [46, 64, 66]. Even less research has been conducted on weight gain in triplet gestations, but case reports indicate that a total gain of 45 to 50 lb, with 36 lb by 24 weeks, is associated with higher birthweights and improved outcomes [69]. These weight gain recommendations are graphed in Fig. 12-5.

Good maternal nutrition is central to achieving optimal fetal growth and development, and to maintaining maternal health and well-being. Through the recommended dietary allowances (RDAs), the

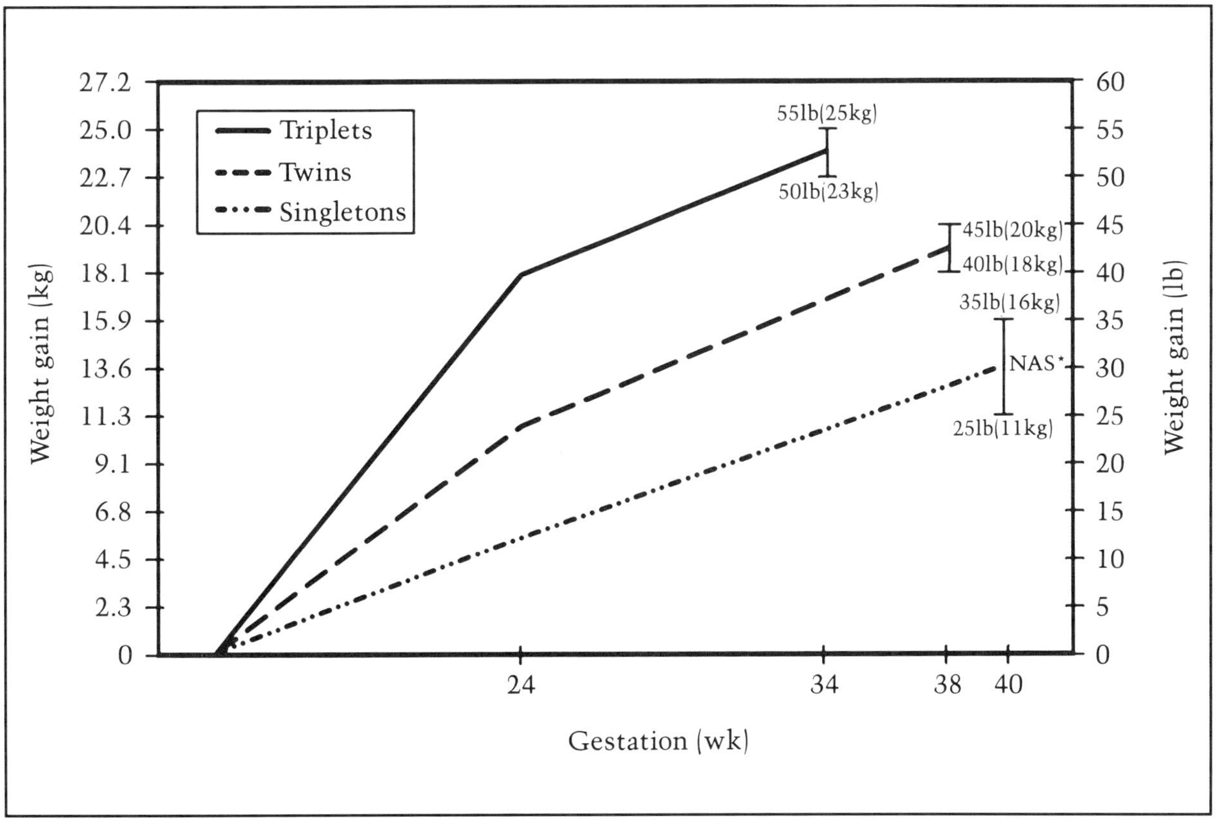

Fig. 12-5
Recommendations for gestational weight gain by plurality.

National Academy of Sciences recommends levels of essential nutrients to meet the additional nutrient demands of a singleton pregnancy (see Chap. 5, The Prenatal Diet). No guidelines have been established for women pregnant with a twin, triplet, or higher-order pregnancy. In the absence of such guidelines and in view of the established need for substantially higher weight gains, it seems reasonable to propose a 50 to 100 percent increase in the RDAs for singleton pregnancy for women pregnant with multiples. Table 12-7 outlines a modified RDA for women pregnant with multiples.

Table 12-7
Summary of RDAs for women aged 25 and older who are pregnant with singletons versus twins

Nutrient	*RDA for singleton pregnancy*	*Modified RDA for twin/triplet pregnancy*	*Dietary sources*
Folic acid	400 mcg	800 mcg	Leafy vegetables, liver
Vitamin D	10 μg	15 μg	Fortified dairy products
Iron	30 mg	50 mg	Meats, eggs, grains
Calcium	1200 mg	1800 mg	Dairy products
Phosphorus	1200 mg	1800 mg	Meats
Pyridoxine	2.2 mg	4.0 mg	Meats, liver, grains
Thiamine	1.5 mg	3.0 mg	Enriched grains, pork
Zinc	15 mg	30 mg	Meats, seafood, eggs
Riboflavin	1.6 mg	3.0 mg	Meats, liver, grains
Protein	60 mg	120 mg	Meats, fish, poultry, dairy
Iodine	175 mcg	300 mcg	Iodized salt, seafood
Vitamin C	70 mg	150 mg	Citrus fruits, tomatoes
Energy	2500 kcal	3000 kcal	Protein, fat, carbohydrate
Magnesium	320 mg	450 mg	Seafood, legumes, grains
Niacin	17 mg	25 mg	Meats, nuts, legumes
Vitamin B_{12}	2.2 mcg	3.0 mcg	Animal proteins
Vitamin A	800 μg	1000 μg	Dark-green, yellow, or orange fruits and vegetables; liver

Source: Adapted from the pregnancy RDAs in the National Academy of Sciences: *Recommended Dietary Allowances* (10th ed.). Washington, DC: National Academy Press, 1989.

Summary and Recommendations

Multiple pregnancy is associated with a greater risk of low birthweight and preterm birth than a singleton pregnancy, with resultant higher risks of neonatal morbidity and mortality. Twins, which comprise 97 percent of all multiple births in the United States, have a slower rate of growth compared to singletons, with significant differences from 35 weeks of gestation onward. Many of these differences are due to zygosity and placental factors, as well as increased incidence in congenital anomalies and complications unique to the twinning process. Maternal factors, such as race, age, height, and weight, all influence the rate of twinning. Length of gestation and twin birthweight are influenced by zygosity, placentation, and gestational weight gain. The highest twin birthweights for gestational age are associated with weight gains of 24 lb by 24 weeks and total gains of 40 to 45 lb, achieved at a rate of gain of about 1.25 lb per week.

References

1. US Dept. of Health and Human Services: *Vital Statistics of the United States, 1979*, Volume 1, *Natality*. Washington, DC: National Center for Health Statistics, 1984.
2. Advance report of final natality statistics, 1989. *Monthly Vital Statistics Report* Vol. 40, No. 8, Suppl. 1, December 12, 1991.
3. Ventura, SJ: Trends in first births to older mothers, 1970–1979. *Monthly Vital Statistics Report* Vol. 31, No. 2, Suppl. 2, May 27, 1982.
4. Luke, B, and Keith, L: The United States Standard Certificate of Live Birth: A critical commentary. *J. Reprod. Med.* 36:587–591, 1991.
5. Kiely, JL: The epidemiology of perinatal mortality in multiple births. *Bull. NY Acad. Med.* 66:618–637, 1990.
6. Leroy, B, Lefort, F, Neveu, P, et al: Intrauterine growth charts for twin fetuses. *Acta Genet. Med. Gemellol.* 31:199–206, 1982.
7. Luke, B, Witter, FR, Abbey, H, et al: Gestational age-specific birthweights of twins versus singletons. *Acta Genet. Med. Gemellol.* 40:69–76, 1991.
8. Wilson, RS: Growth and Development of Human Twins. In F Falkner and JM Tanner (eds.), *Human Growth: A Comprehensive Treatise* (2nd ed.), Vol. 3, *Methodology, Ecological, Genetic, and Nutritional Effects on Growth*. New York: Plenum, 1986. Pp. 197–211.
9. Williams, RL, Creasy, RK, Cunningham, GC, et al: Fetal growth and perinatal viability in California. *Obstet. Gynecol.* 59:624–632, 1982.
10. Gruenwald, P: Environmental influences on twins apparent at birth. *Biol. Neonate* 15:79–93, 1970.
11. Fujikura, T, and Froehlich, LA: Twin placentation and zygosity. *Obstet. Gynecol.* 37:34–43, 1971.

12. Bleker, OP, Oosting, J, and Hemrika, DJ: On the cause of the retardation of fetal growth in multiple gestations. *Acta Genet. Med. Gemellol.* 37:41–46, 1988.
13. Bleker, OP, Breur, W, and Huidekoper, BL: A study of birth weight, placental weight, and mortality of twins as compared to singletons. *Br. J. Obstet. Gynecol.* 86:111–118, 1979.
14. Ramos-Arroyo, MA, Ulbright, TM, Yu, P-L, and Christian, JC: Twin study: Relationship between birth weight, zygosity, placentation, and pathological placental changes. *Acta Genet. Med. Gemellol.* 37:229–238, 1988.
15. Ohel, G, Granat, M, Zeevi, D, et al: Advanced ultrasonic placental maturation in twin pregnancies. *Am. J. Obstet. Gynecol.* 156:76–78, 1987.
16. O'Brien, WF, Knuppel, RA, Scerbo, JC, and Rattan, PK: Birth weight in twins: An analysis of discordancy and growth retardation. *Obstet. Gynecol.* 67:483–486, 1986.
17. Blickstein, I, Shoham-Schwartz, Z, and Lancet, M: Growth discordancy in appropriate for gestational age, term twins. *Obstet. Gynecol.* 72:582–584, 1988.
18. Guaschino, S, Spinillo, A, Stola, E, and Pesando, PC: Growth retardation, size at birth and perinatal mortality in twin pregnancy. *Int. J. Gynaecol. Obstet.* 25:399–403, 1987.
19. Erkkala, R, Ala-mello, S, Piiroinen, O, et al: Growth discordancy in twin pregnancies: A risk factor not detected by measurements of biparietal diameter. *Obstet. Gynecol.* 66:203–206, 1985.
20. Falkner, F: Twin Growth in Relationship to Placentation. In F Falkner and JM Tanner (eds.), *Human Growth: A Comprehensive Treatise* (2nd ed.), Vol. 3. New York: Plenum, 1986. Pp. 213–220.
21. Klebe, JG, and Ingomar, CJ: The fetoplacental circulation during parturition illustrates the interfetal transfusion syndrome. *Pediatrics* 49:112–116, 1972.
22. Tan, KL, Tan, R, Tan, SH, and Tan, AM: The twin transfusion syndrome. Clinical observations on 35 affected pairs. *Clin. Pediatr.* 18:111–114, 1979.
23. Naeye, RL: Human intrauterine parabiotic syndrome and its complications. *N. Engl. J. Med.* 268:804–809, 1963.
24. Rausen, AR, Seki, M, and Strauss, L: Twin transfusion syndrome. A review of 19 cases studied at one institution. *J. Pediatr.* 66:613–628, 1965.
25. Gonsoulin, W, Moise, KJ, Kirshon, B, et al: Outcome of twin-twin transfusion diagnosed before 28 weeks of gestation. *Obstet. Gynecol.* 75:214–216, 1990.
26. Bebbington, MW, and Wittman, BK: Fetal transfusion syndrome: Antenatal factors predicting outcome. *Am. J. Obstet. Gynecol.* 160:913–915, 1989.
27. Ho, SK, and Wu, PYK: Perinatal factors and neonatal morbidity in twin pregnancy. *Am. J. Obstet. Gynecol.* 122:979, 1975.

28. Naeye, RL, Tafari, N, Judge, D, and Marboe, CC: Twins: Causes of perinatal death in 12 United States cities and one African city. *Am. J. Obstet. Gynecol.* 131:267, 1978.
29. McCarthy, BJ, Sachs, BP, Layde, PM, et al: The epidemiology of neonatal death in twins. *Am. J. Obstet. Gynecol.* 141:252, 1981.
30. Keith, L, Ellis, R, Berger, GS, et al: The Northwestern University multihospital twin study. *Am. J. Obstet. Gynecol.* 138:781, 1980.
31. Nylander, PPS: Perinatal mortality in twins. *Acta Genet. Med. Gemellol.* 28:363, 1979.
32. Botting, BJ, MacDonald Davies, I, and MacFarlane, AJ: Recent trends in the incidence of multiple births and associated mortality. *Arch. Dis. Child.* 62:941–950, 1987.
33. Fabre, E, Gonzalez de Aguero, R, de Agustin, JL, et al: Perinatal mortality in twin pregnancy: An analysis of birth weight–specific mortality rates and adjusted mortality rates for birth weight distributions. *J. Perinat. Med.* 16:85–91, 1988.
34. Bronsteen, R, Goyert, G, and Bottoms, S: Classification of twins and neonatal morbidity. *Obstet. Gynecol.* 74:98–101, 1989.
35. Luke, B, Witter, FR, and Johnson, TRB: The effect of higher birthweights for gestational age on length of stay of newborn twins. Presented at the XIII World Congress of Gynaecology and Obstetrics, Singapore, September 1991.
36. Leveno, KJ, Quirk, JG, Whalley, PJ, et al: Fetal lung maturation in twin gestation. *Am. J. Obstet. Gynecol.* 148:405–411, 1984.
37. McCulloch, K: Neonatal problems in twins. *Clin. Perinatol.* 15:141–158, 1988.
38. Luke, B, and Keith, LG: Monozygotic twinning as a congenital defect and congenital defects in monozygotic twins. *Fetal Diagnosis and Therapy* 5:61–69, 1990.
39. Schinzel, AA, Smith, DW, and Miller, JR: Monozygotic twinning and structural defects. *J. Pediatr.* 95:921, 1979.
40. Benirschke, K, and Kim, CK: Multiple pregnancy. II. *N. Engl. J. Med.* 288:1329, 1973.
41. Jones, KL, and Benirschke, K: The developmental pathogenesis of structural defects: The contribution of monozygotic twins. *Semin. Perinatol.* 7:239, 1983.
42. Wyshak, G, and White, C: Genealogical study of human twinning. *Am. J. Public Health* 55:1586–1593, 1965.
43. Taffel, SM: Characteristics of American Indian and Alaska Native births: United States, 1984. *Monthly Vital Statistics Report*, Vol. 36, No. 3, Suppl., June 19, 1987.
44. Taffel, SM: Characteristics of Asian births: United States, 1980. *Monthly Vital Statistics Report*, Vol. 32, No. 10, Suppl., February 10, 1984.
45. MacGillivray, I, and Campbell, DM: The Physical Characteristics and Adaptations of Women with Twin Pregnancies. In L Gedda, P Parisi, and WE Nance (eds.), *Twin Research: Clinical Studies*. New

York: Alan R. Liss, 1978. Pp. 81–86.
46. Brown, JE, and Schloesser, PT: Prepregnancy weight status, prenatal weight gain, and the outcome of term twin gestations. *Am. J. Obstet. Gynecol.* 162:182–186, 1990.
47. Wyshak, G: Reproductive and Menstrual Characteristics of Mothers of Multiple Births and Mothers of Singletons Only: A Discriminant Analysis. In L Gedda, P Parisi, and WE Nance (eds.), *Twin Research 3: Twin Biology and Multiple Pregnancy*. New York: Alan R. Liss, 1981. Pp. 95–105.
48. Campbell, DM, Campbell, AJ, and MacGillivray, I: Maternal characteristics of women having twin pregnancies. *J. Biosoc. Sci.* 6:463–470, 1974.
49. Corney, G, Seedburgh, D, Thompson, B, et al: Multiple and Singleton Pregnancy: Differences between Mothers as well as Offspring. In L Gedda, P Parisi, and WE Nance (eds.), *Twin Research 3: Twin Biology and Multiple Pregnancy*. New York: Alan R. Liss, 1981. Pp. 107–114.
50. Philippe, P: The end of reproductive life in mothers of twins: Epidemiologic analysis of a large data base. *Acta Genet. Med. Gemellol.* 37:249–262, 1988.
51. Bonnelykke, B: Menstrual characteristics of mothers of twins. *J. Biosoc. Sci.* 21:329–334, 1989.
52. Siiteri, PK, Schwartz, B, and MacDonald, PC: Oestrogen receptors and the oesterone hypothesis in relation to endometrial and breast cancer. *Gynecol. Oncol.* 2:228, 1974.
53. Reyes, FI, Winter, JSD, and Faiman, C: Pituitary-ovarian relationships preceding the menopause. I. A cross-sectional study of serum follicle-stimulating hormone, luteinising hormone, prolactin, estradiol, and progesterone levels. *Am. J. Obstet. Gynecol.* 129:557–564, 1977.
54. Campbell, DM: Physiological Changes and Adaptation. In I MacGillivray, DM Campbell, and B Thompson (eds.), *Twinning and Twins*. New York: Wiley, 1988. Pp. 99–109.
55. Tambyraja, RL, and Ratnam, SS: Plasma Steroid Changes in Twin Pregnancy. In L Gedda, P Parisi, and WE Nance (eds.), *Twin Research 3: Twin Biology and Multiple Pregnancy*. New York: Alan R. Liss, 1981. Pp. 189–195.
56. Grennert, L, Gennser, G, Persson, P, et al: Ultrasound and human-placental-lactogen screening for early detection of twin pregnancies. *Lancet* 1:4–6, 1976.
57. Jandial, V, Horne, CHW, Glover, RG, et al: The value of measurement of pregnancy-specific proteins in twin pregnancies. *Acta Genet. Med. Gemellol.* 28:319–325, 1979.
58. Thom, H, Buckland, CM, Campbell, AGM, et al: Maternal serum alpha-feto-protein in monozygotic and dizygotic twin pregnancy. *Prenat. Diagn.* 4:341–346, 1984.
59. Spellacy, WN, Buhi, WC, and Birk, SA: Carbohydrate metabolism in women with a twin pregnancy. *Obstet. Gynecol.* 55:688–691, 1980.

60. Campbell, DM, and MacGillivray, I: Glucose tolerance in twin pregnancy. *Acta Genet. Med. Gemellol.* 28:283–287, 1979.
61. Kohl, SG, and Casey, G: Twin gestation. *Mt. Sinai J. Med. (NY)* 43:523, 1975.
62. Redford, DHA: Uterine growth in twin pregnancy by measurement of total intrauterine volume. *Acta Genet. Med. Gemellol.* 31:145–148, 1982.
63. Campbell, DM, MacGillivray, I, and Tuttle, S: Maternal nutrition in twin pregnancy. *Acta Genet. Med. Gemellol.* 31:221–227, 1982.
64. Pederson, AL, Worthington-Roberts, B, and Hickok, DE: Weight gain patterns during twin gestation. *J. Am. Dietet. Assoc.* 89:642–646, 1989.
65. Konwinski, T, Gerard, C, Hult, AM, and Papiernik-Berkhauer, E: Maternal pregestational weight and multiple pregnancy duration. *Acta Genet. Med. Gemellol.* 22:44–47, 1974.
66. Luke, B, Minogue, J, Abbey, H, et al: The association between maternal weight gain and the birthweight of twins. *J. Maternal-Fetal Med.* 1:267–276, 1992.
67. Hall, MH, Campbell, DM, and Davidson, RJL: Anaemia in twin pregnancy. *Acta Genet. Med. Gemellol.* 28:279–282, 1979.
68. National Academy of Sciences: *Nutrition During Pregnancy*. Washington, DC: National Academy Press, 1990.
69. Gallagher, MW, Gegor, C, Luke, B, and Paine, L: A team approach to management of multifetal pregnancy. Presented at the Armed Forces Section of the American College of Obstetricians and Gynecologists, Bethesda, Maryland, June, 1991.

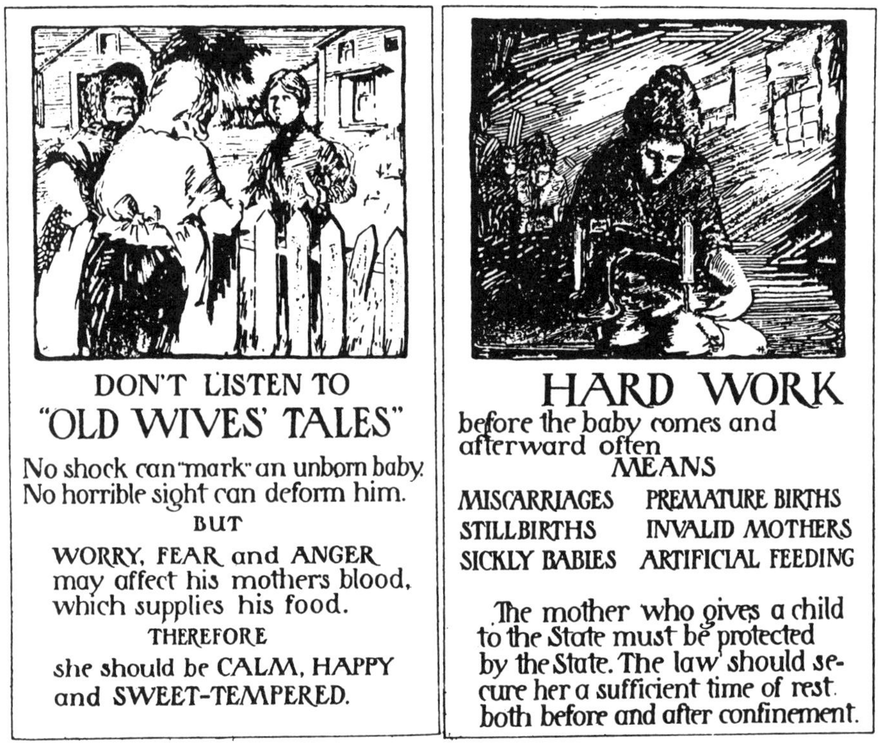

Educational posters for expectant mothers. (Distributed by the National Child Welfare Association, 1919.)

13

Nutrition and Prematurity

Introduction and Historical Evidence

During the 20th century, the majority of research on nutrition and the outcome of pregnancy has focused on three areas: (1) influencing the size of the newborn and facilitating delivery, (2) preventing maternal obesity after delivery, and (3) detecting and preventing pregnancy-induced hypertension [1]. Before the 1980s, few studies evaluated the role of nutritional factors in the etiology of prematurity. In addition, "prematurity" was used to indicate a birthweight of 2500 gm or less as often as it was to describe a gestational age of greater than 25 days before the expected date of confinement [2, 3]. Therefore, in reviewing older literature, it is difficult to differentiate between an outcome of lowered birthweight versus shortened gestation.

Because of these reasons, there is a dearth of research on nutrition and prematurity. An exception to this void are the observational reports of the effects of famine conditions on reproductive performance during World Wars I and II. Although most of these reports also focus on birthweight, they do provide some information on the effect of these "natural experiments" of famine conditions on fertility and length of gestation [4].

World War I

The period of acute deprivation in Germany occurred during the winter of 1916 to 1917. According to the official report to the United Kingdom government by Starling [5], the civil death rate rose from 9.5 percent in 1915 to 37 percent in 1918. The birth rate for Germany during this period was about half the prewar rate, although mean birthweights were not significantly affected. "War amenorrhea" was common, secondary to a shortage of food and the harshness of physical effort and environmental conditions. It has been suggested that several factors were responsible for the relatively high birthweights among the resulting fewer newborns, including the effect of special provisions for pregnant women, a reduction in the proportion of first births, and a rise in the average age and parity of those women who were pregnant [4]. A report from Stockholm [6] indicated that amenorrhea occurred in fewer than 1 percent of hospital patients before the war, but rose to 11 percent by the third quarter of 1918. The maximum incidence of war amenorrhea, predominantly among nulliparas aged 20 to 30, was followed 9 months later by a minimum birth rate.

The data on births are difficult to interpret because of the lack of information on length of gestation, appropriateness of birthweight for gestational age, maturity and vitality, and incidence of stillbirths. Reports from Vienna and Budapest suggest average birthweight reductions of 100 to 200 gm, and indicate that only better-nourished women were having children. The actual condition of perinatal health in Germany during World War I was probably suppressed in the interests of popular morale. The writings of Mossmer in 1916 attest to this [7]: "The sensational statements of Kettner on the frequency at present of small, underdeveloped, fragile, very thin, newborn infants with a 'cerebral' tendency, if they reach the general public, are calculated to cause great anxiety because the alleged inferiority of the children would naturally be attributed to the food shortage."

Although there were no specific reports on the effect of the famine conditions on prematurity, it is likely that a proportion of newborns were both premature and growth retarded.

World War II

Famine conditions also occurred during World War II, and their effect on reproductive outcome was studied in detail in Leningrad and the Netherlands. The siege of Leningrad lasted from August 1941 to August 1943, with famine conditions their worst between September 1941 and February 1942. According to Antonov's description of Leningrad during the siege [8], conditions were worse than during World War I. The city was bombed, there was no heating or public transportation, and the winter of 1941 to 1942 was particularly severe. Bread rations between September 1941 and February 1942 ranged from 250 to 500 gm for manual workers to 125 to 400 gm for clerical workers. Data from the Department for the Newborn of the Leningrad State Pediatric Institute [8] indicate that the birth rate fell and the rates of prematurity, stillbirth, and neonatal death rose in 1942. During the first half of 1942, the stillbirth rate doubled and prematurity rose to 41.2 percent. The average birthweight dropped by 500 to 600 gm, and neonatal mortality rose to 9 percent for term infants and 30.8 percent for premature infants.

In the Netherlands, famine conditions existed from October 1944 until May 1945. Because of the excellent prenatal records and vital statistics maintained by the Dutch before, during, and after the famine, these data have been studied extensively by many researchers [9–13]. Although the dietary and environmental conditions were similar during the famine periods for Leningrad and the Netherlands, the Russian women had been exposed to a much longer period of suboptimal nutrition and extreme physical exertion before the famine. In contrast, the Dutch people had been well nourished and not as physically stressed before the German blockade. Therefore, the results of the effect of wartime famine conditions on reproductive performance in these two areas are not completely comparable. As in Leningrad, war amenorrhea was reported to be as high as 50 percent among urban Dutch women in areas affected by the famine, and the birth rate fell to about one third of normal [10].

Stein and Susser [11–13] conducted the most extensive studies on the effect of the Dutch famine on women and their newborns. They evaluated the prenatal and newborn records from teaching hospitals in Amsterdam, Leiden, and Rotterdam in the famine area, and in Groningen in the north and Heerlen in the south, both areas that were unaffected by famine, although they were receiving reduced food rations. Data on maternal body weight were available only for hospital births in Rotterdam. This measurement, as the postpartum weight, was taken 9 to 10 days after delivery. The greatest reduction in birthweight, birthlength, and head circumference occurred with third-trimester famine exposure. Average length of gestation was reduced by only about 4 days. The effects of the famine on fetal growth were neither mediated nor confounded through shortening of gestation.

A graphic presentation of infant birthweight, birthlength, placental weight, maternal body weight, length of gestation, and caloric rations per day during the 20-month period around the famine is given in Fig. 13-1. Infant birthweight and birthlength, placental weight, maternal body weight, and length of gestation are given in Z-scores (standard deviations from a norm), and caloric rations are given in absolute calories. Maternal body weight was most affected by famine exposure, followed by infant birthweight. Birthlength was much less affected, and length of gestation was affected least of all indices studied.

The dizygotic twinning rate fell in countries affected by malnutrition during World War II, including Norway, France, and Holland [14, 15], and rose after adequate dietary intake was restored. The dizygotic twinning rate may be a reflection of the general maternal nutritional status, and reflect alterations in hormonal factors and reproductive ability caused by chronic malnutrition.

Anthropometric Factors

The most consistent finding in clinical studies is the association between **low pregravid weight** and prematurity [16–23]. **Short mater-**

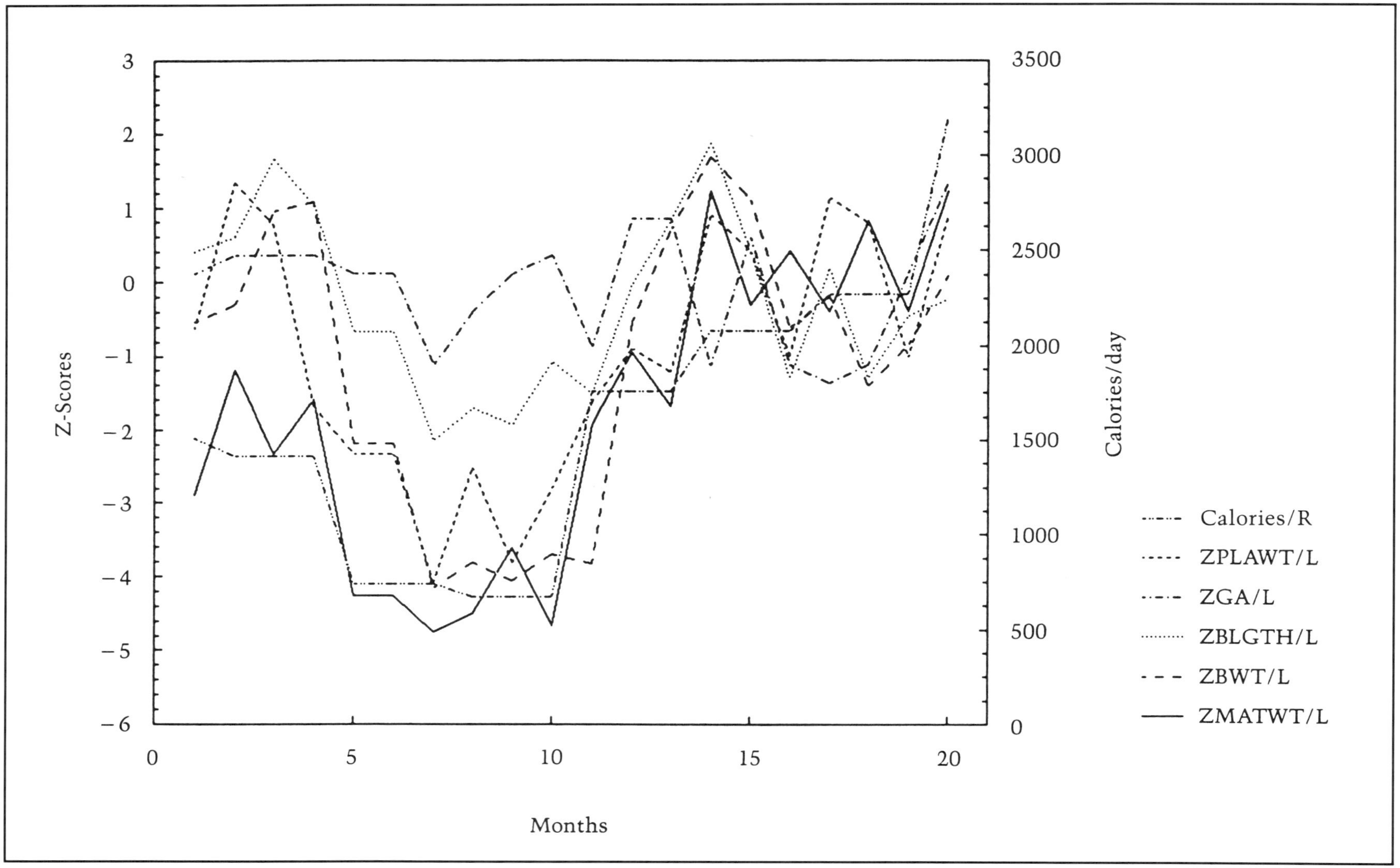

Fig. 13-1
Mean caloric intake and Z-scores of mean maternal body weight (ZMATWT), infant birthweight (ZBWT), birthlength (ZBLGTH), length of gestation (ZGA), and placental weight (ZPLAWT) in Rotterdam, The Netherlands from August 1944 through March 1946. (Adapted from Z. Stein and M. Susser, The Dutch famine, 1944–45, and the reproductive process. II. Interrelations of caloric rations and six indices at birth. *Pediatr. Res.* 9:76–83, 1975.)

nal stature has also been associated with prematurity [18, 21], although its effect is mediated through pregravid weight, as **low weight-for-height**. The effect of increasing height versus increasing pregravid weight is shown graphically in Fig. 13-2, based on data from 17,000 births at the University of Alabama [18]. The incidence of both intrauterine growth retardation (IUGR) and prematurity is inversely proportional to increasing maternal height and pregravid weight, although the effect is much more dramatic with increasing maternal weight. Data from the First British Perinatal Mortality Survey showed that the prematurity rate was nearly twice as great for women who were less than 5 ft tall compared to those 5 ft 8 in. or taller, and the prematurity rate was nearly three times greater among women with pregravid weights of 112 lb or less compared to those weighing 140 lb or more (29.5/1000 live births vs. 10.2/1000 live births) [21]. When viewed together, as weight-for-height, the effect of weight was of much greater importance. Recent research has shown maternal body weight to be equivalent to body mass index [weight/(height)^2] in risk assessment of adverse pregnancy outcome, including prematurity and low birthweight [22, 23].

Mean length of gestation increases with increasing maternal pregravid weight, even within the range of term births. For example, Peckham and Christianson [24] reported increasing mean gestation of 279.2 days to 283.7 days for live births and 273.9 days to 280.7 days for all births with increasing maternal pregravid weight from underweight to overweight. Brown and associates [25] also reported a significant relationship between increasing maternal pregravid weight and length of gestation from 38.9 weeks for very underweight women to 39.5 weeks for normal-weight women. In a study of underweight women matched to normal-weight control subjects, Mitchell and Lerner [26] reported a prematurity rate of 114, 94, and 88 per 1000 live births, respectively, for women less than 81 percent, 81 to 90 percent, and 90 to 110 percent weight-for-height. Frentzen and colleagues [27] reported prematurity rates of 158 and 115 per 1000 live births, respectively, for normal-weight and overweight women.

The second most important nutritional factor associated with prematurity is **low gestational weight gain**, as inadequate total gain or rate of gain. Low gestational weight gain is one of the few risk factors for prematurity that may be susceptible to intervention. These two direct causes, low pregravid weight and low gestational weight gain, act indirectly in the other nutritionally related factors associated with prematurity (Table 13-1). Those studies that have controlled for gestational age while examining the association between maternal

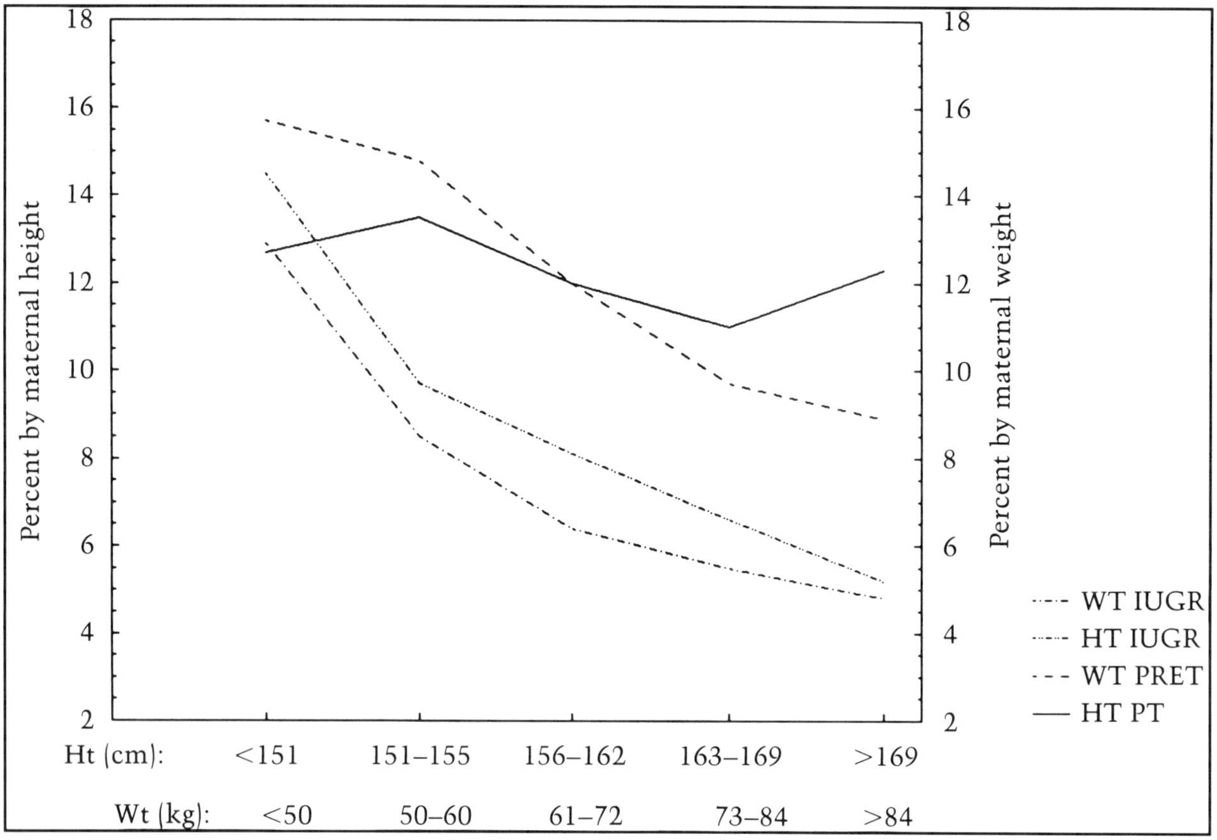

Fig. 13-2
Percent intrauterine growth retardation (IUGR) and preterm (PRET) birth by maternal pregravid weight (WT) and height (HT) categories. (Adapted from SW Wen et al, Intrauterine growth retardation and preterm delivery: Prenatal risk factors in an indigent population. *Am. J. Obstet. Gynecol.* 162:213–218, 1990.)

gestational weight gain and prematurity have reported a significant relationship between gestational weight gain and prematurity [18, 19, 28–32]. Papiernik and Kaminski [28] demonstrated a significant association between premature birth and maternal weight gain of less than 5 kg (11 lb) by 32 weeks' gestation. Van den Berg and Oechsli [29] reported that preterm birth was more likely to occur when the rate of weight gain was 0.23 kg (0.5 lb) or less after 20 weeks' gestation. Hediger and associates [30] reported a significantly increased risk of prematurity with inadequate late weight gain (<4.3 kg or 9.5 lb after 24 weeks' gestation). Using multivariate analysis of risk factors for prematurity, Berkowitz [31] reported an odds ratio of 4.28 for inadequate weight gain, adjusted for pregnancy duration.

Table 13-1
Nutrition-related factors associated with prematurity

1. *Anthropometric*
   Low pregravid weight
   Low body fat
   Low total gestational weight gain
   Low rate of gestational weight gain
   Inadequate late weight gain (after 24 wk)
2. *Dietary*
   Fasting/starvation
   Chronic malnutrition/undernutrition
   Inadequate vitamin A
   Inadequate folate
   Inadequate iron
   Inadequate magnesium
   Inadequate calcium
   Inadequate zinc
   Inadequate essential fatty acids
   Inadequate essential amino acids
3. *Lifestyle*
   Smoking
   Alcohol use

Abrams and associates [32] reported a 60 percent increased risk of spontaneous preterm birth in women with a low rate of gain (<0.27 kg or 0.6 lb/wk), compared with those with an average rate (0.27–0.52 kg or 0.6–1.15 lb/wk). Women with a low rate of gain were more than twice as likely to deliver prematurely as those with a high rate of gain (>0.52 kg or 1.15 lb/wk). A subsequent report using the same study population indicated that only low maternal weight gain was significantly associated with both IUGR and prematurity [19].

In twin gestations, higher maternal weight gain is significantly associated with higher birthweight and longer length of gestation. Luke and associates [33] demonstrated that, regardless of maternal pregravid weight, total weight of 40 to 45 lb and rate of gain of 1.25 lb/wk were associated with a lower incidence of low birthweight and prematurity in twin gestations.

Maternal pregravid weight, alone or in combination with gestational weight gain, may exert its effect on pregnancy outcome (as length of gestation and birthweight) through the presence (or absence) of maternal nutrient reserves, particularly **maternal body fat**. According to Frisch [34], there are at least four mechanisms by which maternal body fat may directly affect ovulation, menstruation, fertility, and gestation. First, it serves as a significant extragonadal source of estrogen, accounting for a third of the circulating estrogen of premenopausal women. Second, body weight (and therefore body fat) influences the direction of estrogen metabolism to more potent or less potent forms, with very thin women having an increase in the relatively inactive 2-hydroxylated form of estrogen and heavier women having an increase in the more potent 16-hydroxylated form. Third, overweight women and young girls who are fatter have a diminished capacity for estrogen to bind to serum sex hormone–binding globulin (SHBG), resulting in an elevated percentage of free serum estradiol. Through changes in the proportion of body fat, SHBG regulates the availability of estradiol to the brain and other target tissues, influencing reproductive performance. Fourth, because maternal body fat stores steroid hormones, changes in the proportion of body fat affect reproductive ability indirectly through hypothalamic regulation of body temperature, energy balance, and response to luteinizing hormone–releasing hormone.

As a buffer against environmental stresses and fluctuations in dietary intake, maternal body fat may also play an important role in the hormonal and biochemical aspects of gestation. In addition to paralleling longer length of gestation [25], increasing pregravid weight (an indirect measure of increasing body fat) is associated with better intrauterine growth, as reflected in higher birthweights, longer birth-lengths, and larger head circumferences [25, 35–37]. This interrelationship was demonstrated in the studies of well-nourished women whose pregnancies coincided with the Dutch famine of 1944 to 1945 [11–13]. Maternal body weight absorbed the first impacts of the famine, preceding a decline in placental weight and newborn measures. Only after a lower threshold limit of maternal weight was reached, representing a depletion of maternal body fat, did nutritional deprivation significantly directly affect the products of conception (first the placenta, then birthweight). With the provision of food after the liberation, the metabolic needs of the mother and the placenta took priority; maternal body weight and placental weight were quicker to recover, with birthweight increasing only after a time lag (see Fig. 13-1).

The effect of **fasting** on preterm birth may have a hormonal basis, also mediated through maternal body fat. A doubling of the birth rate following a 24-hour total food and water fast, termed the *Yom Kippur effect*, has been reported [38] (Fig. 13-3). The hormonal basis of this phenomenon has been demonstrated in the rhesus monkey [39]. The fast results in an initial decrease in maternal whole blood glucose,

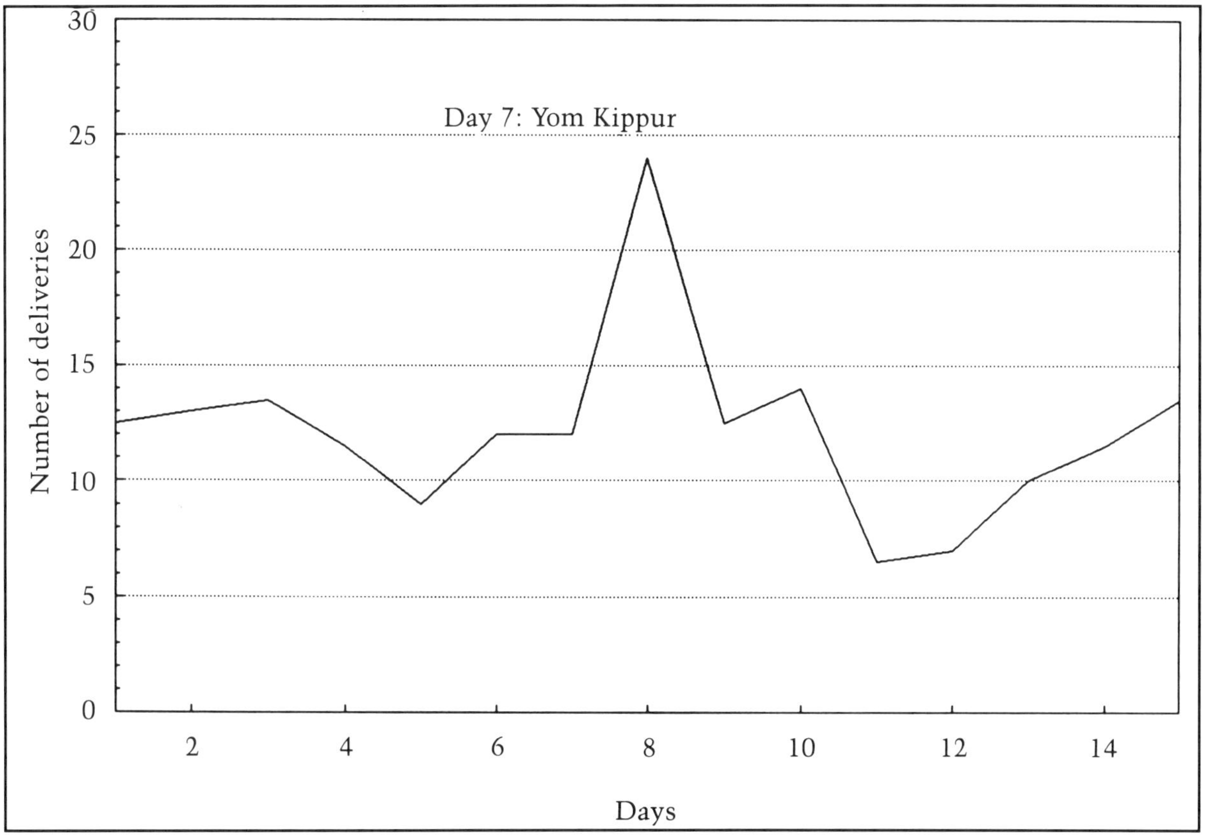

Fig. 13-3
Mean deliveries per day before, during, and after the 24-hour fast of Yom Kippur. (Adapted from M Kaplan et al, Fasting and the precipitation of labor: The Yom Kippur effect. *J.A.M.A.* 250:1317–1318, 1983.)

followed by an increase in the maternal arterial plasma prostaglandin concentration, and results in increased frequency of nocturnal myometrial contractions.

Research on **skinfold changes during pregnancy**, estimating the accretion and utilization of body fat during gestation, reflects this concept of optimal maternal reserves associated with better pregnancy outcome (as longer gestation and higher birthweight) [40–42]. In studies of healthy women with term pregnancies, total maternal body fat increased during pregnancy, reaching a peak between 24 and 28 weeks, followed by a decrease during the remaining 12 weeks [40, 43]. By 6 to 8 weeks postpartum, amount of total body fat was similar to that at 10 weeks of gestation. Increases in total body fat were less for multiparas compared to primiparas and for overweight women compared to normal weight or underweight women [43].

In a series of studies comparing anthropometric changes during pregnancy in Asian and European mothers who had small-for-gestational-age (SGA) infants versus appropriate-for-gestational-age (AGA) infants, Bissenden and associates [41, 42] demonstrated the effect of the accretion of body fat on length of gestation and birthweight. Asian women with SGA infants had gained less weight and fat during the second trimester, and had pregnancies that averaged 1.6 weeks shorter than those of European women with SGA infants [41]. Asian women with AGA infants had comparable length of gestation and weight gains, but double the increase in body fat compared to European women with AGA infants [42].

Dietary Factors

The increase in body weight (and therefore body fat) associated with optimal pregnancy outcomes is the theoretical basis behind programs and studies using **nutritional supplementation** during pregnancy. Despite differences in the nutritional status of the populations studied and their living conditions, the results of studies of nutritional supplementation in Guatemala [44], Africa [45], Peru [46], and Taiwan [47] have been strikingly consistent, reporting a modest increase in average birthweight (about 100 gm), but a substantial reduction in the incidence of low birthweight (<2500 gm). Unfortunately, although data on length of gestation are obtained as part of most studies, and its effect on birthweight controlled for, most studies fail to evaluate the association between the use of the nutritional supplement and duration of gestation.

One of the most famous randomized controlled trials of prenatal nutritional supplementation was conducted in New York City between 1970 and 1976 [48]. This study included black women with low pregravid weight, low gestational weight gain, a history of having at least one low-birthweight infant, and a current low-protein intake. The study included three groups: The first group received a high-protein (40 gm), high-calorie (470 kcal), vitamin-mineral fortified beverage; the second group received a low-protein (6 gm), lower-calorie (322 kcal), vitamin-mineral fortified beverage; and the third group received the vitamin-mineral equivalent as a prenatal tablet (nonintervention, control group). The surprising results of this study included a significant increase in very preterm births (25–30 weeks' gestation) and associated neonatal deaths and growth retardation among the remaining pregnancies up to 37 weeks of gestation among women in the high-protein supplement group. Length of gestation was increased for women in the low-protein supplement group, and the growth-retarding effects of smoking on birthweight were reduced for both high- and low-protein supplement groups.

A nonresearch prenatal nutritional supplementation program was initiated in the United States in 1975 as an addition to the food stamp program. The Special Supplemental Food Program for Women, Infants, and Children (known as WIC) is administered by the US Department of Agriculture. Authorized as an amendment to the Child Nutrition Act of 1966, the WIC program is for pregnant and lactating women, infants, and children up to 4 years of age who have a demonstrated financial and nutritional need. For pregnant, postpartum, and lactating women and for children aged 1 to 4, the special monthly food coupons provide for 31 qt. vitamins A and D fortified milk or equivalent; cheese as a milk substitute (1 lb = 3 qt); 2.5 dozen eggs; four 8-oz packages of iron-fortified cereal; and six 46-oz. cans or equivalent of fruit juices. These food packages were designed to correct reported inadequacies of iron, vitamin A, and vitamin C in the diets of low-income individuals in the United States. The effects of the WIC program on maternal anemia, birthweight, length of gestation, and childhood growth are periodically evaluated [49–51]. One of the earliest studies prospectively evaluated the effects of WIC participation between 1973 and 1976 for 19 projects located in 14 states [49]. Among pregnant women in the program, there was an increase in maternal weight gain and infant birthweight, a reduction in maternal iron-deficiency anemia, and an increase in length of gestation. After adjustment for potentially confounding variables, length of gestation was significantly associated with duration of WIC participation.

The effect of WIC participation from midpregnancy was evaluated in a prospective, randomized controlled trial [50]. WIC participation significantly increased mean birthweight and had a positive effect on the birthweight of women who smoked. Length of gestation was not significantly different between WIC participants and nonparticipants.

A third evaluation of WIC participation was conducted as a longitudinal study [51]. In addition to higher birthweight, WIC participation was associated with lower rates of very-preterm (<33 wk) and preterm (<37 wk) birth, although problems with study design may reduce the difference.

Other studies have examined the association between individual nutrients and prematurity; these nutrients include **vitamin A** [52],

folate [53], **magnesium** [54], **calcium** [55–57], **long-chain n-3 fatty acids** [58–62], and **iron** [63, 64]. Vitamin A deficiency, alone and in combination with protein-calorie malnutrition, is widely prevalent in developing countries. In a case-control study comparing pregnancy outcome by income and social class in India, Shah and Rajalakshmi [52] reported a significant association between both growth retardation and prematurity and reduced **vitamin A** levels in the affected infants and their mothers compared to adequately grown term infants and their mothers. Hibbard [53] reported the results of a prospective study of low **erythrocyte folate** on subsequent adverse pregnancy outcomes in Cardiff, Wales. Low erythrocyte folate concentrations were found among 13 percent of women who subsequently had normal, term pregnancies, compared to 83 percent of women who subsequently aborted, 61 percent who had malformed newborns, 18 percent who delivered preterm, and 49 percent whose infants were SGA. The results of a double-blind randomized trial of magnesium prenatal supplementation was reported by Spatling and Spatling [54]. Women supplemented with 15 mmol per day magnesium-aspartate-hydrochloride had significantly fewer preterm births and longer median length of gestation than women given the placebo of 13.5 mmol per day aspartic acid. The magnesium supplementation was also associated with lower maternal and newborn morbidity.

Recent studies on prenatal **calcium supplementation** have demonstrated a significant effect in reducing adverse pregnancy outcomes [55–57]. In a randomized, double-blinded controlled clinical trial of calcium supplementation (2 gm elemental calcium as calcium carbonate), Villar and Repke reported significant reductions among the calcium group versus the placebo group in prematurity (7.4 vs. 21.1%), low birthweight (9.6 vs. 21.1%), mean length of gestation (39.2 vs. 37.9 wk), and mean birthweight (3129 gm vs. 2939 gm). The calcium group also had lower incidences, although not statistically significant, of preeclampsia and pregnancy-induced hypertension (0 vs. 3.4% and 3.3 vs. 5.7%, respectively), in agreement with previous studies [56, 57]. Significantly higher birthweights and longer length of gestation have also been reported in other studies of calcium supplementation [56, 57]. Villar and Repke hypothesize that the effect of calcium supplementation is mediated by a reduction in uterine smooth-muscle contractility.

Length of gestation has also been studied in regard to differences in the **fatty acid component of the diet**. Dietary **long-chain n-3 fatty acids** inhibit the formation of the dienoic prostaglandins from arachidonic acid. Recent studies have hypothesized that a high maternal intake of marine foods rich in long-chain n-3 fatty acids increases birthweight and duration of pregnancy through this inhibition of prostaglandin synthesis [58–60]. Evaluating differences in pregnancy outcome between two geographically distinct areas (the Faroe Islands and Denmark), Olsen and associates [58] compared the ratio of n-3 fatty acids to arachidonic acid in maternal erythrocytes in Faroese and Danish women during the postpartum period. Faroese women had significantly higher average ratio compared to Danish women (0.73 vs. 0.61). This 20 percent difference was associated with an increase in pregnancy duration of 5.7 days, as well as higher mean birthweight. The only other controlled trial of n-3 fatty acid intake during pregnancy was conducted in London in 1938 to 1939; in this study pregnant women were given either no supplement or a supplement with vitamins, minerals, and halibut liver oil [61]. The results of this 50-year-old trial, which has recently been reviewed as scientifically sound [62], included significantly smaller proportion of pregnancies with short durations among the supplemented group.

Several large studies evaluating the effect of maternal **iron status** have shown a significant association between extremes of maternal hemoglobin and prematurity. Garn and associates [63] evaluated the hematologic and pregnancy outcome data on more than 50,000 pregnancies from the Collaborative Perinatal Project conducted in 1959 to 1965. As shown in Figs. 13-4 and 13-5, there is a "U-shaped" relationship between maternal hematologic levels and adverse pregnancy outcomes. High hemoglobin and hematocrit, like low hemoglobin and hematocrit, increase the probabilities of fetal death, prematurity, low birthweight, and low Apgar scores. Data from nearly 55,000 births in the Cardiff Births Survey, conducted in 1970 to 1982, confirmed these findings, indicating the same relationship between extremes of maternal hematologic levels and adverse pregnancy outcome, including prematurity [64]. Low hemoglobin and hematocrit levels probably reflect inadequate dietary iron intake and poor iron stores, while high hematologic values indicate inadequate plasma volume expansion.

Lifestyle Factors

Other factors, which may be mediated through alterations in nutritional status, may also affect length of gestation. Studies of **cigarette smoking** and **alcohol use** have reported a significant adverse effect on the incidence of prematurity. Current estimates of the prevalence of

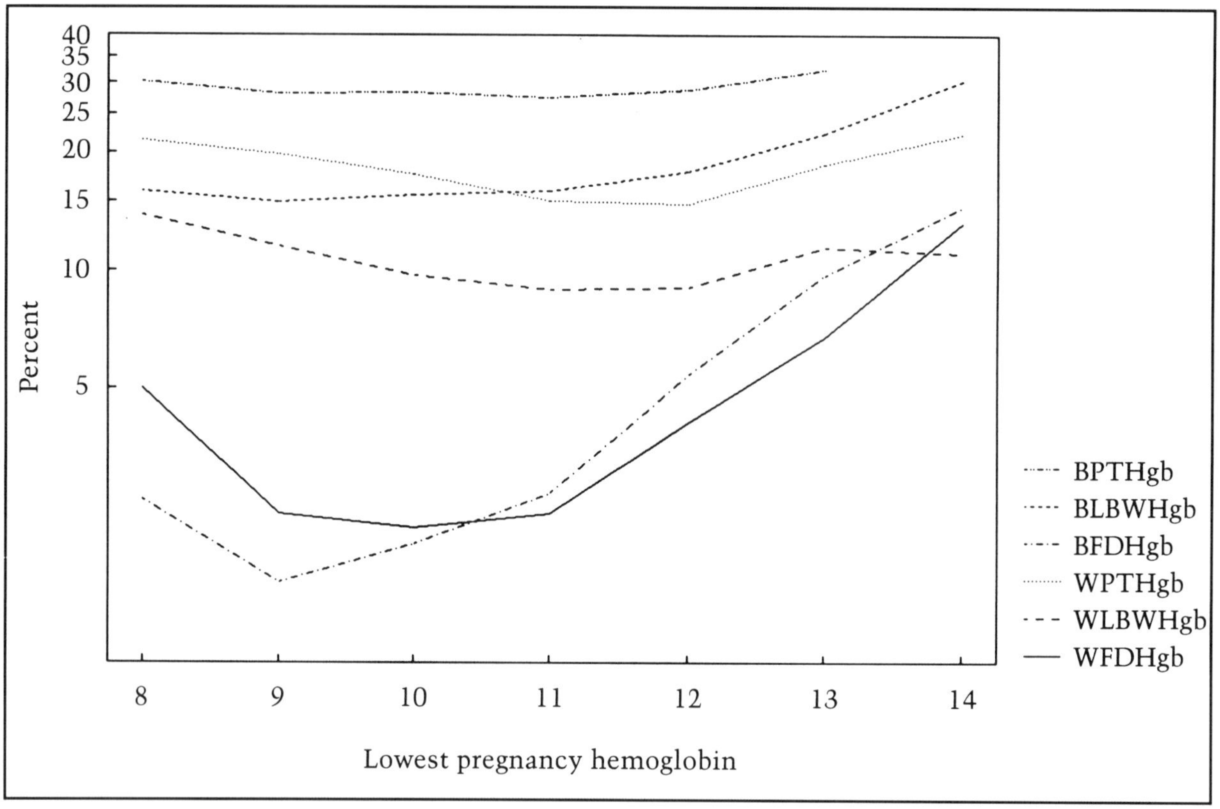

Fig. 13-4
Percent fetal death (FD), preterm (PT), and low birthweight (LBW) by maternal race (W, white; B, black) and lowest pregnancy hemoglobin (Hgb). (Adapted from SM Garn et al, Maternal hematologic levels and pregnancy outcome. *Semin. Perinatol.* 5:155–162, 1981.)

smoking during pregnancy range from 25 percent for whites versus 23 percent for blacks and 36 percent for unmarried women versus 18 percent for married women [65]. The relative risk of prematurity for smokers versus nonsmokers ranges from 1.1 to 2.4, with 4 to 14 percent of preterm births attributable to maternal smoking [21, 66]. In a report of more than 30,000 births between 1974 and 1977 in the Kaiser-Permanente Birth Defects Study, the likelihood of very-preterm delivery (<33 wk) was increased 60 percent in women who smoked 20 or more cigarettes per day, with 4 percent of preterm (<37 wk) and 9 percent of very-preterm births attributable to smoking [67].

The adverse effects of maternal smoking on intrauterine growth and duration of gestation are independent of other factors, such as race, parity, socioeconomic status, pregravid weight, and gestational weight gain. Smoking may exert its effects directly or indirectly, influenc-

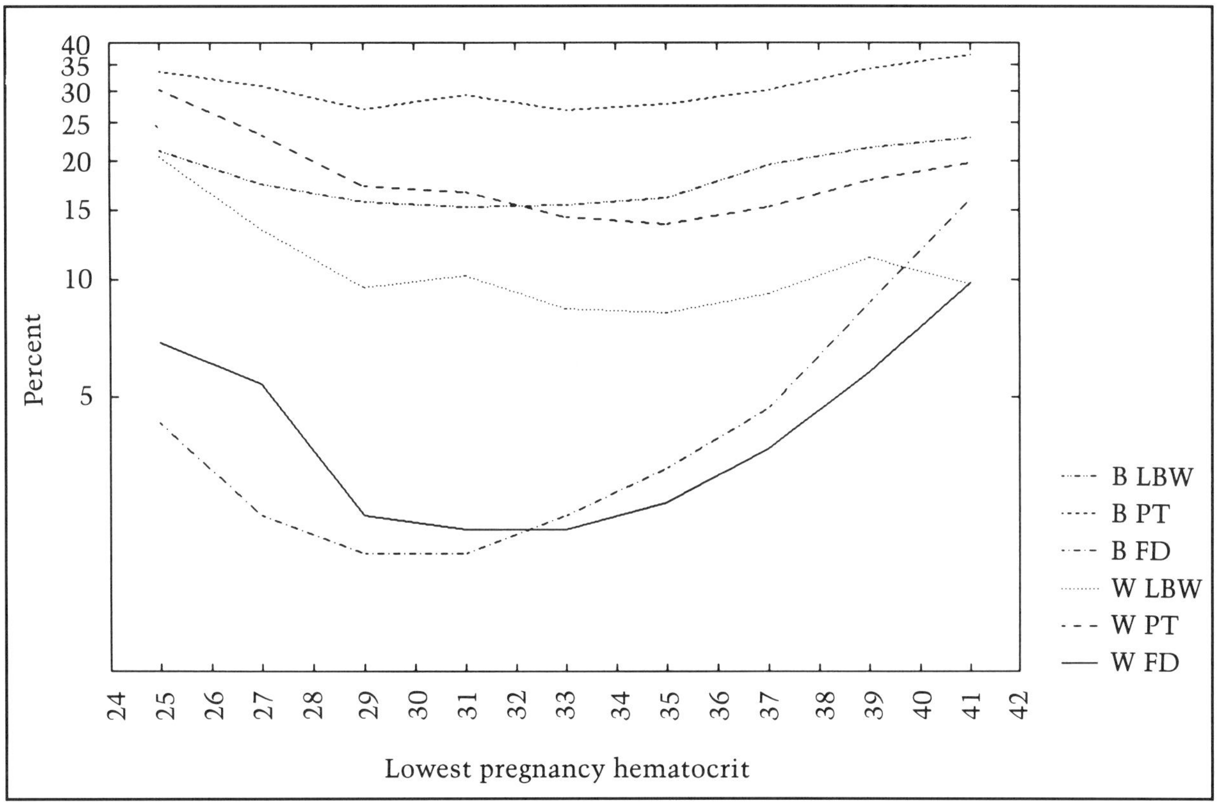

Fig. 13-5
Percent fetal death (FD), preterm (PT), and low birthweight (LBW) by maternal race (W, white; B, black) and lowest pregnancy hematocrit (Hct). (Adapted from SM Garn et al, Maternal hematologic levels and pregnancy outcome. *Semin. Perinatol.* 5:155–162, 1981.)

ing oxygenation, hemoglobin and hematocrit levels, placental structure, and maternal nutritional status. Several nutrients have been identified as being reduced by maternal smoking, including vitamins B_{12}, A, and C; zinc; folate; and essential amino acids (see Chap. 8). The exact mechanism by which maternal smoking causes an increase in prematurity is not well established, but it is probable that nutritional factors play an important role.

The cause-and-effect relationship between maternal alcohol consumption and prematurity is not as clear. The alcohol-related adverse effects on pregnancy outcome are caused by a combination of the toxic effects of alcohol and its metabolic by-products, nutritional factors, and genetic predisposition. As with smoking, specific nutrients, including vitamin A, zinc, and folate, are adversely affected by maternal alcohol consumption (see Chap. 9). Few studies have evaluated the association between maternal alcohol consumption and prematurity. Sokol and associates [68] reported significant increases in mean birthweight and birthweights below 2500 gm and 2000 gm with maternal alcohol consumption, but comparable mean length of gestation and rates of prematurity. Shiono and colleagues [67] reported that maternal alcohol consumption was associated with preterm birth, but this risk was more pronounced for moderately preterm infants (33–36 wk) than for infants born before 33 weeks' gestation. In addition, after adjustment for other confounding variables, the association was only of borderline significance. Hingson and co-workers [69] reported that, after controlling for potentially confounding variables, the level of maternal alcohol consumption before conception was significantly related to shorter gestation.

Conclusions and Recommendations

Although the scientific evidence between nutritional factors and length of gestation is not as strong as it is for birthweight, several important factors indicate a relationship. First, pregravid nutritional status, as pregravid weight, amount of body fat, and reserves of iron and folate, appears to influence both intrauterine growth and duration of gestation. Chronic malnutrition, from famine conditions or personal habits (smoking and alcohol), adversely affects these measures of nutritional status, resulting in compromised pregnancy outcome. Specific nutrients may help overcome the adverse effects of chronic malnutrition on pregnancy outcome through hormonal or physiologic mechanisms. Low pregravid weight, representing a generalized compromised nutritional state, has the strongest association with prematurity, followed by low gestational weight gain. If pregravid weight and other nutrient deficits, such as iron and folate, cannot be corrected before conception, higher gestational weight gain may compensate. Dietary intake to achieve this gain should be through nutrient-rich foods, particularly those high in protein; vitamins A, C, and B_{12}; folate; calcium; and trace minerals (i.e., zinc and magnesium), as well as carbohydrates and calories. These factors are particularly important in primiparas, because there is a strong tendency to repeat gestational ages and birthweights in subsequent pregnancies [70]. Bakketeig and associates [70] have estimated that 19.3 percent of all premature births are due to a history of premature births, and 28 percent of all low-birthweight infants are due to a history of low birthweight. Nutrition plays an important role in pregnancy outcome for all populations, and is a powerful, although often unrecognized, mechanism by which to augment intrauterine growth and enhance duration of gestation.

References

1. Luke, B, and Johnson, TRB: Nutrition and pregnancy: A historical perspective and update. *Women's Health Issues* 1:177–186, 1991.
2. Thomson, AM, and Billewicz, WZ: Clinical significance of weight trends during pregnancy. *Br. Med. J.* 1:243–247, 1957.
3. Jeans, PC, Smith, MB, and Stearns, G: Incidence of prematurity in relation to maternal nutrition. *J. Am. Dietet. Assoc.* 31:576–581, 1955.
4. Chapter 15, Childbearing under adverse conditions. In FE Hytten and I Leitch, *The Physiology of Human Pregnancy* (2nd ed.). London: Blackwell, 1971. Pp. 441–459.
5. Starling, EH: *Report on Food Conditions in Germany*. London: Her Majesty's Stationary Office, 1919 (in [4]).
6. Nilsson, A: Uber sog. Kriegsamenorrhoe. *Zbl. Gynak.* 44:684, 1920 (in [4]).
7. Mossmer, D: Uber 'Kriegsneueborene.' *Zbl. Gynak.* 40:684, 1916 (in [4]).
8. Antonov, AN: Children born during the siege of Leningrad in 1942. *J. Pediatr.* 30:250–259, 1947.
9. Smith, CA: The effect of wartime starvation in Holland upon pregnancy and its product. *Am. J. Obstet. Gynecol.* 53:599–608, 1947.
10. Smith, CA: Effects of maternal undernutrition upon the newborn infant in Holland (1944–1945). *J. Pediatr.* 30:229–243, 1947.
11. Stein, Z, Susser, M, Saenger, G, and Marolla, F: *Famine and Human Development: The Dutch Hunger Winter of 1944–1945*. New York: Oxford, 1975.
12. Stein, Z, and Susser, M: The Dutch famine, 1944–1945, and the reproductive process. I. Effects on six indices at birth. *Pediatr. Res.* 9:70–76, 1975.
13. Stein, Z, and Susser, M: The Dutch famine, 1944–1945, and the reproductive process. II. Interrelations of caloric rations and six indices at birth. *Pediatr. Res.* 9:76–83, 1975.
14. Bulmer, MG: Twinning rate in Europe during the war. *Br. Med. J.* 1:29–30, 1959.
15. Torgersen, J: Hereditary and environmental factors in twinning. *Am. J. Phys. Anthropol.* 9:441–454, 1951.
16. Kramer, MS: Intrauterine growth and gestational duration determinants. *Pediatrics* 80:502–511, 1987.
17. Mitchell, MC, and Lerner, E: Factors that influence the outcome of pregnancy in middle class women. *J. Am. Dietet. Assoc.* 87:731–735, 1987.
18. Wen, SW, Goldenberg, RL, Cutter, GR, et al: Intrauterine growth

retardation and preterm delivery: Prenatal risk factors in an indigent population. *Am. J. Obstet. Gynecol.* 162:213–218, 1990.
19. Abrams, B, and Newman, V: Small-for-gestational age birth: Maternal predictors and comparison with risk factors of spontaneous preterm delivery in the same cohort. *Am. J. Obstet. Gynecol.* 164:785–790, 1991.
20. Edwards, SE, Alton, JR, Barrada, I, and Hakanson, JY: Pregnancy in the underweight woman. *Am. J. Obstet. Gynecol.* 135:297–302, 1979.
21. Fedrick, J, and Anderson, ABM: Factors associated with spontaneous preterm birth. *Br. J. Obstet. Gynecol.* 83:342–350, 1976.
22. Wolfe, HM, Zador, IE, Gross, TL, et al: The clinical utility of maternal body mass index in pregnancy. *Am. J. Obstet. Gynecol.* 164:1306–1310, 1991.
23. Garn, SM, and Pesick, SD: Relationship between various maternal body mass measures and size of the newborn. *Am. J. Obstet. Gynecol.* 36:664–668, 1982.
24. Peckham, CH, and Christianson, RE: The relationship between prepregnancy weight and certain obstetric factors. *Am. J. Obstet. Gynecol.* 111:1–7, 1971.
25. Brown, JE, Jacobson, HN, Askue, LH, and Peick, MG: Influence of pregnancy weight gain on the size of infants born to underweight women. *Obstet. Gynecol.* 57:13–17, 1981.
26. Mitchell, MC, and Lerner, E: Weight gain and pregnancy outcome in underweight and normal weight women. *J. Am. Dietet. Assoc.* 89:634–641, 1989.
27. Frentzen, BH, Dimperio, DL, and Cruz, AC: Maternal weight gain: Effect on infant birthweight among overweight and average-weight low-income women. *Am. J. Obstet. Gynecol.* 159:1114–1117, 1988.
28. Papiernik, E, and Kaminski, M: Multifactorial study of the risk of prematurity at 32 weeks of gestation. I. A study of the frequency of 30 predictive characteristics. *J. Perinatol. Med.* 2:30–36, 1974.
29. van den Berg, BJ, and Oechsli, FW: Prematurity. In MB Bracken (ed.), *Perinatal Epidemiology*. New York: Oxford, 1984. Pp. 69–85.
30. Hediger, ML, Scholl, TO, Belsky, DH, et al: Patterns of weight gain in adolescent pregnancy: Effects on birthweight and preterm delivery. *Obstet. Gynecol.* 74:6–12, 1989.
31. Berkowitz, GS: An epidemiologic study of preterm delivery. *Am. J. Epidemiol.* 113:81–92, 1981.
32. Abrams, B, Newman, V, Key, T, and Parker, J: Maternal weight gain and preterm delivery. *Obstet. Gynecol.* 74:577–583, 1989.
33. Luke, B, Minogue, J, Abbey, A, et al: The association between maternal weight gain and the birthweight of twins. *J. Maternal-Fetal Med.* 1:267–276, 1992.
34. Frisch, RE (ed.): *Adipose Tissue and Reproduction*. Basel: Karger, 1990.
35. Luke, B, and Petrie, RH: Intrauterine growth: Correlation of infant birthweight and maternal postpartum weight. *Am. J. Clin. Nutr.* 33:2311–2317, 1980.

36. Luke, B, Dickinson, C, and Petrie, RH: Intrauterine growth: Correlations of maternal nutritional status and rate of gestational weight gain. *Europ. J. Obstet. Gynecol. Reprod. Biol.* 12:113–121, 1981.
37. Luke, B, Jonaitis, MA, Petrie, RH: A consideration of height as a function of prepregnancy nutritional background and its potential influence on birthweight. *J. Am. Dietet. Assoc.* 84:176–181, 1984.
38. Kaplan, M, Eidelman, AI, and Aboulafia, Y: Fasting and the precipitation of labor: The Yom Kippur effect. *J.A.M.A.* 250:1317–1318, 1983.
39. Binienda, Z, Massmann, A, Mitchell, MD, et al: Effect of food withdrawal on arterial blood glucose and plasma 13,14-dihydro-15-keto-prostaglandin F concentrations and nocturnal myometrial electromyographic activity in the pregnant rhesus monkey in the last third of gestation: A model for preterm labor? *Am. J. Obstet. Gynecol.* 160:746–750, 1989.
40. Taggart, NR, Holliday, RM, Billewicz, WZ, et al: Changes in skinfolds during pregnancy. *Br. J. Nutr.* 21:439–451, 1967.
41. Bissenden, JG, Scott, PH, King, J, et al: Anthropometric and biochemical changes during pregnancy in Asian and European mothers having light for gestational age babies. *Br. J. Obstet. Gynaecol.* 88:999–1008, 1981.
42. Bissenden, JG, Scott, PH, Hallum, J, et al: Anthropometric and biochemical changes during pregnancy in Asian and European mothers having well grown babies. *Br. J. Obstet. Gynaecol.* 88:992–998, 1981.
43. Pipe, NGJ, Smith, T, Halliday, D, et al: Changes in fat, fat-free mass, and body water in human normal pregnancy. *Br. J. Obstet. Gynaecol.* 86:929–940, 1979.
44. Lechtig, A, Martorell, R, Delgado, H, et al: Food supplementation during pregnancy, maternal anthropometry and birthweight in a Guatemala rural population. *J. Trop. Pediatr.* 24:217–222, 1978.
45. Prentice, AM, Whitehead, RG, Watkinson, M, et al: Prenatal dietary supplementation of African women and birthweight. *Lancet* 1:489–492, 1983.
46. Mora, JO, de Paredes, B, Wagner, M, et al: Nutritional supplementation and outcome of pregnancy. I. Birthweight. *Am. J. Clin. Nutr.* 32:455–462, 1979.
47. Adair, LS, and Pollitt, E: Outcome of maternal nutritional supplementation: A comprehensive review of the Bacon Chow study. *Am. J. Clin. Nutr.* 41:948–978, 1985.
48. Rush, D, Stein, Z, and Susser, M: A randomized controlled trial of prenatal nutritional supplementation in New York City. *Pediatrics* 65:683–697, 1980.
49. Metcoff, J, Costiloe, P, Crosby, WM, et al: Effect of food supplementation (WIC) during pregnancy on birth weight. *Am. J. Clin. Nutr.* 41:933–947, 1985.
50. Edozien, JC, Switzer, BR, and Bryan, RB: Medical evaluation of the special supplemental food program for women, infants, and children. *Am. J. Clin. Nutr.* 32:677–692, 1979.

51. Rush, D, Sloan, NL, Leighton, J, et al: Longitudinal study of pregnant women. *Am. J. Clin. Nutr.* 48:439–483, 1988.
52. Shah, RS, Rajalakshmi, R: Vitamin A status of the newborn in relation to gestational age, body weight, and maternal nutritional status. *Am. J. Clin. Nutr.* 40:794–800, 1984.
53. Hibbard, BM: Folates and the fetus. *South Afr. Med. J.* 49:1223–1226, 1975.
54. Spatling, L, and Spatling, G: Magnesium supplementation in pregnancy: A double-blind study. *Br. J. Obstet. Gynaecol.* 95:120–125, 1988.
55. Villar, J, and Repke, JT: Calcium supplementation during pregnancy may reduce preterm delivery in high-risk populations. *Am. J. Obstet. Gynecol.* 163:1124–1131, 1990.
56. Villar, J, Repke, J, Belizan, JM, and Pareja, G: Calcium supplementation reduces blood pressure during pregnancy: Results of a randomized controlled clinical trial. *Obstet. Gynecol.* 70:317–322, 1987.
57. Lopez-Jaramillo, P, Narvaez, M, Weigel, RM, and Yepez, R: Calcium supplementation reduces the risk of pregnancy-induced hypertension in an Andes population. *Br. J. Obstet. Gynaecol.* 96:648–655, 1989.
58. Olsen, SF, Hansen, HS, Sommer, S, et al: Gestational age in relation to marine n-3 fatty acids in maternal erythrocytes: A study of women in the Faroe Islands and Denmark. *Am. J. Obstet. Gynecol.* 164:1203–1209, 1991.
59. Olsen, SF, and Joensen, HD: High liveborn birthweights in the Faroes: Comparison between birthweights in the Faroes and in Denmark. *J. Epidemiol. Community Health* 39:27–32, 1985.
60. Olsen, SF, Hansen, HS, Sorensen, TIA, et al: Intake of marine fat, rich in n-3 polyunsaturated fatty acids, may increase birthweight by prolonging gestation. *Lancet* 2:367–369, 1986.
61. The People's League of Health: The nutrition of expectant and nursing mothers in relation to maternal and infant mortality and morbidity. *J. Obstet. Gynaecol. Br. Emp.* 53:498–509, 1946.
62. Olsen, SF, and Secher, NJ: A possible preventive effect of low-dose fish oil on early delivery and preeclampsia: Indications from a 50-year-old controlled trial. *Br. J. Nutr.* 64:599–609, 1990.
63. Garn, SM, Ridella, SA, Petzold, AS, and Falkner, F: Maternal hematologic levels and pregnancy outcome. *Semin. Perinatol.* 5:155–162, 1981.
64. Murphy, JF, Newcombe, RG, O'Riordan, J, and Coles, EC: Relation of haemoglobin levels in first and second trimesters to outcome of pregnancy. *Lancet* 1:992–995, 1986.
65. Williamson, DF, Serdula, MK, Kendrick, JS, and Binkin, NJ: Comparing the prevalence of smoking in pregnant and nonpregnant women, 1985 to 1986. *J.A.M.A.* 261:70–74, 1989.
66. Meyer, MB, Jonas, BS, and Tonascia, JA: Perinatal events associated with maternal smoking during pregnancy. *Am. J. Epidemiol.* 103:464–476, 1976.

67. Shiono, PH, Klebanoff, MA, and Rhoads, GG: Smoking and drinking during pregnancy: Their effects on preterm birth. *J.A.M.A.* 255:82–84, 1986.
68. Sokol, RJ, Miller, SI, and Reed, G: Alcohol abuse during pregnancy: An epidemiologic study. *Alcoholism: Clinical and Experimental Research* 4:135–145, 1980.
69. Hingson, R, Alpert, JJ, Day, N, et al: Effects of maternal drinking and marijuana use on fetal growth and development. *Pediatrics* 70:539–546, 1982.
70. Bakketeig, LS, Hoffman, HJ, and Harley, EE: The tendency to repeat gestational age and birth weight in successive births. *Am. J. Obstet. Gynecol.* 135:1086–1103, 1979.

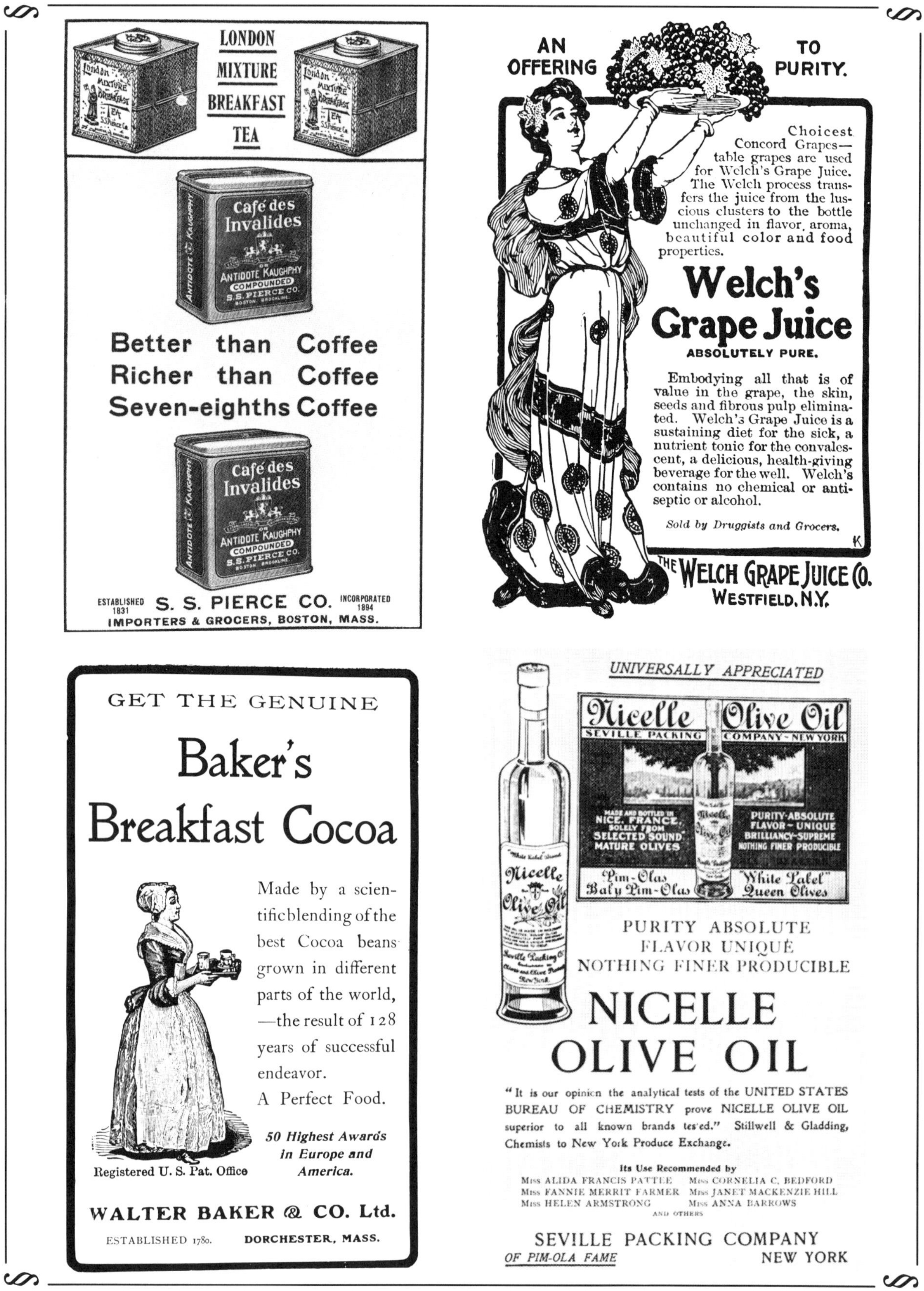

Advertisements in *Practical Dietetics with Reference to Diet in Disease.* (From AF Pattee. *Practical Dietetics with Reference to Diet in Disease.* [5th ed.]. New York: Pattee, 1905.)

Appendix: Sources of Nutrition Information

Organizations

American College of Obstetricians and Gynecologists
409 12th Street, SW
Washington, DC 20024

American Diabetes Association
18 East 48th Street
New York, New York 10017

American Dietetic Association
216 West Jackson Boulevard, Suite 800
Chicago, Illinois 60606-6995

American Dietetic Association
National Center for Nutrition and Dietetics
Consumer Nutrition Hotline
1-800-366-1655
(9 AM–4 PM, Central Standard Time, Mon–Fri)

American Heart Association
7320 Greenville Avenue
Dallas, Texas 75231

La Leche League International
9616 Minneapolis Avenue
Franklin Park, Illinois 60131

National Dairy Council
63000 North River Road
Rosemont, Illinois 60019-9922

National Livestock and Meat Board
444 North Michigan Avenue
Chicago, Illinois 60611

Nutrition Foundation
1122 16th Street, NW
Washington, DC 20036

Office of Disease Prevention and Health Promotion
Mary E. Switze Building, Room 2132
330 C Street, SW
Washington, DC 20201

Books

Albert, MB, and Calloway, CW: *Clinical Nutrition for the House Officer*. Baltimore: Williams & Wilkins, 1992. Softcover, 248 pp. $19.00.

American Dietetic Association:
Hmong Food Customs, Practices, and Holidays
Mexican American Food Customs, Practices, and Holidays
Jewish Food Customs, Practices, and Holidays
Navajo Food Customs, Practices, and Holidays
Chinese Food Customs, Practices, and Holidays
Chicago: American Dietetic Assoc.: 1992. $5.75 each ($5.00 for members).

*Baskette, M, and Mainella, E: *The Art of Nutritional Cooking*. New York: Van Nostrand Reinhold, 1992. Softcover, 258 pp. $36.95.

*Berning, JR, and Steen, SN (eds.): *Sports Nutrition for the 90s: The Health Professional's Handbook*. Gaithersburg, MD: Aspen Publishers, 1991. Hardcover, 299 pp. $45.00.

*Brown, JE: *Everywoman's Guide to Nutrition*. Minneapolis: University of Minnesota Press, 1991. Hardcover, 364 pp. $19.95.

Combs, GE, Jr: *The Vitamins: Fundamental Aspects in Nutrition and Health*. San Diego, CA: Academic Press, 1992. Hardcover, 519 pp. $49.95.

*Franz, MJ, Etzwiler, DD, Joynes, JO, and Hollander, PM (eds.): *Learning to Live Well with Diabetes*. Minneapolis: DCI Publishing, 1991. Softcover, 511 pp. $24.95.

*Hamilton, M, Kolotkin, RL, Cogburn, DF, et al: *The Duke University Medical Center Book of Diet and Fitness*. New York: Fawcett Columbine, 1990. Hardcover, 417 pp. $19.95.

*Herbert, V, and Subak-Sharpe (eds.): *The Mount Sinai School of Medicine Complete Book of Nutrition*. New York: St. Martin's Press, 1990. Hardcover, 796 pp. $35.00.

Hines, JH (ed.): *Anthropometric Assessment of Nutritional Status*. New York: Wiley-Liss, 1991. Hardcover, 431 pp. $99.95.

*For both lay and professional audiences.

Hollingsworth, DR: *Pregnancy, Diabetes and Birth: A Management Guide* (2nd ed.). Baltimore: Williams & Wilkins, 1992. Hardcover, 288 pp. $70.00.

*Jacobson, MF, and Fritschner, S: *Fast-Food Guide* (2nd ed.). New York: Workman Publishing, 1991. Softcover, 331 pp. $7.95.

Kanarek, RB, and Marks-Kaufman, R: *Nutrition and Behavior: New Perspectives*. New York: Van Nostrand Reinhold, 1991. Hardcover, 308 pp. $42.95.

MacDonald, I (ed.): *Monitoring Dietary Intakes*. Berlin: Springer-Verlag, 1991. Hardcover, 259 pp. $89.00.

*Minirth, F, Meier, P, Hemfelt, R, and Sneed, S: *Love Hunger: Recovery from Food Addiction*. Nashville, TN: Thomas Nelson Publishers, 1990. Hardcover, 336 pp. $17.95.

*Rolfes, SR, and De Bruyne, LK (Whitney, ER, ed.): *Life Span Nutrition: Conception Through Life*. St. Paul: West Publishing, 1990. Hardcover, 528 pp. $42.25.

Schaub, J, Van Hoof, F, and Vis, H (eds.): *Inborn Errors of Metabolism*. Nestle Nutrition Workshop Series, Vol. 24. New York: Raven Press, 1991. Hardcover, 298 pp. $62.00.

*Small, DM, and Adams, AS: *The Healthy Meat Eater's Cookbook*. Boston: Adams Publishing Group, 212 pp. $14.95.

Wallace, HM, Ryan, GM, and Oglesby, AC (eds.): *Maternal and Child Health Practices* (3rd ed.). Oakland, CA: Third Party Publishing, 1988. Softcover, 738 pp. $29.95.

*For both lay and professional audiences.

Index

Note: Page numbers followed by f *indicate illustrations; those followed by* t *indicate tables.*